REACH and the Environmental Regulation of Nanotechnology

REACH and the Environmental Regulation of Nanotechnology presents a thorough and comprehensive legal analysis on the status of nanoscale chemicals under the EU's REACH (Registration, Evaluation, Authorisation, and Restriction) regulation, asking whether it effectively safeguards human health and environmental protection.

This book examines the European Commission's claim that REACH offers the best possible framework for the risk management of nanomaterials. Through a detailed and meticulous analysis of the four phases of REACH, Kuraj assesses the capacity of the Regulation to protect human health and the environment against the potential harms associated with exposure to nanomaterials, and draws attention to the ways in which the specificities of nanoscale chemicals are (not) tackled by the current REACH framework. Overall, this book is an innovative and timely contribution to the ongoing debate on how to best address the unprecedented risks posed by the growing pursuit of nanotechnological innovation by the EU and global policy agenda.

REACH and the Environmental Regulation of Nanotechnology will be of great interest to advanced students and scholars of environmental law and policy, environmental governance, science and technology studies, and environment and health.

Nertila Kuraj is a Postdoctoral Research Fellow at the Department of Public and International Law, University of Oslo, Norway, and a Visiting Scholar at UC Berkeley School of Law.

T0399530

Routledge Studies in Environment and Health

The study of the impact of environmental change on human health has rapidly gained momentum in recent years, and an increasing number of scholars are now turning their attention to this issue. Reflecting the development of this emerging body of work, the *Routledge Studies in Environment and Health* series is dedicated to supporting this growing area with cutting edge interdisciplinary research targeted at a global audience. The books in this series cover key issues such as climate change, urbanisation, waste management, water quality, environmental degradation and pollution, and examine the ways in which these factors impact human health from a social, economic and political perspective.

Comprising edited collections, co-authored volumes and single author monographs, this innovative series provides an invaluable resource for advanced undergraduate and postgraduate students, scholars, policy makers and practitioners with an interest in this new and important field of study.

Environmental Health Risks
Ethical Aspects
Edited by Friedo Zölzer and Gaston Meskens

Climate Change and Urban Health
The Case of Hong Kong as a Subtropical City
Emily Ying Yang Chan

Environmental Health and the U.S. Federal System
Sustainably Managing Health Hazards
Michael R. Greenberg and Dona Schneider

REACH and the Environmental Regulation of Nanotechnology
Preventing and Reducing the Environmental Impacts of Nanomaterials
Nertila Kuraj

For more information about this series, please visit: www.routledge.com/Routledge-Studies-in-Environment-and-Health/book-series/RSEH

REACH and the Environmental Regulation of Nanotechnology

Preventing and Reducing the Environmental Impacts of Nanomaterials

Nertila Kuraj

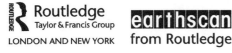 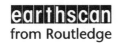

Routledge
Taylor & Francis Group

LONDON AND NEW YORK

earthscan
from Routledge

First published 2020
by Routledge
2 Park Square, Milton Park, Abingdon, Oxon OX14 4RN

and by Routledge
605 Third Avenue, New York, NY 10017

First issued in paperback 2021

Routledge is an imprint of the Taylor & Francis Group, an informa business

British Library Cataloguing-in-Publication Data
A catalogue record for this book is available from the British Library

Library of Congress Cataloging-in-Publication Data
A catalog record has been requested for this book

ISBN 13: 978-0-367-78499-7 (pbk)
ISBN 13: 978-0-367-18964-8 (hbk)

Typeset in Bembo
by Wearset Ltd, Boldon, Tyne and Wear

This book is dedicated to Professor Hans Christian Bugge, and to him only – in the unshaken believe that *Care*, the unifying element of life on Earth, remains the sole and ultimate revolutionary act.

March 2019
UC Berkeley School of Law

Contents

Acknowledgements

This book is based on my PhD thesis which I defended at the Faculty of Law, University of Oslo (UiO), Norway, in May 2017. I owe a debt of gratitude to many people whose presence and support was essential in the process of turning a thesis into an academic volume.

Special thanks of infinite gratitude go to my PhD supervisors, Professors Hans Christian Bugge and Christina Voigt for their seemingly endless patience and constant trust in me and my academic pursuits. I feel proud and privileged to be their student.

I am grateful to my PhD reviewing committee, Professors Elen Stokes, Steffen Foss Hansen, and Hans Petter Graver, for positively evaluating my thesis and contributing thus to the publishing of this book. Thank you!

Thanks are to be extended to the Norwegian Ministry of Education and Research (Kunnskapsdepartementet) for generously funding my PhD position, which was based at the Department of Public and International Law, UiO. At the Law Faculty in Oslo, I would like to thank Professors Inger Johanne Sand and Dag Michalsen for their assistance during the many stages of this long process.

Many thanks also to Guro Frostestad and Marianne Gjerstad for their administrative support.

In Oslo I had the great fortune of meeting wonderful people that have brought joy and richness to my life. Without the genuine friendship and the academic inspiration precious Amrei Müller provides, this book would simply not have been possible. My research has greatly benefited from our many academic debates, her invaluable feedback on my work, and the sharing of nice food and coffee during beautiful summer evenings and crispy winter days in lovely Oslo. I am grateful to her also for showing me that strength resides in kindness and that integrity is everything. My environmental-sister and wonderful colleague, Eléonore Maitre-Ekern, has been a trusted and precious friend from the very beginning and I am grateful she has remained such during all these stormy years. Her excellent academic feedback and her profound humanity and uncompromising attitude have been a great source of strength. This book would not have been finished without her. I look forward to exciting collaborations in our common field of research and in the shared commitment for a better and greener planet.

To fantastic Marte Guttulsrød, the green girl par excellence, I owe special thanks for being always a true friend. Her deeply caring nature has been a balm of courage and healing even in the most difficult of moments. The Babette's feasts we often shared and the time spent in picturesque spots of the breath-taking Norwegian nature, are moments I cherish and look forward to repeating again soon.

I would like to thank also the amazing Froukje Maria Platjouw for being an inspiring colleague and friend at UiO, and for the encouragement with my project(s).

Special thanks go also to colleagues Eivind Junker, Luca Tosoni, Michelle Q Zang, Tone Linn Wærstad, Kevin McGillivray and Professors Beate Sjåfjell, Kirsti Strøm Bull, Endre Stavang, and brilliant scholar and courageous woman, Isabel Mota Borges.

Many thanks to my mentor at UiO, Professor Lutz Bachmann, with whom I had the luck to cross paths and whose precious advice and generous support have been vital during the final stages of this book.

Besides being based on my PhD, the book is also the fruit of a long process unfolding in many countries and institutions. The initial idea germinated at the Law Faculty, at the University of Pisa, in Italy, where I completed my Master thesis on nanotechnology regulation in the Food Law area, under the supervision of Professor Eleonora Sirsi. Her dedicated teaching and cutting-edge scholarship have strongly influenced and deeply inspired my inclination to research on the 'law of the future' and new technologies. I will always be indebted to her for initiating and guiding me on the intriguing and exciting path I currently walk. Always in Pisa, my special thanks go also to Professor Eleonora Bennati, for her encouragement and trust during my undergraduate studies.

Splendid Dr Sandrine Blanchemanche deserves special thanks for hosting me at INRA, Paris, during my Master thesis's writing, and for the great support and trust she has always shown towards me and my research.

Many thanks to Professor Mariagrazia Alabrese for hosting me as a visiting scholar at the Sant'Anna School of Advanced Studies, in Pisa.

Special gratitude is due to Professor Nilgün Cılız, at the Institute of Environmental Sciences, at Boğaziçi University, in Turkey, for hosting me there as a visiting PhD. Thanks to her I had the chance to conduct research on Turkish chemicals legislation, which is included in this book. The days on the beautiful campus by the turquoise waters of the Bosporus were flavoured by the aroma of fresh simit and taze kahve shared with my dear friends Pakize Şeker and Başak Burcu Yiğit, whom I thank for making my stay in Istanbul an authentic one.

The University of California, Berkeley, has a special place in my heart and research. The time I spent there in 2014 as a visiting PhD was an enriching and life-changing experience. Thanks to a FRIPRO mobility grant from the Research Council of Norway (Norges forskningsråd), to which I take the chance here to express my deepest gratitude, I am lucky to be back as a Post-doctoral Researcher at Berkeley. The joy of finalising my book at Berkeley, writing in the Law School open terrace, under a cobalt Californian sky, is almost indescribable.

I owe a special depth of wholehearted gratitude to Professor Daniel Farber, who has hosted me at Berkeley, both times, and whose innovative work in environmental law continues to inspire generations of environmentalists worldwide.

Many thanks to the UC Berkeley School of Law for generously allowing me to work and research while using its excellent library services and premises on campus, and to the Director of the Berkeley Law Visiting Scholars Program, Farrah Fanara, for facilitating my stay and work here. Always at Berkeley I would like also to thank Professor Shigeo Miyagawa, of the Waseda University Law School, in Tokyo, for introducing me to Japanese law and helping me arrange a research stay at Waseda, and Professor Tadashi Otsuka for hosting me there.

My colleague and brilliant friend Hadassa Noorda, now at NYU, is also a treasured gift from Berkeley. I thank her for sharing her love for truth and beauty and for practicing authenticity as a way of being.

Fantastic Lisa Findley and Oda Charlotte Sebusæter deserve all my gratitude for helping me with the editing technicalities involved in writing a thesis and a book. Thank you!

My friends and family, scattered over four continents, remain the essence of my life. Fantastic Eri and Marco: thank you for always being there for me. Misa, Iva, Alba, Claudia, Anna L, Xiaobo, Ela, Mersi, Eriona Sh, Ashi, Albana, Klara, Brikena, Farid, Ina N, Ashi, Erida, Prof. Berti, Michael K and Randy, Evita, Najada, Adriana, Ina S, Rodi, Bulut, Endri, Leta, Tatjana, Valentina, Bardha, Millani, Mamica, Laura, Matilda, Mela, Bajamja, Diana, Gazi, Tefta, Tea, Ragnhild K, Per H, Shefqeti (aka Edi), Natalia, Paul, Alexa, Aybike, daj Çimi: thank you!

Finally, I want to thank the two most precious people in my life whom I love dearly and endlessly. My sister Sabina has always encouraged me in my academic pursuits and believed in my ideas and the publishing of this book even when my own trust was vacillating. I thank her for the bubbly Nordic summers, for sharing the love of opera, art, and everything beautiful – and for being into my life, always. The most beautiful creature I know, my mother Afërdita, is the reason for anything worthwhile I might be or do. She is a true kind warrior and a tireless caregiver, capable of making life bearable and meaningful even under the most arduous of circumstances. From her I have learned that the only way to go through this short dream we call life is by paying attention to and deeply caring about anything – from cooking to writing a book on nanotechnology – or anyone we commit to. True to the name she bears, she is the personification of love and I thank her for lavishing such love on me: O jet!

Abbreviations

AD	analytic-deliberative
ADI	acceptable daily intake
ADME	absorption, distribution, and excretion
AG	Advocate General
AIHA	American Industrial Hygiene Association
ATM	atomic force microscope
BoA	Board of Appeal
CA	competent authority
CAS	Chemical Abstracts Service
CCSA(s)	Certified Chemical Safety Assessor(s)
CEF	Panel on Food Contact Materials, Enzymes, Flavourings, and Processing Aids
CEFIC	European Chemical Industry Council
CFREU	Charter of Fundamental Rights of the European Union
CIEL	Centre for International Environmental Law
CJEU	Court of Justice of the European Union
CLP	Classification, Labelling, and Packaging
CMR	carcinogenic, mutagenic, or toxic to reproduction
CNT(s)	carbon nanotube(s)
CoRAP	Community Rolling Action Plan
CSA	chemical safety assessment
CSR	chemical safety report
CTPHT	coal tar pitch, high temperature
DDT	dichlorodiphenyltrichloroethane
DE	dossier evaluation
DEFRA	Department for Environment, Food, and Rural Affairs
DG	directorate-general
DNEL	derived no-effect level
EAP	Environmental Action Programme
EC	European Community
ECHA	European Chemicals Agency
EDCs	endocrine disrupting chemicals
EEA	European Environmental Agency

EEC	(Treaty establishing the) European Economic Community
EFSA	European Food Safety Authority
EINECS	European Inventory of Existing Commercial Substances
ELINCS	European List of Notified Chemical Substances
EMA	European Medicines Agency
ENMs	engineered nanomaterials
EPA	Environmental Protection Agency
EU	European Union
FCM(s)	food contact material(s)
FDA	Food and Drug Administration
GAARN	Group Assessing Already Registered Nanomaterials
GDs	Guidance Documents
GHS	Globally Harmonized System of Classification and Labelling of Chemicals
GLP	good laboratory practice
HPV	high production volume
HSE	Health and Safety Executive
HSE	health, safety, and environment
IPCS	International Programme on Chemical Safety
IPPD	Integrated Pollution Prevention and Control Directive
IRSST	Institut de recherche Robert-Sauvé en santé et en sécurité du travail
ISO	International Organization for Standardization
IUCLID	International Uniform Chemical Information Database
IUPAC	International Union of Pure and Applied Chemistry
JRC	Joint Research Centre
KEK/CICR	Kimyasalların Envanteri ve Kontrolü Hakkında Yönetmelik/ Chemicals Inventory and Control Regulation
KETs	key enabling technologies
KKDIK	Kimyasalların Kaydı, De erlendirmesi, zni ve Kısıtlanması Yönetmelik/Turkish Regulation on the Registration, Evaluation, Permission, and Restriction of Chemicals
LC	lethal concentration
LD	lethal dose
LO(A)EL	lowest-observed-(adverse)-effect level
MAD	mutual acceptance of data
MMT	methylcyclopentadienyl manganese tricarbonyl
MoEUP	Turkish Ministry of Environment and Urban Planning
MS(s)	Member State(s)
MSC	Member States Committee
MWCNTs	multi-walled carbon nanotubes
NEL	no-effect level
NGOs	non-governmental organisations
NO(A)EL	no-observed-(adverse)-effect level
NOEL	no-observed-effect level

NRC	National Research Council
OECD	Organisation for Economic Co-operation and Development
OR(s)	only representative(s)
PBT/vPvB	persistent, bioaccumulative, and toxic/very persistent and very bioaccumulative
PCBs	polychlorinated biphenyls
PEC	predicted environmental concentration
PET	polyethylene terephthalate
PNEC	predicted no-effect concentration
POD	point of departure
POPs	persistent organic pollutants
PP	precautionary principle
(Q)SARs	(quantitative) structure-activity relationships
QMV	qualified majority voting
RA	risk assessment
RAAF	Read-Across Assessment Framework
RAC	Committee for Risk Assessment
RC	Royal Commission
RC	risk characterisation
RCR	risk characterisation ratio
REACH	Registration, Evaluation, Authorisation, and Restriction of Chemicals
RIP-oN	REACH Implementation Project
RM	risk management
RMM	risk management measures
RMO	risk management options
RoI	Registry of Intentions
ROS	reactive oxygen species
RPS	regulatory procedure with scrutiny
RS	British Royal Society
RT	regulatory toxicology
SAE/SEA	Turkish by-law on the Classification, Labelling, and Packaging of Substances and Mixtures
SAICM	Strategic Approach to International Chemicals Management
SCCS	Scientific Committee on Consumer Safety
SCENIHR	Scientific Committee on Emerging and Newly Identified Health Risks
SDS	safety data sheets
SDS/GBF	Turkish by-law on Safety Data Sheets on Hazardous Substances and Mixtures
SEA	socio-economic analysis
SEAC	Committee for Socio-Economic Analysis
SIN	Substitute It Now
SLIM	simpler legislation for the internal market
SMEs	small and medium-sized enterprises

SP	substitution principle
STM	scanning tunnelling microscope
SVHC(s)	substance(s) of very high concern
SWCNTs	single-walled carbon nanotubes
SWD	Staff Working Document
TD	technical dossier
TDMA	Titanium Dioxide Manufacturers Association
TEC	Treaty establishing the European Community
TEU	Treaty on European Union
TFEU	Treaty on the Functioning of the European Union
TGs	Test Guidelines for the Chemicals
TiN	titanium nitride
TiO_2	titanium dioxide
TKTD	toxicokinetic-toxicodynamic
TSCA	Toxic Substances Control Act
UA	uncertainty analysis
UFs	uncertainty factors
UVCB	unknown or variable composition, complex reaction products or of biological materials
VSSA	volume-specific surface area
WeE	Weight of Evidence
WFD	Water Framework Directive
WHO	World Health Organization
WP	White Paper
WPN	Working Party on Nanotechnology
WTO	World Trade Organization

1   Introduction

From *Silent Spring* to planetary boundaries

They are everywhere. Most of our food contains a cocktail made of their long and uneasy names. We drink them normally with our drinking water. We constantly inhale them too. Our bodies have become a storage place for dozens of types of them, although not necessarily as a consequence of a deliberative choice to host them in our tissues and organs. And yet they have found a way to enter the bloodstream, to contaminate mothers' milk. Even unborn babies carry their burden, as more than 200 of them have been found to show up in umbilical cord blood. Each and every one of us is hence likely to come into contact with more than 100,000 man-made synthetic chemicals which we know, at best, very little about.

Nature, too, is subjugated to the constant application of these 'elixirs of death'[1] to an extent that our modern lives unfold in a 'synthetic environment'.[2] Rivers and ground-waters are loaded with several types of chemicals like pesticides and agro-chemicals substances. Heavy metals and microplastics have pervaded seas and oceans. Man-made chemicals have proved also to bioaccumulate and persist in soil for many decades after they have been deposited. Essentially, there hardly are places or creatures on this planet that have not already been contaminated by pesticide and herbicide residues, heavy metals pollutants, and other synthetic chemicals.

Indeed, chemical pollution knows no geographical boundaries: organochlorines, chlorinated hydrocarbons, and heavy metals have been detected in the otherwise pristine and fragile ecosystems of the High North, notwithstanding the fact that this region is not a major producer of these chemicals.[3] Long-range transport by air and water currents is known to cause toxic substances to move across and beyond national borders, contributing to the *global* dimension of chemical pollution. The types of hazards and risks chemicals pose and the soaring levels of this type of pollution, are such that chemical pollution actually is considered to represent a *planetary boundary*.

'Planetary boundaries' is a concept coined in 2009 by Rockström et al., referring to nine entities, which define the safe operating space for humanity with respect to the Earth system and are associated with the planet's biophysical subsystems or processes.[4]

Beside chemical pollution, the other identified boundaries include: *climate change; rate of biodiversity loss (terrestrial and marine); interference with the nitrogen and phosphorus cycles; stratospheric ozone depletion; ocean acidification; global freshwater use; change in land use;* and *atmospheric aerosol loading.*

For some of these boundaries, scientists were able to identify thresholds that ought not to be crossed, lest the impacts to the Earth system might be deleterious with potential disastrous consequences for humans. Regretfully for the state of the planet, three of the nine identified boundaries' safe thresholds have already been crossed: climate change, biodiversity loss, and nitrogen cycle.[5] As far as the chemical pollution boundary is concerned, no safe threshold could be determined by Rockström et al., so in this case *we don't know what we don't know* and, therefore, we are dealing with ignorance.

The ignorance on the effects and impact of chemical pollution, other authors have suggested, can be better addressed through the concept of *planetary boundary threats.*[6] These authors argue that the concept of chemical pollution as a planetary boundary is poorly defined. Rather, they suggest, the chemical pollution planetary boundary can be seen as a 'placeholder for all chemical pollution–related planetary boundary problems that we are currently ignorant about'.[7] Three conditions must be met *simultaneously* for a chemical to pose a planetary boundary threat:

(C1) – The chemical or mixture of chemicals has a disruptive effect on a vital earth system process;

(C2) – The disruptive effect is not discovered until it is, or inevitably will become, a problem at a planetary scale;

(C3) – The effects of the pollutant in the environment cannot be readily reversed.[8]

REACH, the new EU chemicals law, and the hazard-based procedures therein, are identified as an appropriate regulatory approach to confront chemical pollution ignorance.[9] In a more recent paper, additional criteria were set to identify chemicals, which in the light of the three conditions mentioned above, are considered to be planetary boundary threats.[10]

In the last update to the planetary boundary framework, Steffen et al. suggest that the introduction of novel entities – consisting of new substances, new forms of existing substances, and modified life-forms that have the potential for unwanted geophysical and/or biological effects,[11] can be considered as posing planetary boundary threats.

Nanomaterials are explicitly mentioned in this regard, as adding to the existing large burden of 100,000 chemicals already contributing to the boundary of chemical pollution.[12] But what exactly are nano-chemicals? Broadly speaking, nano-chemicals are substances with a size range of 1–100 nanometres (nm). One nanometre is one billionth of a metre (10^{-9}). To put it into perspective, it is on the same scale as a virus. One billionth of a metre is also the size of ten hydrogen atoms side by side and about one thousandth of the length of a typical bacterium.[13] It is one hundred thousand times smaller than the diameter of a human hair, a thousand times smaller than a red blood cell, or about half the size of the diameter of DNA.[14] But why is there a growing concern about their effects on human health and ecosystem integrity? What makes them so special? And, importantly, are the laws currently in place, e.g. the REACH Regulation, able to offer a good oversight and an effective regulatory coverage for nano-related environmental pollution?

The overall aim of this book is to examine the legal status of nanoscale chemicals under the REACH regulatory framework. More broadly, the book explores the appropriateness of the existing risk assessment methodologies that uphold modern and technically complex laws regulating chemicals risk as a legitimate basis for decision-making in the face of uncertainty.

Before addressing the specific nature of nanoscale chemicals and their peculiar risk profiles, an overview of the REACH framework is necessary in order to understand the approach and aim of this monograph concerned.

Tackling the problem: a brief introduction to REACH

In 2006, the EU passed what is considered to be 'the most controversial and complex piece of regulation in European history'.[15]

The REACH[16] Regulation sets forth the legal regime governing the **R**egistration, **E**valuation, **A**uthorisation and **R**estriction of **Ch**emicals, either on their own or in articles and preparations. The four phases of REACH each rest on a set of detailed legal and administrative provisions, which are tightly harnessed to and informed by the regulatory science in the area of chemicals legislation, that of regulatory toxicology (RT).[17] While the legal and administrative provisions are contained in the 235 pages and 141 Articles of the Regulation, the test methods and technical requirements for data generation, in accordance with RT make up for the remaining 614 pages of this massive 849-page flagship of EU chemical policy. To this almost intimidatingly large official text of REACH, add the further 5,000 pages of Guidance Documents produced by the European Chemicals Agency.[18]

The conspicuous size of this unprecedented legal endeavour and amount of its regulatory requirements, correspond to, or rather, are owed to, the exceptionally ambitious aim[19] REACH seeks to attain: ensuring a high level of protection of human health and the environment, including the promotion of alternative methods for assessment of hazards of substances, as well as the free circulation of substances on the internal market while enhancing competitiveness and innovation.[20]

In practical terms, REACH intends to achieve this by addressing the so-called 'burden of the past'. The term refers to the failure of the previous EU piecemeal and inconsistent chemicals legislation, which didn't require any safety data for 'existing chemicals', i.e. chemicals placed on the market prior to 1981. As a consequence, for 99 per cent of such substances, amounting to more than 100,000 chemicals, there was virtually no available information regarding their toxicity for human health and the environment.[21] Moreover, the burden of proof lay entirely with the authorities which meant they had to demonstrate the existence of hazard and risk before being able to adopt regulatory measures. In such a situation, the need for better regulation in order to counter and prevent environmental and human health risks of chemicals, became a priority for the EU legislator. This is how REACH came along.

Industry, according to REACH, must bear the burden for generating safety data on both *new* and *existing* chemicals, otherwise no access to the EU market is to be granted. Known also as the 'no data, no market' principle, this provision, which to some extent shifts the duty to gather and assess toxicity data to private entities, is one of the main features of the new framework.[22] Along with the *producer responsibility principle*, REACH is based on the principle of substitution – an essential corollary of the principle of sustainable development – and, most importantly, on the *precautionary principle*, which is said to underpin the REACH provisions.[23]

More concretely, the framework that REACH puts in place for remedying 'toxic ignorance'[24] consists of four semi-independent but interrelated phases.

(1) Registration represents the gateway into the REACH system. It stipulates that chemicals, both *new* and *existing*, manufactured and/or imported in quantities over 1 tonne per producer or importer per year (hereafter t/y), are to be registered with the European Chemicals Agency (ECHA).[25] The duty to register is a tiered one. REACH foresees four tiers based on the volume of production. Each tier, and the requirements it entails, is analysed in Chapter 3. Suffice to say here that the duty to provide data for registration purposes is incremental: the higher the quantity of production, the wider the data set and testing on health and environmental risks to be submitted to the ECHA. In addition, at the 10 t/y of volume of production, the obligation to prepare a chemical safety report (CSR) is triggered. This report must contain a *chemical safety assessment* (CSA) of the chemical, meaning that the producer shall provide information to all the users of the chemical through transparent and reliable information on the exposure scenarios used in assessing the chemical hazard.

(2) Evaluation is the second phase of REACH, concerned with the assessment of the quality and correctness of the data submitted by the registrants. This aspect of REACH is administered mainly by the ECHA, which is in charge of the correct implementation of REACH. Three types of evaluation can be performed within REACH: dossier evaluation,[26] substance evaluation,[27] and evaluation of intermediates.[28] One important outcome of the

substance evaluation procedure is the identification of substances of very high concern (SVHCs). The term refers to chemicals possessing particularly hazardous properties for human health and/or the environment which, as such, cannot be commercialised and used unless their specific uses are authorised.

(3) Authorisation, the true novelty of the REACH reform, is a stepwise process consisting of the identification of SVHCs; their placement in the Candidate List of substances requiring authorisation; and the final inclusion, by Commission decision, of such hazardous chemicals in Annex XIV of REACH, which contains substances that are de facto banned *unless* authorised. A major advantage of the Authorisation phase in terms of environmental protection is that it is mainly a hazard-based procedure, transcending minimum thresholds (like the 1 t/y one for Registration). In other words, the sole potential of the intrinsic properties of a given chemical to harm human health and/or the environment is sufficient to trigger Authorisation. As this book will show, particularly in Chapter 5, this procedure is particularly relevant for those chemicals, such as endocrine disrupters (EDCs) and nano-scale chemicals, which do not respond to the current golden rule of RT where 'dose makes the poison'. In addition, Authorisation fosters innovation by encouraging the substitution of SVHCs with less harmful alternatives, in line with the substitution principle endorsed by REACH.

(4) Restriction, the fourth and last phase of REACH, provides for the restriction of chemicals that pose an unacceptable risk to humans and/or the environment and which at the same time need to be addressed on a Community-wide basis. Labelled as the 'safety net' of REACH, Restriction represents a limited number of novelties when compared to the pre-REACH procedure for restricting dangerous chemicals, where the burden of proof lay completely with authorities.[29]

It is important to stress here that REACH is overarching legislation, set to provide the input toxicity data that might be used also in other sectoral legislation – i.e. single media-based environmental directives and even international environmental treaties – in order to analyse risks of chemicals in their specific areas of application. In addition, its procedures for limiting the use of the most dangerous chemicals can create an 'upstream filter', which should reduce the overall use of dangerous chemicals, easing hence the control of problematic substances in sector-specific law.

As far as complex chemicals are concerned though, REACH presents two elements that might appear problematic. First, the threshold for triggering registration is set at 1 t/y, and significant data requirements are only triggered at 10 t/y of production volumes. Chemicals that have a mode of toxic action not dependent on the quantity of exposure will hardly be captured by REACH, even though they might be harmful at quantities well below the 1 t/y minimum threshold. The only phase able to provide a regulatory option would in principle be that of Authorisation. Second, REACH is *technologically neutral*. Although the term of technology neutrality was conceptualised in the realm of information and telecommunication technologies,[30] it is used here to designate the absence in REACH of any reference to the technological process of producing/using chemicals. More specifically, the concept of substance, which constitutes the very object of regulation in REACH, is silent on the mode of production and/or use under the technological profile. But while technological neutrality can represent a statutory drafting technique aimed at ensuring that the laws will be flexible enough to operate in diverse technological contexts, such laws can lag behind in a rapidly evolving realm of technology.[31] This book will take a closer look at how technological neutrality is framing the present and prospected options for an appropriate regulation of nanoscale substances in REACH.

Hence, the question naturally arises: what is so special about the products of nanotechnology application, e.g. nanoscale chemicals, to ask for their specific and targeted regulatory coverage within (a reformed) REACH?

Introducing the nano-world: an overview of the tiny particles

Nano, from Greek *dwarf*, has become a buzzword in the last decade. The prefix (whose symbol is *n*), denotes a size range of 10^{-9} or one billionth of a metre (or 0.000000001), generally designating materials/substances of the size between 1 and 100 nm.[32] Note that the terms 'nanosubstances', 'nanochemicals', 'nanomaterials', 'chemicals in nanoscale', and 'materials in nanoscale' are used interchangeably throughout this book.

Nano is increasingly associated with all different sorts of consumer products, ranging from cleaning detergents to antibacterial training clothes and from miraculous cosmetics to smart food and intelligent food contact materials and labelling. Nanotechnology is considered to be the next technological revolution, which is about to radically affect the way we live and the environment we inhabit. For instance, it has been argued that not only will nanotechnology improve food security by enabling us to produce more food in a more sustainable way (e.g. using less harmful pesticides and fertilisers), but it will also enhance food safety by enabling more hygienic food processing packaging and storage on the one hand, and the creation of intelligent labelling, which changes colour to signal the presence of pathogens or allergens, on the other.[33] Also remarkable is the fact that nanotechnology prospects include the production of healthy and nutritious foods that allegedly have an even better taste, flavour, and mouth feel than their traditional version. In addition, nano-encapsulated food additives and supplements will enhance the uptake and bioavailability of nutrients and supplements through food.[34] What better solution for a constantly hungry, yet severely obese planet?

It is also argued that nanotechnology can be used to advance environmental protection and sustainable development to an extent that nanotechnology is considered a key component for green innovation,[35] able to offer arguably inexpensive and sound solutions to some of the most pressing global crises. In this regard, prospected green nanotechnology applications include:

water filtration and purification systems; sensors for the detection and the removal of pathogens and chemical pollutants in all environmental compartments; applications for the production of clean and renewable energies such as next-generation solar cells and electric cars with nanotechnology-enabled batteries. The advocated advantages of nanotechnology also include nano-solutions for sustainable agriculture such as the development of environmentally friendly nano-agrochemicals and nano-sensing systems for real-time monitoring of crop growth and field conditions;[36] and even creative solutions to combat climate change, i.e. by lofting *nano titanium dioxide* particles in the stratosphere in order to scatter sunlight back to space and thus cause temperatures to drop – in case the currently pursued methods of reducing CO_2 might go wrong.[37]

Last but not least, rapidly advancing applications of nanotechnology include targeted drug delivery and diagnostic, theranostic, and regenerative medicine. The European Medicines Agency (EMA) has currently granted authorisation for 7 nano-based medicines[38] while its American counterpart, the Food and Drug Administration (FDA), has approved more than 20 nanoparticle-based drugs.[39]

However, enthusiasm about the potentially infinite applications of nanotechnology is tempered by concerns related to the negative impacts and risks yet to be understood that come with the growing diffusion of man-made nanosubstances. Mineral-based cosmetic products, for example, might pose significant risks related to the subsequent uptake of nanoparticles in the systemic circulation, metabolism, and potential accumulation in secondary target organs.[40] In addition, due to their special nature, nano-chemicals have the ability to absorb other toxic substances and carry them into living organisms. As far as human health risks are concerned, nanomaterials have been associated with long-term inflammation in different tissues and organs, cardiovascular effects, and even the potential to cross the blood-brain barrier under certain circumstances.[41] The European Food Safety Authority (EFSA) also contends that little is known on the fate of nanoscale particles after they enter the human body. Their contact with intestinal sub-mucosal tissue enables nanoparticles to enter the capillaries and hence, through portal circulation, reach the liver, the lymphatic system, and other internal organs.[42] In this regard, the Scientific Committee on Emerging and Newly Identified Health Risks (SCENIHR) states:

> The hypothesis that smaller means more reactive and thus more toxic cannot be substantiated by the published data. In this respect nanomaterials are similar to normal substances in that some may be toxic and some may not.[43]

As will be shown in this book, a case-by-case risk assessment of *each* nanoscale chemical and its use is thus suggested by scientific bodies. However, a major hindrance in carrying out reliable risk assessments for toxicity evaluations of nanoscale materials is the lack of adequate test methods and protocols to this end. Current documents, designed for traditional (bulk) chemicals, are generally considered to be applicable to risk assessment of nanoscale chemicals. At the same time, a need to update and modify them in the light of nanotoxicity's special features is repeatedly advocated by the SCENIHR and EFSA, but also by the scientific community at large.

In light of these considerations, one might ask: is the science and application of nanotechnology providing us with a sort of panacea to cure most modern evils, or is it just offering us a peek into a Pandora's box of new and unparalleled risk, including that of wiping out our own existence from the Earth[44] and/or reducing Earth to a lifeless mass of grey goo?[45] And what coverage do the existing risk regulatory frameworks offer in terms of risk prevention and minimisation of the negative impact of nanoscale chemicals on human health and the environment?

As is often the case with new technologies, the existing laws and regulations offer some oversight and coverage for nanotechnology and the early products of its application. However, as Elen Stokes points out, 'regulatory coverage is no guaranty of regulatory adequacy'.[46] This holds to be particularly true for laws dealing with novel and fast-paced developing technologies in a context of great scientific uncertainty and ignorance. Notwithstanding these concerns, the European Commission seems to assume that the existing regulatory frameworks, chiefly the REACH Regulation, are adequate. In its last Communication on the regulatory status of nanotechnology, the Commission stated that it 'remains convinced that REACH sets the best possible framework for the risk management of nanomaterials'.[47] This book will scrutinise the validity and viability of this assumption in an attempt to examine the ability of REACH's provisions to ensure a high level of human health and environmental protection for chemicals in nanoscale. Since nanoscale chemicals are currently nowhere defined in REACH, it is helpful to elaborate to some detail on the peculiar nature of such chemicals given that, as will be shown, it is this very nature that warrants special attention on the regulatory plan.

The rest of this introductory chapter (and a good part of Chapter 7) provides the relevant techno-scientific background against which the legal rules are called to establish risk management measures. This is necessary because we hold that understanding the nature of nano-chemicals is key to understanding whether the current regulatory frameworks are adequate in addressing risks associated with nanosized chemicals, or whether they offer merely a false sense of security, overlooking risks instead of *specifically* tackling and addressing them.

There is plenty of room at the bottom – how it all started

In this general introduction, to put it in Richard Feynman's words, 'I would like to describe a field, in which little has been done, but in which an enormous amount can be done in principle.'[48] In his influential essay, 'There's Plenty of Room at the Bottom', Feynman set out the foundational concepts for what was going to become a buzzword in the following decades: nano-technology. However, the word 'nanotechnology' does not appear in his ori-ginal lecture where he instead talks about a 'strange particle' in the context of 'manipulating and controlling of things at very small scale'.[49] In his visionary presentation, Feynman explored ways we might write the entire *Encyclopedia Britannica*, and possibly all the books in the world, on a pinhead. He dwelled on the methods, the materials, and even the tools that could be used to this aim and how, more generally, to overcome problems and limitations that might halt this process of miniaturisation. Feynman had no doubt that, in principle, the laws of physics allow for a drastic decrease in the size of things in a practical way. The main obstacles to the concretisation of such an endeavour, as Feynman saw them, were related to the lack of appropriate tools, e.g. those needed to assemble and operate tiny machines that could be used in medicine, and powerful electron microscopes that would allow scien-tists to actually *see* the arrangement of atoms in these miniaturised assemblies. The most revolutionary idea advanced by Feynman was the possibility of (re) arranging atoms 'one by one in the way we want them'.[50] Through such customised atomic design, Feynman theorised, we will get a vastly greater range of possible properties that substances can have and of different things that we can do with them. The marvellous biological system (i.e. the cells of an organism) and its ability to write information on a small scale and use it for a determinate function inspired Feynman's ideas.[51] Other scholars have fol-lowed up on the nature-inspired manipulation of matter, most notably Eric K. Drexler, who suggests the possibility of protein design.[52]

However, the term nanotechnology does not appear in Feynman's work. It was used for the first time in 1974 by Japanese scientist Norio Taniguchi in the realm of ultra-fine products and ultra-fine machining.[53] The term was then popularised by Drexler in his book from 1986. It is worth remembering here that besides the utopian promise of 'nanotechnology allowing people to manufacture anything they need by feeding waste material into a box that would use nanoscale assemblers to re-configure it into the necessary form, e.g. an automobile or a piece of beef', Drexler is also widely known for his dysto-pian warning on the risks nanotechnology conceals. Most notably he warns against the possibility of an accidental release of nano-machine replicators that could devour all carbon in the biosphere and hence transform the natural and man-made world, by turning everything into what he calls a 'grey goo'.[54] On the road to nanotechnological revolution, this sort of accident that would obliterate life is one 'we cannot afford'.[55] Indeed, Drexler holds, to prevent it is to 'prove our evolutionary superiority'.[56]

An important parenthesis to be opened here concerns the creation of tools in the 1980s and beginning of the 1990s that would be fundamental to nanote-chnology's progress. Feynman lamented in his paper from 1959 that the elec-tron microscopes were not good enough to allow for a rapid development of the nano-based machines and that an electronic microscope that was at least 100 times better, would enable a more rapid progress as it would allow scientists to see individual atoms distinctly.[57] In 1986 Gerd Binnig and Heinrich Rohrer were awarded the Nobel Prize for their work on the *Scanning Tunnelling Microscope* (STM). Just as Feynman had hoped, the STM allowed scientists to gaze at the atomic-world level. Relying on the quantum property of quantum tunnelling, STMs enable an accurate probing and measuring of the configuration of electrons circling individual atoms.[58] A few years later, Binning and his colleagues invented the *Atomic Force Microscope* (ATM). The main novelty of this tool is the possibility to 'touch' the atoms on different chemical surfaces, allowing not only the imaging of atoms, but most importantly, their manipulation and rearrangement into the desired configurations. Using such techniques, Donald Eigler of IBM Research managed to arrange several Xenon atoms in a vacuum to spell out 'IBM'.[59] In the following years the discovery of the *buckminsterfullerenes* – soccer-ball-shaped molecules of 60 carbon atoms – would pave the way for the first widely celebrated application of nanotechnology: the discovery of *carbon nanotubes* (CNTs). CNTs can be both single-walled (SWCNTs) and multi-walled (MWCNTs). CNTs represent also the first nanosubstance to be considered under the REACH framework. Due to having the same molecular composition of bulk-size carbon, CNTs were initially exempted by the REACH Regulation requirements as substances on which sufficient information is known and of minimum risk because of their intrinsic properties.[60] However, the question arises as to why a different arrangement of carbon atoms in nanoscale, while maintaining the *same molecular composition* of larger-scale carbon, is not to be considered similar, in terms of risks for human and environmental health, as compared to the arrangement of the same atoms in the bulk form of carbon? This question leads us to the brief but necessary exploration of the principal physicochemical laws that govern the nanosize realm and their implication for the toxicological profiles of chemicals in nanoscale.

This book takes the view that a thorough elucidation and understanding of such properties bolsters the argument for specific and tailored regulatory measures for nanoscale chemicals, which the book ultimately advocates.

A small matter of definition?

As already mentioned, nanotechnology refers to the design, characterisation, production, and application of structures, devices, and systems by controlling shape and size at the nanometre scale.[61] However, it is important to elaborate in some detail on the distinctive features of nanosubstances, where special attention ought to be devoted to their 'universal parameter': size.[62] This is necessary due to the fact that there is an ongoing debate on how nanosubstances should be defined for regulatory purposes, and size is at the centre of this debate. Also, as long as a clear definition is missing, it is difficult to enact tailored regulatory responses to the risks posed by nano-chemicals.

As the definition above suggests, nanomaterials incorporate an element of intentionality: they are manufactured/engineered at this tiny scale in order to be used for specific purposes and/or fulfil certain functions. Some scholars and regulatory bodies will hence use the term *engineered nanomaterials* (ENMs) to distinguish them from both *naturally occurring* nanosize substances and *incidentally* produced ones. The latter are present in different environmental compartments. There is an ongoing debate about the differences between the naturally occurring nano-chemicals and the manufactured ones in terms of risks for humans and the environment. Given the focus on REACH, this book is concerned with nanosubstances intentionally produced as such. Note that this is not to say that naturally occurring nanoparticles do not represent serious risks for health and the environment, but that such risks would need to be addressed under other media-specific environmental legislation.

Although in general there is no officially agreed binding definition on what precisely is to be considered a nanomaterial, a great part of the scientific community and regulatory bodies take the view that nanomaterials fall within the size range of 1 to 100 nm. However, disagreement exists on the upper-limit of 100 nm, as this fails to encompass aggregates and agglomerates of nanomaterials, which still exhibit nano-related physicochemical properties. Discussion surrounds also the 1 nm lower limit, especially because below that limit, we enter the atomic realm. As we shall see, the definitions so far adopted or suggested by regulatory agencies and scientific bodies, do provide for derogation from such limits and/or the concomitant use of characterisers other than size, whenever such characterisers correlate to the emergence of toxicity profiles of nanomaterials. Currently, the scientific uncertainties on the physicochemical properties and the risks these entail for human and environmental health, are profound and permeating. Scientific uncertainty and ignorance have, to some extent, also contributed to the impossibility of reaching a legally binding definition of nanosubstances. Considering that the possibility to define the subject of a regulation is the first necessary step towards the development of effective legislation, the controversy on definition parameters is certainly holding back the regulatory process on nanoscale substances.[63]

In this regard, while the EU has been at the forefront of efforts to establish a science-based definition to be used for regulatory purposes, other regulatory regimes, such as the US, have opted not to define nanomaterials. The American Food and Drug Administration (FDA) recognises that while the adoption of a definition for a 'nanoscale material' might offer meaningful guidance in one context, that definition may be too narrow or broad to be of use in another. On these grounds, the FDA does not recommend adopting 'formal, fixed definitions for such terms [nanotechnology and nanoscale material] for regulatory purposes'.[64] Nonetheless, in 2014 the FDA issued a guidance, which, while upholding the policy choice not to establish 'regulatory definitions',[65] suggests a number of points to be considered when evaluating if an FDA-regulated product involves the application of nanotechnology:

1   Whether a material or end product is engineered to have at least one external dimension, or an internal or surface structure, in the nanoscale range (*approximately 1 nm to 100 nm*);

2   Whether a material or end product is *engineered to exhibit properties or phenomena, including physical or chemical properties or biological effects, that are attributable to its dimension(s)*, even if these dimensions fall outside the nanoscale range, up to one micrometre (1,000 nm).[66]

The difficulty in providing a formal and fixed definition for a rapidly developing scientific discipline and the products of its applications reflects the limits of knowledge and the scientific ignorance surrounding the understanding of the very nature of such chemicals. Therefore, to adopt a formal codification of definitions that are not backed by reasonable scientific evidence might impair the regulatory progress to the same degree as the lack of a formal definition. In addition, an inflexible definition at a time of uncertainty could seriously undermine the possibilities to assess the nature and degree of risks posed by nanosubstances; it could exclude certain nanosubstances, which, despite not corresponding to the rigid parameters of a definition, nonetheless display modes of toxic action owed to their nanoscale.

It is not surprising that the EU legislature has been struggling with similar issues. In 2009, the EU Parliament called on the Commission to:

> [introduce] a comprehensive *science-based definition* of nanomaterials in Community legislation as part of nano-specific amendments to relevant horizontal and sectoral legislation; and promote the adoption of a harmonised definition of nanomaterials at the international level and to adapt the relevant European legislative framework accordingly.[67]

The Commission answered such calls by adopting a Recommendation which tries to strike a balance between leaving a definitional vacuum and adopting an arbitrary definition of the term *nanomaterial*, not grounded in scientific consensuses.[68] The scientific bases for the elaboration of such definition offered in the Recommendation are to be found in the reports prepared by the SCENIHR[69] and the Joint Research Centre (JRC).[70] Both documents concur that size as a measurand is universally applicable to the identification of nanomaterials. For the SCENIHR, although size is the 'most suitable measurand',[71] that alone does *not* explain the novel properties and the risks emerging as a consequence of the nanoscale. Thereby, a number of other specific characterisers such as the *number size distribution* or the *volume-specific surface area (VSSA)* may be used to define nanomaterials.[72] In addition, all three known types of nanomaterials – natural, accidental or by-products, and the internationally engineered ones – shall be covered by the definition. More specifically on the size range, the SCENIHR provided that while the lower limit of 1 nm shall be maintained as a valid one, for the upper limit it suggested 'using 500 nm as high upper threshold and 100 nm as low upper threshold'.[73]

Similarly, the JRC suggested that size (in the range of 1–100 nm) should be used as the only defining property.[74] However, other characterisers such as size distribution, and shape and state of agglomeration and aggregation were also singled out as relevant characterisers that should be addressed specifically in subsequently developed legislation on nanomaterials. Such considerations, the JRC further clarified, do not distinguish between naturally occurring nanomaterials and manufactured ones. If such a distinction is thought to be relevant, it should be included in specific regulations by using additional qualifiers such as 'engineered' or 'manufactured'.[75] Finally, the JRC suggested that a better term to use at this state of research would be that of 'particulate nanomaterial'.[76]

Notwithstanding this suggestion, the adopted Commission Recommendation retains the term 'nanomaterial', which it defines as

> a *natural, incidental or manufactured material* containing particles, in an unbound state or as an aggregate or as an agglomerate and where, for 50% or more of the particles in the number size distribution, one or more external dimensions is in the size range 1 nm–100 nm.[77]

Hence, besides size, the number size distribution and the specific surface area by volume can be used in defining nanomaterials.[78] Contextually, some room for derogation and flexibility is provided for. For instance, the definition allows for derogations from the number size distribution criterion[79] and from the cut-off size values for larger (aggregates and agglomerates) or smaller particles (SWCNTs and graphene flakes) which nonetheless might display hazardous profiles.[80] Ultimately, the recommended parameters of the Commission's definition are subject to review and update in light of experience with nanomaterials and in light of scientific and technological developments. As we shall see, the recommended definition has been incorporated into a number of pieces of binding secondary legislation, albeit with minor variations. Doubts about the legitimacy of such incorporation have been raised.

As far as the updating of the definition is concerned, four years after the definition's adoption, a new report from the JRC was issued in 2015. The report suggested different scenarios/options on how to bring the definition in line with the latest developments in the field.[81] It followed that in September 2017, the Commission began a public consultation on the revision of the 2011 Recommendation, with the intention of reviewing the definition in light of new scientific progress, and by so doing, achieving a more consistent application of this definition across EU legislation.[82] The Commission states that the review is not expected to bring major alteration to the existing text of the definition, but rather, will mainly consist of clarifications of the 2011 formulation and ways to aid its implementation. Importantly, the Commission declares that the main elements, i.e. definition centred on size and the additional qualifiers, e.g. particle number size distribution, are planned to remain unaltered (see Chapter 3 for details). The adoption of the modified text, expected by the end of 2018,[83] was delayed and the process is currently ongoing.

It should also be noted that other private international bodies have contributed significantly to developing harmonised terminology for nanoscale materials. Most notably, the International Organization for Standardization (ISO) was the first to provide a definition of the term nanomaterial in 2010.[84] The OECD has also carried out substantial work with regard to the understanding of the nature and risks posed by substances in nanoscale. Starting from 2008, a number of documents have been published by its internal special Working Party on Nanotechnology (WPN).[85]

In sum, there is little doubt that size, ranging between 1 and 100 nanometres, represents one agreed parameter by which a multitude of actors and documents define nanotechnology and the products of its applications. However, due to the legal nature of these documents – they all remain instruments of *soft law* – the quest for legal certainty and coherence remains a daunting task. This is so in particular if we consider that for regulatory purposes, a definition should be not only as clear and simple as possible, but also unambiguous and comprehensive.[86] This seems not to be the case with nanoscale substances. Notwithstanding some clarity and guidance provided by the definition endorsed by the Commission, inconsistency remains if the repercussions of a definition embedded in a soft law instrument are closely scrutinised on the legal plan. The first problem concerns the possibility for a definition endorsed in a soft law instrument to be incorporated *ex novo* in newly enacted legally binding documents; or to modify the definitions contained in existing legal instruments. Indeed, before the Recommendation by the Commission was adopted, the cosmetics regulation and some food-related legislation were already addressing nanomaterials. They contained a clear reference to substances in nanoscale and provided a definition of these substances so as to distinguish them from bulk materials. Is there a legal duty to update the definitions in these earlier instruments in accordance with the changes that might be made to the definition of the 2011 Recommendation? Similar questions arise with regard to incorporating the Commission's definition *ex novo* in EU horizontal legislation. The focus here is on REACH, as the Regulation is the fulcrum of this book. Chapter 3 provides an in-depth analysis on the question of definition of nanomaterials in REACH. It is nevertheless relevant to mention at this point that nothing in REACH, and especially nothing in the definition of 'substance' therein, refers to the size of a chemical or any of the nano-relevant characterisers thus far mentioned. The only documents where a reference to the term 'nanomaterial' currently appears in the REACH context are the guidance documents (GDs) drafted by the European Chemicals Agency (ECHA). The objection here is that although the ECHA is one of the few regulatory agencies with decision-making powers, its GDs are not legally binding.[87] As a result, there has been constant pressure on the Commission by the Parliament and by civil society at large, to intervene so as to include a reference to nanomaterials within the REACH framework. The process for doing so has been a long and difficult one, culminating in April 2018, in the adoption of a Draft Regulation that will amend REACH so as to include nano-specific requirements to some of its Annexes and which are expected to come into force in 2020.

However, as this book will try to demonstrate, the lack of any nano-specific terminology in the REACH's legal text, and particularly the lack of a definition for nanoscale substances as *new* and *distinct* from their bulk counterparts, is worrisome from an environmental and human health standpoint. This definition lacuna is creating confusion and legal inconsistency on the status of such chemicals in REACH. As a consequence, the very existence of a legal duty to register nano-chemicals under the REACH framework is unclear. In the current absence of nano-specific provisions in REACH, particularly in the Articles composing its legal body, one major risk is that because of this loophole, nanoscale chemicals will slip through the regulatory grid of the Regulation. Without any specific testing and data requirements on their toxicity profiles in REACH, nanomaterials will basically be treated as another, smaller version of their bulk counterpart. In practical terms, there is a risk that a producer can, for example, place nano silver on the market without providing data on its specific risks on humans and the environment, on the assumption that bulk silver has already been granted authorisation because of the lack of safety issues. However, as this book will demonstrate, this is one of the most dangerous assumptions to be made. The following section tries to demonstrate why the idea that nanoscale materials are just a tiny version of conventional chemicals is not only misleading but also scientifically flawed.

Why size matters under the risk profile

There is little doubt that the defining feature of nanomaterials is their size, ranging from 1 to 100 nm at least in one dimension. Why not, then, treat nanoscale chemicals just as a new miniaturised version of known bulk chemicals? The answer this book substantiates in the following chapters is that nanosubstances, far from being similar to their bulk counterparts, are new entities, in need of specific consideration, both under a toxicological and a legal profile.

To begin with, nanoscale chemicals behave like nothing in macroscale. Size, albeit being the most straightforward and important characteriser, is reductive – if the amazing range of physicochemical properties that emerge as a consequence of size reduction are not properly understood. It is precisely thanks to their different properties and behaviour that nano-chemicals are pursued and used in order to fulfil a particular function or have a specific effect. These very same properties, though, are responsible for the emergence of unprecedented risks for human health and ecosystems. As a consequence, there is an urgent need to delineate the criteria determining when a nanoscale substance 'is *"new for legal and regulatory purposes"* and *"new for safety evaluation purposes"*',[88] including within the existing legal frameworks like REACH.

The American Environmental Protection Agency (EPA) defines nanotechnology as the manipulation of matter for use in particular applications through certain chemical and/or physical processes to create materials with specific properties.[89] Such processes can be *bottom-up* (by assembling smaller subunits through chemical synthesis or crystal growth)[90] or *top-down* (by milling or lithographic etching of a large sample to obtain nanoparticles).[91] But as already stated, the emergence of unique properties as a consequence of size reduction is at the same time the source of unknown and unexpected risks for humans and the environment. What does this mean concretely?

The first thing worth mentioning is that at nanoscale, we are operating at the border between classical and quantum physics. At this realm, the properties displayed by the substances are not only novel and unique, but at the same time unexpected.[92] As a consequence it is virtually impossible to make predictions about the environmental fate of such chemicals or their general impact on ecosystems and human health.[93] Nonetheless, making sense of their peculiar physicochemical properties, responsible for the unique behaviour they display, can foster a deeper understanding of their toxicity mechanisms and the correlated risks. To put it differently, understanding why silver or gold in nanoscale need a specific tailored regulatory coverage, backed by specific toxicity testing for the nanoform, is an essential preliminary step towards taking effective risk management measures.

Kimberly A. Gray offers a brilliant and exhaustive account of why the behaviour and consequently the risk profiles of chemicals in nanoscale are different for those of chemicals in the macroscale. The following draws significantly on her elaboration.[94] The starting point is the fact that size matters. And it matters greatly. As size approaches the nanoscale, mechanical, electronic, chemical, biological, optical, and other physicochemical properties change dramatically.[95] For instance, metal oxides such as iron oxide and titanium dioxide at nanoscale do not scatter light and are transparent, which makes them particularly attractive for the cosmetic industry.[96] Changes in colour and other fundamental properties such as conductivity and melting point are also observable. For instance, nano gold loses its metallic nature and, depending on the exact size, can appear red or blue.[97] There are two main reasons for the emergence of these unique properties.

The first concerns the exponential increase of the surface area per unit of volume, as size decreases. This is known as *the surface area effect*. By a way of example, Trudy E. Bell explains that if the surface area of a cubic centimetre of a solid material is 6 square centimetres, the surface area of a cubic centimetre of 1 nm particles in an ultrafine powder is 6,000 square metres! Or, more concretely, if 10 g of silver in the form of spherical nanoparticles with a diameter of 10 nm exhibit a total surface area of about $570\,m^2$, a single solid silver sphere with the same mass has a surface area of about $4.7\,cm^2$. This means that size-reduction *for the same mass* of the same substance, gives an increase in total surface area for the nanomaterial form, of more than a factor of 1,200,000.[98] This enormous surface increase causes nanomaterials to be extremely reactive.[99] Other factors such as surface coating and surface shape contribute to the reactivity of a nanomaterial and its behaviour in the human body and in the environmental media. The reason why this happens is that as size decreases, more atoms will be located on the surface of a chemical. Given that surface atoms tend to form more bonds with other materials and melt at a lower temperature, the behaviour of chemicals reduced in this way will change dramatically.[100] Paradoxically though, the large surface area is what makes nanosubstances attractive in terms of environmental solutions and remedies, given the ability of nanosize particles to sorb organic and inorganics chemicals from various contaminated environmental compartments.[101] As a result, the development of sensors capable of detecting biological and chemical contaminants in environmental media such as water and soil, represents one of most prominent areas of nanotechnology application. However, the same surface area that enables the cleaning-up function, can also pose considerable threats given that nanoscale materials can bind with dangerous chemicals and transport them deeper into subcellular organs, creating the so-called *Trojan horse effect*.[102] The small size also enables deeper penetration into organs' tissues or the nucleus of cells and mitochondria, or even the crossing of the blood-brain barrier, causing among other things oxidative stress and DNA damaging, i.e. elevated cancer risks.[103]

The other important effect verifiable at nanoscale is the *quantum effect*. For the details of the science upholding the quantum effect we refer to Gray.[104] Here suffice it to mention that the quantum effect, which is size-dependent and takes place starting at around 100 nm, is responsible for the whole set of characterising properties such as transparency, colour, electrical conductivity, etc.[105] The quantum effect is also responsible for the unpredictable behaviour of nanoscale materials and the discontinuity of propriety-displaying: hence nano gold is catalytically reactive in the size range 3–5 nm but essentially inert outside this range.[106]

Concluding on the importance of size under the risk profile, the following points constitute a condensed manifesto on nanotechnology and its science, to be consulted in parallel with the legal analysis unfolding in the remaining chapters of this book:

1   Volume and/or weight are the incorrect units of measurement for nano-materials. Rather, the surface area which increases by orders of magnitude for the same weight, is the most important measurand, albeit not the only one. Other factors such as surface reactivity, shape, and encapsulation are responsible for the emergence of the amazing, yet highly hazardous, properties in nanoscale substances. It is currently *not* possible to determine safe levels of exposure for nanomaterials.

2   Nanoscale chemicals are not just a tiny version of their bulk counterpart. Although the atomic-molecular composition might be the same, the way atoms are 'packed' in nanoscale leads to a completely different behaviour in terms of physicochemical properties and risks. Hence, because of the

unique arrangement of their atoms (i.e. the location on the surface, the bonding patterns, and the greater number of surface atoms), nanosubstances are new substances. Their behaviour is governed by new laws of physics: those of quantum mechanics.

3   The fact that nano-chemicals are used in consumer products in quantities well below those of bulk materials, does not mean that risks of diffuse pollution are negligible. In addition, nanomaterials exhibit cytotoxicity which might cause serious disruption of ecosystem processes. From this, coupled with what is stated in points 1 and 2, i.e. that such effects do not depend on the quantity/mass, it becomes obvious that it is necessary to prevent/control the emission of nanoscale chemicals into the environment, as the only effective way to contain risks.

4   There are no data to demonstrate that nanomaterials will aggregate into larger particles in the environment, therefore becoming more inert and depositing in soil or sediments. There is instead a great need to develop appropriate methodologies for ecotoxicity and cytotoxicity of nanomaterials' risk assessment.

5   There is also a need for a tiered approach to comprehensive toxicity risk assessment which should take place at the same time as the development of nano-enhanced products progresses. This is a fundamental step that cannot be obscured by lamenting about the high costs for such a comprehensive assessment.[107]

Delimiting the field of inquiry

Although touching upon general questions related to the ability of REACH's legal framework to lessen negative environmental impacts of rapid technological development, the focus of this book is narrowed down to nanotechnology and precisely to the first generation of its applications: nanosubstances.

The technological complexity of nanotechnology development has been classified by the EPA as encompassing four stages of development resulting in progressively complex applications.[108] According to the EPA, the first generation of nanotechnology applications, 'passive nanostructures', include:

> [n]ano-structured coatings, nanoparticles, nanostructured metals, polymers, ceramics, Catalysts, composites, displays.[109]

Given that the basic concept on which REACH builds its set of rules is that of 'chemical substance', either on its own or in mixtures and preparations, it seems pertinent to circumscribe our analysis to this category of nanotechnology application. In addition, the confinement to this first category is owed to the fact that polymers, catalysts, and composites are dealt with under the REACH structure through rules significantly different from those applicable to chemical substances. Hence, under the assumption of the applicability of the REACH system to *passive nanostructures* as a whole, legal differentiations arise depending on whether a chemical in nanoscale fulfils the criteria for being considered a chemical substance or a polymer, for example. Pointing out such differences is important, and a reference to the exemption regimes in REACH is relevant as they might have significant consequences in terms of environmental protection rules. For instance, while REACH exempts polymers from registration requirements, it does nevertheless impose an obligation to register for monomer units forming the polymer. Therefore, nano titanium nitride used in *polyethylene terephthalate* (PET) bottles as a fortifier will have to be registered in REACH if tonnage bands and hazard criteria are met, although the polymer it forms falls out of the REACH scope.[110]

The other three categories of nanotechnology development envisaged by the EPA – *active nanostructures, 3-D nanosystems and systems of nanosystems*, and *molecular nanosystems* – are not part of this book's subject. With the exemption of active nanostructures, which have already crossed laboratory borders in the form of, for example, target delivery drugs, sensors, and solar cells, the last two advanced products are still in their infancy. In addition, the three complex applications in question represent peculiarities that are difficult to capture under the REACH legal framework, which was designed for chemicals. This way, self-assembly and molecule-to-molecule nanosystems will probably pose unique health, safety, and environmental (HSE) concerns which would need to be addressed under tailored regulations. It is legitimate to think that the task of regulating complex nano-products would trigger targeted and specific intervention of the EU legislator through innovative legal instruments. To put it differently, although REACH rules might be flexible and adaptive enough (albeit through pertinent amendments) for the first generation of nanotechnology, it is difficult to assert the same for the future generations of the science of the very small. As the EPA foresees: 'integration of these fourth-generation nanotechnologies with information, biological, and cognitive technologies will lead to products which can now only be imagined'.[111]

Therefore, no reference will be made to legal challenges and environmental issues springing from such applications in this book. Nevertheless, the awareness of the future development of nanoscience and nanotechnology is relevant to the delimitation of the scope and subject matter of this book by exclusion, in the sense that the present analysis is concerned only with the first generation of nanotechnology applications. To do otherwise would demand significant legal and scientific understanding and research – well beyond the REACH realm of application, exclusively concerned with chemicals substances.[112] Additionally, this book is built upon the presumption that the current concepts of hazard and risk, as well as the methodologies designated to measure and assess them embodied in REACH can *maybe* be applied – although intervention and review are needed also in this case – only to the first generations of nanotechnology applications, mainly to nano-chemicals. Complex future developments in the sector, such as *nano-robots* and *synthetic biology*, might require us to develop completely new measures and tools in order to manage an entirely new concept of risk, known as *infinite risk*.[113] It thus falls outside the REACH area of competence to deal with future complex and infinite risks and our focus is rather on nano-chemicals and their environmental impacts.

In addition, the main focus of this book is on the prevention and reduction of nano-related *environmental* risks. Human health risks are not dismissed entirely though, as it is virtually impossible to separate the study of environmental and human health risks presented by chemical pollution in a clear-cut manner. And yet, peculiarities persist with regard to each area. It is generally recognised for instance, that the study of chemical harm on the environment is a less developed area of toxicology as compared to that of human health risks. Lack of clinical data, impossibility of testing chemical-cocktails, and the ignorance concerning the way chemicals affect ecosystems in their integrity, make the study of environmental risks regulation a priority.

Scope of the study and methodology

On the basis of the preliminary observation and with the subject matter finally defined, the *raison d'être* of this book is the position of the Commission on the status of nanomaterials in REACH. This position is set out in the following communications, adopted respectively in 2008 and 2012, shedding light on the Commission's understanding of the regulatory status of nanomaterials in REACH and beyond. The Commission affirmed:

> There are no provisions in REACH referring explicitly to nanomaterials. However, *nanomaterials are covered by the 'substance' definition in REACH.*[114]

Overall the Commission remains convinced that *REACH sets the best possible framework for the risk management of nanomaterials* when they occur as substances or mixtures but more specific requirements for nanomaterials within the framework have proven necessary. The Commission envisages modifications in some of the REACH Annexes and encourages ECHA to further develop guidance for registrations after 2013.[115]

The focus on REACH is built on several considerations. First, REACH represents not only the ultimate effort of the EU legislator to set up a legal framework for addressing potential environmental and health impacts of chemical substances *upstream*, directly at the very source of their manifestation (the production and use of chemicals as such) but also, due the overarching nature of the regulation:

> data generated under REACH will serve as input to other regulation, such as worker protection, cosmetics and environmental protection. It complements product legislation (e.g. general product safety) to the extent that this does not cover environmental aspects.[116]

Second, REACH endorses a number of environmental principles, which might play a central role in the early regulation of nanotechnology and their first-generation products, nanosubstances/nanomaterials. The precautionary principle,[117] the polluter pays principle,[118] and the substitution principle[119] are core elements of the REACH law and policy. Hence, when questioning the effectiveness of REACH in regulating nano-chemicals, the potential application of such principles to this category of chemicals will also be questioned. Lastly, although REACH was conceptualised so as to contain few overlaps with other sector-specific legislation, e.g. medicine and cosmetic regulations,[120] this book holds that when REACH supplements such legislation, interesting legal cross-fertilisation can take place.

But does REACH actually (and as the Commission claims), as it currently stands, appropriately and exhaustively cover nanoscale substances so that high levels of human health and environmental protection are ensured for this class of chemicals? This book sets out to answer this question through a detailed legal (chiefly Chapters 2–6) and techno-scientific (chiefly Chapter 7) analysis. In the attempt to answer this question, we shall keep in mind that REACH is a modern environmental law. Therefore, the assessment of its effectiveness in regulating nanoscale chemicals is necessarily centred on the concept of risk in general, and the element of uncertainty in the specific. Put differently, the inquiry into the effectiveness of REACH's provisions to offer high levels of protection against the human health and environmental risks of nanomaterials, is an inquiry into whether the risk regulation models delineated in REACH, can also be applied to highly uncertain nano-risks.

On such premises, the methodological approach employed throughout this book is necessarily an interdisciplinary one. Although interdisciplinarity is not an easy task for lawyers, it must be recalled here that the shift towards interdisciplinarity in legal research was born first and foremost out of the practical need to keep pace with the complex socio-economic developments taking place in the real world around us. And nowhere is this better observable than in the realm of environmental law. Many of the critical problems that environmental law tries to address involve considerations of a great number of factors and interactions beyond law. Concepts such as sustainability, human health and environmental protection, and more in general ecosystem and biodiversity preservation, cannot be properly understood through legal lenses alone. Instead, in order to be able to grapple with the substantial core of such concepts, legal scholars must move away from their tendency to be 'natural luddites'.[121] In a nutshell thus 'the separate efforts of social and natural sciences are unlikely to fully illuminate the fabric of or fashion solutions to environmental problems'.[122] Moreover, what seems to be often neglected is the fact that environmental law – and chemicals regulation as part of it – is in practice highly interdisciplinary.[123] It is relevant to recall here that environmental law as an independent legal branch emerged primarily in response to the work of environmentalist scientists such as Rachel Carson,[124] whose ideas inspired the adoption of specific legal rules to counter some of the most pressing factors of pollution and ecosystems degradation. Interdisciplinarity affects also the environmental models used in decision-making, which often incorporate a wide range of information from different fields of expertise.[125]

Furthermore, the legal research on the regulation of the environmental risks of nanotechnology applications, cannot and should not overlook the distinctive nature of nanotechnology, which is in itself an intrinsically interdisciplinary *scientific* subject. Having a firm grasp of the physicochemical properties that emerge at nanoscale can aid the understanding of the risks that the regulators are called to manage. In other words, placing our analysis on the science-law juncture is necessary both for a constructive critique of the shortcomings of the existing regulatory models and for the elaboration of effective future regulatory options. This is so because we take the view that 'collaboration between environmental lawyers and scientists is essential in the development of sustainable solutions to environmental problems'.[126]

Already from the preliminary introduction of REACH here presented, it is easy to notice that the Regulation is a massive endeavour of law-and-science, to the extent that for many of its cornerstone concepts, it is virtually impossible to separate the science from the law. Hence, any sort of legal scholarship in an area like REACH requires a certain literacy in natural sciences such as chemistry, physics, biology,[127] and, importantly, regulatory toxicology.

The law-science dialogue is also important to the work of advisory bodies for the way advisory science is used by policy-makers. This, in turn, has a direct impact on the democratic dimension of decision-making in terms of participation, transparency, and the right to know.[128] As this book will show, these are all crucial elements in order to trigger a precautionary ruling. In line with the interpretation of precaution as *Care*, the final chapter (Chapter 8) of this book advocates for the creation of a new theory of responsibility for regulators legislating on potentially catastrophic risks. Using Hans Jonas's ideas[129] on the new imperative of responsibility, the eighth chapter and the book as a whole call for new ethical principles to guide regulatory measures in the (nano)technological age.

Notes

1 Rachel Carson, *Silent Spring* (Houghton Mifflin 1962, Reprinted in Penguin Classics 2000) 31.
2 Murray Bookchin, *Our Synthetic Environment* (Harper & Row 1974).
3 See in general: T.N. Savinova, G.W. Gabrielsen, and S. Falk-Petersen, The Joint Norwegian-Russian Commission on Environmental Cooperation, The Seabird Expert Group, 'Chemical Pollution in the Arctic and Sub-Arctic Marine Ecosystems: an Overview of Current Knowledge' (Report no. 3: 1994/95, NINA 1995).
4 Johan Rockström et al., 'A Safe Operating Space for Humanity', (2009) 461 Nature 472, 472.
5 Ibid. 473.
6 Linn M. Persson et al., 'Confronting Unknown Planetary Boundary Threats from Chemical Pollution' (2013) 47 Environ. Sci. Technol. 12619.
7 Ibid. 12620.
8 Ibid. 12620.

9 Ibid. 12621.
10 Matthew MacLeod et al., 'Identifying Chemicals That Are Planetary Boundary Threats' (2014) 48 Environ. Sci. Technol. 11057.
11 Will Steffen et al., 'Planetary Boundaries: Guiding Human Development on a Changing Planet' (2015) 347 Science 1259855, 1259855–1259886.
12 Ibid. 1259855–1259856.
13 Geoffrey Hunt and Michael D. Mehta (eds), *Nanotechnology: Risk, Ethics and Law* (Earthscan 2006) 3.
14 Science Policy Council, Nanotechnology Workgroup, 'EPA Nanotechnology White Paper' (EPA100/B-07/001 2007) (hereafter, (EPA 2007)) 5.
15 Elizabeth Fisher, 'The "Perfect Storm" of REACH: Charting Regulatory Controversy in the Age of Information, Sustainable Development, and Globalization' (2008) 11 Journal of Risk Research 541, 541.
16 Council Regulation (EC) 1907/2006 of 18 December 2006 concerning the Registration, Evaluation, Authorisation and Restriction of Chemicals (REACH), establishing a European Chemicals Agency, amending Directive 1999/45/EC and repealing Council Regulation (EEC) No. 793/93 and Commission Regulation (EC) No. 1488/94 as well as Council Directive 76/769/EEC and Commission Directives 91/155/EEC, 93/67/EEC, 93/105/EC and 2000/21/EC [2006] OJ L396/1 (hereafter, REACH).
17 This book uses the term regulatory toxicology (RT) to refer both to toxicology and ecotoxicology. Regulatory toxicology governs the toxicological risk analysis involving effects on human health and the environmental pollution. However, RT does not equate with toxicology which it takes as a basis but at the same time simplifies for risk management purposes. See in general H. Paul A. Illing and Timothy C. Marrs 'Regulatory Toxicology' in Bryan Ballantyne, Timothy C. Marrs, and Tore Syversen (eds), *General and Applied Toxicology: Vol. 6* (3rd edn, Wiley 2009) and Chapter 7 of this book for a detailed analysis on the subject.
18 Steven Vaughan, 'EU Chemicals Regulation New Governance, Hybridity and REACH' (Elgar 2015) 2.
19 Magnus Breitholtz et al., 'Improving the Value of Standard Toxicity Test Data in REACH' in Johan Eriksson, Michael Gilek, and Christina Rudén (eds), *Regulating Chemical Risks: European and Global Challenges* (Springer 2010) 86.
20 REACH, Article 1(1).
21 See: Commission, 'Strategy for a Future Chemicals Policy' COM (2001) 88 final.
22 Fisher 2008 (n 15) 548.
23 REACH, Article 1(3).
24 The term was coined by the US Environmental Defense Fund in its report from 1997, 'Toxic Ignorance. The Continuing Absence of Basic Health Testing for To-Selling Chemicals in the United States' which denounced the problem and the dimension of a nearly total lack of data on the toxic profiles of widely used chemicals. Available at: www.edf.org/sites/default/files/243_toxicignorance_0. pdf accessed 22.02.2019; See also Nertila Kuraj, 'Complexities and Conflict in Controlling Dangerous Chemicals: The Case of Regulating Endocrine Disruptors in EU Law' in Eléonore Maitre-Ekern, Carl Dalhammar, and Hans Christian Bugge (eds), *Preventing Environmental Damage from Products: An Analysis of the Policy and Regulatory Framework in Europe* (CUP 2018) 281–282.
25 REACH, Article 75(1).
26 REACH, Articles 40–43.
27 REACH, Articles 44–48.
28 REACH, Article 49.
29 Kuraj (n 24) 282–284.

30 See Council Directive 2002/21/EC of the European Parliament and of the Council of 7 March 2002 on a common regulatory framework for electronic communications networks and services (Framework Directive) OJ L108/33.

31 See Lyria B. Moses, 'Recurring Dilemmas: The Law's Race to Keep Up with Technological Change' (2007) UNSW Law Research Paper 21/2007.

32 See SCENIHR, 'Scientific Basis for the Definition of the Term "Nanomaterial"' (6 July 2010); EPA 2007 (n 14).

33 See in general: FAO, 'International Conference on Food and Agriculture Applications of Nanotechnologies: Report of Technical Round Table Sessions' (NANOAGRI 2010) 18.

34 Ibid. 46.

35 See in general: OECD, 'Nanotechnology for Green Innovation' (2013) No. 5 OECD Science, Technology and Industry Policy Papers.

36 FAO (n 33) 18.

37 Peter Davidson, 'Up and Away' (*TEC Magazine*, May 2012) www.tcetoday. com/~/media/Documents/TCE/Articles/2012/851/851geoengineering.pdf accessed 11.10.2016.

38 For a complete list of such applications, including the names of the substances and the therapeutic uses see the assessment reports by EMA at: www.ema. europa.eu/ema/ accessed 21.02.2019.

39 C. Lee Ventola, 'The Nanomedicine Revolution: Part 2: Current and Future Clinical Applications' (2012) 37 Pharmacy and Therapeutics T 582.

40 See in general: SCENIHR, 'Preliminary Opinion on Safety of Nanomaterials in Cosmetic Products' (19 June 2007).

41 SCENIHR, 'Opinion on the Appropriateness of the Risk Assessment Methodology in Accordance with the Technical Guidance Documents for New and Existing Substances for Assessing the Risk of Nanomaterials' (21–22 June 2007) 51.

42 EFSA, 'The Potential Risks Arising from Nanoscience and Nanotechnologies on Food and Feed Safety' (2009) 958 The EFSA Journal 1, 15.

43 SCENIHR, 'Risk Assessment of Products of Nanotechnologies' (19 January 2009) 10.

44 Dennis Pamlin and Stuart Armstrong, '12 Risks that Threaten Human Civilisation: The Case for a New Risk Category' (Global Challenges Foundation 2015).

45 Eric K. Drexler, *Engines of Creation: The Coming Era of Nanotechnology* (Anchor Books 1986).

46 Elen Stokes, 'Nanotechnology and the Products of Inherited Regulation' (2012) 39 Journal of Law and Society 93, 94.

47 Commission, 'Second Regulatory Review on Nanomaterials' (Communication) COM (2012) 572 final, 11.

48 Richard P. Feynman, 'There's Plenty of Room at the Bottom: An Invitation to Enter a New Field of Physics' (1960) 23 (5) Engineering and Science 22, 22.

49 Ibid.

50 Ibid. 34.

51 He writes:

> Biology is not simply writing information; it is doing something about it. A biological system can be exceedingly small. Many of the cells are very tiny, but they are very active; they manufacture various substances; they walk around; they wiggle; and they do all kinds of marvelous things – all on a very small scale. Also, they store information. Consider the possibility that we too can make a thing very small which does what we want – that we can manufacture an object that maneuvers at that level!
>
> Feynman (n 48) 25

52 Drexler (n 45).

53 See in general: Norio Taniguchi et al., *Nanotechnology: Integrated Processing Systems for Ultra-precision and Ultra-fine Products* (OUP 1996).
54 Drexler (n 45) 147–148.
55 Ibid. 147.
56 Ibid.
57 Feynman (n 48) 24.
58 See UNESCO 'The Ethics and Politics of Nanotechnology' (2007) 38–41.
59 Ibid. 42.
60 REACH, Article 2(7)(a).
61 The Royal Society and The Royal Academy of Engineering, *Nanoscience and Nanotechnologies: Opportunities and Uncertainties* (The Royal Society 2004) 5.
62 SCENIHR 2010 (n 32) 24.
63 On such issue see: Andrew D. Maynard, 'Don't Define Nanomaterials' (2011) 475 Nature 31.
64 FDA, 'Nanotechnology: A Report of the U.S. Food and Drug Administration Nanotechnology Task Force' (25 July 2007) 6–7, emphasis added.
65 FDA, 'Guidance for Industry: Considering Whether an FDA-Regulated Product Involves the Application of Nanotechnology' (June 2014) 5.
66 Ibid. 6, emphasis added. The same position was reconfirmed in the latest document from the Administration: FDA, 'Guidance for Industry Use of Nanomaterials in Food for Animals' (August 2015).
67 Parliament resolution of 24 April 2009 on regulatory aspects of nanomaterials (2008/2208(INI)), P6_TA(2009)0328 [2009] OJ C184E/82, 87.
68 Commission Recommendation 2011/696/EU of 18 October 2011 on the definition of nanomaterial [2011] OJ L275/38.
69 SCENIHR 2010 (n 32).
70 Göran Lövestam et al., 'Considerations on a Definition of Nanomaterial for Regulatory Purposes' (European Commission JRC 2010).
71 SCENIHR 2010 (n 32) 33.
72 Ibid.
73 Ibid.
74 Lövestam et al. (n 70) 26.
75 Lövestam et al. (n 70) 26–27.
76 Lövestam et al. (n 70) 31.
77 Commission Recommendation 2011/696/EU, (1).
78 Ibid.
79 'In specific cases and where warranted by concerns for the environment, health, safety or competitiveness the number size distribution threshold of 50% may be replaced by a threshold between 1 and 50%.' Ibid.
80 'By derogation from point 2, fullerenes, graphene flakes and single wall carbon nanotubes with one or more external dimensions below 1 nm should be considered as nanomaterials.' Ibid.
81 See Hubert Rauscher et al., 'Towards a Review of the EC Recommendation for a Definition of the Term "Nanomaterial": Part 3: Scientific-Technical Evaluation of Options to Clarify the Definition and to Facilitate its Implementation' (European Commission JRC 2015).
82 'EC Begins Consultation on Revising Recommendation on Definition of Nanomaterial' (*Bergeson & Campbell*, 20 September 2017) https://nanotech.lawbc.com/2017/09/ec-begins-consultation-on-revising-recommendation-on-definition-of-nanomaterial/ accessed 28.02.2019.
83 'Definition of a Nanomaterial' (*EC*) http://ec.europa.eu/environment/chemicals/nanotech/faq/definition_en.htm accessed 22.02.2019.
84 ISO, 'Nanotechnologies – Vocabulary – Part 1: Core Terms' (ISO/TS 80004–1:2010).

85 Available at: www.oecd.org/sti/nano/reports.htm accessed 01.03.2019.
86 Lövestam et al. (n 70) 10.
87 This was confirmed in a very recent case law on REACH, where the Court of Justice of the European Union (CJEU) stated that the ECHA documents (a Technical Guidance in this case) 'cannot be of a legally binding nature' in as much they are not part of the binding Union acts mentioned by Article 288 TFEU. See Case C-106/14 – *FCD and FMB* [2015] ECLI:EU:C:2015:576, para 28.
88 Michael R. Taylor, 'Regulating the Products of Nanotechnology: Does FDA Have the Tools it Needs?' (PEN5 2006) 7, emphasis added.
89 Ibid. 7.
90 Kimberly A. Gray, 'Five Myths about Nanotechnology in the Current Public Policy' in David A. Dana (ed.) *The Nanotechnology Challenge Creating Legal Institutions for Uncertain Risks* (CUP 2011) 7.
91 Trudy E. Bell, 'Understanding Risk Assessment of Nanotechnology' (National Nanotechnology Initiative 2007).
92 Hunt and Mehta (n 13) 5.
93 Gray (n 90) 12.
94 Ibid. 12.
95 Bell (n 91) 2.
96 Gray (n 90) 15.
97 Ibid.
98 The nano silver example is provided by the JRC, 'REACH Implementation Project Substance Identification of Nanomaterials (RIP-oN 1)', Advisory Report (European Commission JRC March 2011) 21.
99 Bell (n 91) 2.
100 Gray (n 90) 18.
101 EPA 2007 (n 14) 37.
102 See, with regard to nano silver: Eun-Jung Park et al., 'Silver Nanoparticles Induce Cytotoxicity by a Trojan-Horse Type Mechanism' (2010) 24 Toxicol In Vitro 872.
103 SCENIHR 2009 (n 43).
104 Gray (n 90) 18–20.
105 Bell (n 91) 3.
106 Gray (n 90) 20.
107 Gray (n 90) 46–49.
108 See EPA 2007 (n 14) 13.
109 Ibid.
110 Nano TiN, as a fortifier in PET bottles, has already been approved by the EFSA in 2008 and the authorisation was extended to similar uses of the substance in 2012. In this regard see: EFSA Panel on Food Contact Materials, Enzymes, Flavourings and Processing Aids (CEF), 'Scientific Opinion on 21st List of Substances for Food Contact Materials' (2008) The EFSA Journal 888–890, 1–14; and EFSA Panel on Food Contact Materials, Flavourings, Enzymes and Processing Aids, 'Scientific Opinion on the Safety Evaluation of the Substance, Titanium Nitride, Nanoparticles, for Use in Food Contact Materials' (2012) 10(3):2641 EFSA Journal 1–8.
111 EPA 2007 (n 14) 12.
112 See also IRGC Policy Brief 'Nanotechnology Risk Governance Recommendations for a Global, Coordinated Approach to the Governance of Potential Risks' (International Risk Governance Council 2007) 7.
113 Catastrophic scenarios of infinite risks are better illustrated here: Pamlin and Armstrong (n 43).
114 Commission, 'Regulatory Aspects of Nanomaterials' (Communication) COM (2008) 366 final 4.

115 COM (2012) 572 final, 11.
116 COM (2008) 366 final, 5.
117 REACH, recital (9) and (69); REACH Article 1(3).
118 Through the '*no data, no market*' leitmotiv introduced in Article 5 of REACH, the intention of the EU legislature is that of shifting forward the producer's responsibility at the very first stage of the chemicals' production and, through cost allocation on industry for the generation of safety data, to anticipate the polluter pays concept.
119 Reference to the substitution of dangerous chemicals with less dangerous alternatives – both chemical and technological – is often found throughout the text of REACH, for example recitals (12) and (70)–(74). However, it is the Authorisation phase, Title VII of REACH, that represents the fulcrum of the substitution principle, given that the final aim of Authorisation is that of fostering substitution and the phasing out of highly hazardous chemicals.
120 See in general: Commission, 'General Report on REACH' (Staff Working Document) SWD (2013) 25 final, 4–15.
121 C.P. Snow, *The Two Cultures* (CUP 1961) 22.
122 David N. Wear, 'Challenges to Interdisciplinary Discourse' (1999) 2 Ecosystems 299, 299.
123 Dave Owen and Caroline Owen, 'Interdisciplinary Research and Environmental Law' (2015) 41 Ecology L.Q. 887, 890.
124 Ibid. 894.
125 For an overview on the role and importance of environmental models in decision-making, see Elizabeth Fisher, Pasky Pascual, and Wendy Wagner, 'Understanding Environmental Models in Their Legal and Regulatory Context' (2010) 22 J Environmental Law 251.
126 John McEldowney and Sharron McEldowney, 'Science and Environmental Law: Collaboration across the Double Helix' (2011) 13 Environmental Law Review 169, 169.
127 Jack M. Balkin and Sanford Levinson, 'Law and the Humanities: An Uneasy Relationship' (2013) 18 Yale Journal of Law and the Humanities 155, 161.
128 McEldowney and McEldowney (n 126) 173.
129 Hans Jonas, *The Imperative of Responsibility: In Search of an Ethics for the Technological Age* (University of Chicago Press 1984).

2   Why REACH?

Investigating REACH's history of
adoption and the early question of
nanotechnology regulation therein

Introduction

In light of the aim and object of this study, as laid out in Chapter 1, the
present chapter focuses on the early legal discourse concerning the status of
nanoscale chemicals in REACH. The analysis that follows seeks to contextualise such discourse on two levels.

First, it presents a brief introduction to the emergence and evolution of
EU environmental law, where chemicals risk regulation belongs. Attention
will be here drawn to the (constitutional) significance of choosing the appropriate legal basis for environmental measures and how this affects the powers
of the EU institution and, particularly, of Member States (MSs), to enact
more stringent environmental measures. Second, a detailed analysis of the EU
chemicals policy in the pre-REACH period will be presented in order to
understand why and how the REACH reform came about. The EU chemicals regulation represents one of the earliest legal regimes for the control of
technological risk and its transformation has taken place parallel to that of
general EU environmental law. Inevitably, therefore, chemicals regulatory
regimes, which REACH epitomises, reflect the emergence and consecration
of a number of principles and approaches that have been shaping EU environmental policy for the last four decades.[1]

The close relationship between chemicals risk regulation and the consecration of the EU as a leading global actor in environmental protection policies
is best reflected in the history of the adoption of REACH, which this chapter
examines in detail. As will be shown, REACH's lengthy and uneasy process
of negotiation is a symptom of the deeply divergent interests affected by regulatory measures on risk prevention and control. The classical bifurcation of
conflicting interests sees trade, economic growth, and technological leader-
ship objectives as colliding with or even opposed to the high levels of protection of human and environmental health aims. Interestingly, nanotechnology
and the products of its application are placed exactly on the intersection
between these conflicting interests.

As Tanja Ehnert evocatively puts it, both a 'nanomania' and a contextual
'nanophobia' have characterised the approach of the EU chemical sector to

nanotechnology and the products of its applications.[2] In the same vein, if on the one hand, the promotion of R&D activities and nano-enhanced products is fully supported and promoted in the EU, particularly by the Commission, on the other hand, the same institution is generally reluctant to introduce nano-specific provisions or amendments to relevant pieces of legislation.[3] Such reluctance is observable not only for existing legal frameworks which were affected by the advent of nanotechnology *after* they were adopted but also for newly enacted regulations such as REACH, which could have been rendered nano-specific before being enacted. The proposed provisions pertaining to nano-chemicals coverage in REACH will be analysed here with some preliminary consideration on the failure to incorporate them in the final text of REACH. Said failure appears particularly regrettable in light of the fact that REACH is gradually becoming a global standard-setter in chemicals regulation well beyond the EU, as the final part of this chapter will demonstrate by using the post-Brexit UK and Turkey's approach to chemical regulation in relation to and as influenced by REACH.

Overall, this chapter starts challenging the prevailing idea that REACH is deemed to also cover nano-scale chemicals – even in the complete absence of any reference to nano-chemicals in its legal texts. The underpinning idea is that in any event, regulatory coverage is no guarantee of regulatory adequacy.[4]

Evolution of EU environmental law and its chemical policy

From the emergence of EU environmental law to post-Lisbon novelties

Until the adoption of the Single European Act (SEA) in 1986, there was no formal basis for environmental policy in the EU.[5]

The lack of a legal basis in the EEC Treaty[6] meant that environmental measures only incidentally emerged in the decision-making process during *this first phase* of environmental law development.[7] Directive 67/548/EEC[8] is a clear example. Based on Article 100 EEC, the Directive was primarily pre-occupied with the removal of the hindrances deriving from different national regimes in the (then) six Member States regarding the classification, packaging, and labelling of dangerous substances and preparations aiming at ensuring a good functioning of the internal market.[9] Protecting 'the public, and in particular workers'[10] was seen as an indirect consequence of harmonisation.

During the *second phase* of EU environmental law development, starting with the adoption in 1973 of the first EU Environmental Action Programme (EAP),[11] most of the legal acts were based on Article 100 EEC (now Article 115 TFEU) such as the Directive concerning the lead content in petrol[12] and that on toxic and dangerous waste.[13] However, the clear-cut nature of Article 100 EEC, concerned exclusively with the internal market functioning, made it difficult for the provision to be invoked widely as a legal basis for environmental policies. Therefore, the complementary powers the Council was bestowed with under Article 235 (now Article 352 TFEU) were necessary for the adoption of environmentally oriented acts.[14]

Although environmental protection was considered to represent one of the objectives of the community by extensive interpretation of Article 2 EC,[15] the consecration of such Article as a legitimate basis for environmental legislation was made possible only after the *ADBHU* case.[16] In this case, the CJEU ruled that environmental protection was one of the Community's 'essential objectives'.[17] Hence, the restrictive measures challenged in front of the Court were found to be legitimate[18] for so long as they are neither 'discriminatory nor go beyond the inevitable restrictions which are justified by the pursuit of the objective of environmental protection, which is in the general interest'.[19] As a result, Article 235 EEC could be invoked not only in concomitance to Article 100 EEC as a valid legal basis for environmental policy, but also on its own. The Wild Birds Directive[20] and the Directive on a limit value for lead in the air[21] are a clear example of this legitimation as they were all based on Article 235 EEC.[22]

Environmental measures taken based on Article 235 EEC had to be adopted by the Council by unanimity. However, as Ingmar von Homeyer notices, this formal requirement was 'softened' by the technocratic decision-making mode, especially at the Commission level where scientific knowledge constituted the main basis as well as the most important justification for environmental measures at EU level.[23] Despite the tensions created by the coexistence of unanimity voting in the Council with a science-based technocratic approach in the Commission, a number of commendable top-down measures were adopted in this period, e.g. a number of water quality directives and the Air Quality directive.[24]

The adoption of the SEA[25] in 1986 marked the beginning of the *third phase* of environmental law development in the EU. Significant changes occurred in the EEC Treaty structure and, for the first time, environmental considerations were explicitly incorporated in the Treaty. A new Environmental Title was added and the new Articles 130r–130t EEC (now Articles 191–193 TFEU) establishing a series of environmental objectives, empowering the Council to implement those objectives, and, interestingly, permitting MSs to adopt stricter standards in determinate circumstances.[26] Although the SEA introduced a specific legal basis for Community environmental measures, Article 130s, the formulation of Article 100a EEC (now Article 114 TFEU) made this article the preferred basis for environmental measures. Article 100a required the *high level of protection aim to be included* in all harmonising measures relating to the creation of the internal market.[27] Unlike the Articles 130–130s, Article 100a allowed for qualified majority voting (QMV) in the Council and for the MSs to maintain stricter national measures.[28] The consequence was that the internal market regime reflected the majoritarian voting rule, in both building of qualified majorities and blocking minorities.[29]

There is, in other words, a shift from the environmental focus of the second phase to the economic completion-based focus of the third phase of environmental law development within the EU. Consequently, the justification for environmental measures relied less on science and more on the technical feasibility and economic implications of such measures.[30]

Henceforth the recourse to Article 235 EEC was extremely rare.

During *the fourth* phase, marked with the entry in force of the Treaty on European Union (the Treaty of Maastricht),[31] environmental concerns were no longer merely found in Title VII but were included in Articles enshrining the objectives of the Community. The new Article 2 referred to 'sustainable and non-inflationary growth respecting the environment' while the new Article 3(k) lists 'a policy in the sphere of the environment' among the activities and common polices that the Community shall implement pursuant to Article 2(1) TEC.[32]

Perhaps the major novelty of this phase was the introduction of the QMV also for environmental measures under the new Article 175 TEC (former Article 130s and current Article 192 TFEU) strengthening in particularly the Parliament's role in certain environmental policy areas. In its role as a co-legislator, the Parliament also had the possibility to veto the decisions on environmental measures.[33] What is also distinctive of this phase is the shift from the harmonisation approach of the internal market regime, towards a more integrated one where both economic efficiency and environmental effectiveness are important. This resulted in a more inclusive policy network where both science experts and other stakeholders were included in the decision-making process.[34] It must be pointed out that the concept of sustainable development that emerged with the Rio Summit of 1992, provided an impetus to the need to integrate the environmental protection aim in the economic policies at EU level.

Typical of this phase is the adoption of framework directives such as the Air Quality Framework Directive, the creation of the European Environmental Agency (EEA), and the increase of the role of the public information in environmental issues.[35]

The novelties of the *fifth* phase introduced by the Treaty of Amsterdam in 1997[36] concerned mainly the constitutional status of environmental protection, introducing the task to pursue 'a high level of protection and improvement of the quality of the environment'.[37] Besides, the duty to integrate environmental protection into other policies was elevated to the rank of a general principle and endorsed in Article 6 TEC (today Article 11 TFEU). The co-decision procedure became the ordinary one, putting the Parliament on equal footing with the Council, which no longer had a final chance to adopt the first text of an act if the Parliament disagreed on it.[38] Importantly during this phase, the concept of sustainable development became central to the EU environmental policies with a special emphasis on the structural problems of various economic sectors that have created *persistent* environmental problems.[39] Persistent environmental problems are characterised by complex causes, delay of effects, scientific uncertainty, and low visibility[40] – all factors that make the recourse to scientific and technological arguments less appealing on a political plan as compared to other areas of EU environmental governance regimes.[41] The main instrument for adopting environmental measures remained the framework directive, like the Water Framework Directive. The peculiarity of the framework directives of this phase, as compared to those of the fourth phase, is that they are more reflexive, operating through a number of institutional and instrumental features (e.g. development of protocols and indicators) that support cross-national comparison and mutual learning.[42]

All these Treaties, including the Nice Treaty of 2000,[43] were renegotiated under the Lisbon Treaty, in 2009, which re-moulded the EU legal landscape through the creation of two main bodies: the Treaty on European Union (TEU)[44] and the Treaty on the Functioning of the European Union (TFEU).[45]

With this *sixth and last phase* of development, the EU environmental law enters a new era of important procedural and substantial changes. Notably, Article 3 TEU, in establishing the internal market, stipulates that the Union shall work for the *sustainable development of Europe*, with particular emphasis on 'a *high level of protection* and *improvement of the quality* of the environment'. The Union shall also 'promote scientific and technological advance'.[46] Whereas the old Article 2 TEC referred to the sustainable development of economic activities, the new Article 3 TEU refers to the 'sustainable development of Europe', making sustainable development a horizontal objective that can well relate to technological development, among other things.

Currently, the environmental integration principle is found in three provisions of the TFEU Treaty[47] and its prominent role in the law and policy of the Union is undisputable.

Perhaps what might be regarded as the main novelty of the Lisbon Treaty for the regulation of environmental impacts of nanotechnology in REACH (and beyond) is the right of initiative granted to EU citizens pursuant to the new Article 11(4) to submit legal proposals directly to the Commission. This new provision constitutes a way for bringing certain new issues into the political agenda of the EU, when enough support is found to exist among the EU citizens,[48] and nanotechnology might be one such issue.

The new Articles 191–193 TFEU in the environmental title are a verbatim transcription of the old Articles 174–175 TEC.

Against this general background on the EU environmental law, the following section turns to the relevance of the legal basis for the adoption of environmental measures and the implications for the MSs' rights to maintain/introduce stricter measures aimed at the protection of health and the environment.

The constitutional relevance of the legal basis for environmental measures and the MSs' derogatory powers to adopt stricter measures

In the light of the considerations made so far, it is clear that EU environmental measures pursue a double objective. Such measures are aimed at the attainment of the environmental objectives set out in the Treaty, while seeking to achieve at the same time a smooth functioning of the internal market and avoiding distortions to competition.[49]

Given that the EU institutions can only act *according to* and *within* the boundaries of powers conferred by the Treaties,[50] the choice of a legal basis for environmental measures is important. It influences among others:

- the competences in the subject, thus the validity of the measures;
- the decision-making procedure and the degree of involvement of various EU institutions;
- the degree to which Member States can enact stricter environmental measures on a national level.[51]

Consequently, 'the choice of an appropriate legal basis has a constitutional significance'.[52]

Considering that environmental measures have a direct bearing on other freedoms and prerogatives of the Union – such as the free movement of goods, the internal market, health, and consumers' rights, etc. – different Treaty provisions may serve as a legal basis for a given environmental measure.[53] Note that the environment has been listed among the 11 shared competences between the EU and the Member States by Article 4(2)(e) TFEU.

As Ludwig Krämer puts it:

> The choice of the correct legal basis is important because the elaboration of the proposal, the participation of other Union institutions, the intensity of these participation [Articles 293–294 TFEU] and the residual rights for Member States are different from one provision to another.[54]

One of the most important things affected by the choice of the legal basis concerns the derogatory powers of MSs, that is their ability to adopt more stringent measures for controlling environmental (chemicals) risks. Environmental secondary legislation is commonly based on Article 114(3) TFEU (Approximation of laws Title) or Articles 191–193 TFEU (Environment Title). In exceptional cases, a measure can have a double basis, if it pursues two policy objectives that have exactly the same weight. Notwithstanding this eventuality, it is currently impossible to base an environmental measure on both Articles 114 and 192 TFEU.[55]

Regardless of the basis chosen for an environmental measure, these measures should not conflict with the functioning of the internal market principle enshrined in Article 26 TFEU and the free circulation of goods and services objective therein. Essentially, two institutional mechanisms have been promoted in order to protect the unity of the internal market in the light of national divergent measures.

The first one consists of a *negative harmonisation* and is based on the requirements of Articles 34 and 35 TFEU, which prohibit unjustified quantitative restrictions on imports and exports between MSs as well as measures *of equivalent effect*.[56] In this case, national authorities might seek to regulate chemicals more strictly using Article 36 TFEU as a justification of such measures. However, a number of conditions must be fulfilled:

- the subject matter shall not be *completely* harmonised by the EU measure;
- Article 36 measures must be justified in the light of non-economic reasons;[57]
- they are necessary for the attainment of the aim and at the same time are proportionate and non-discriminatory; and,
- such measures need not be notified to the Commission and are not subject to time limits.[58]

The second mechanism, known as *positive harmonisation*, consists of directives and regulations, which harmonise rules and practices for the free circulation of certain goods (e.g. chemicals), in order to resolve upfront the tension that might arise between the free trade and environmental aims.[59] However, even in the case of a positive harmonisation, MSs are still left with some room for manoeuvre – provided that national measures do not concern the harmonised standards and that they are in any case proportionate.

Importantly, in the *Toolex* case[60] the Court of Justice of the European Union (CJEU) had to decide whether Sweden was allowed to restrict the industrial use of *trichloroethylene* when secondary legislation harmonising the restrictions on the marketing and use of certain dangerous substances and preparations[61] existed on the EC level. The Court held that although the Swedish legislation constituted, in principle, a measure having an effect equivalent to a 'quantitative restriction within the meaning of Article 30 [now Article 34 TFEU] of the Treaty',[62] it was nevertheless 'justified under Article 36 of the Treaty [now Article 36 TFEU] on grounds of protection of health of humans'.[63] Moreover, the Court stated that 'the health and life of humans rank foremost among the property or interests protected by Article 36 of the Treaty'.[64]

It must be stated here that the (positive) harmonisation operated by EU rules might be *complete* or *partial*. In case of a partial harmonisation, MSs will have a greater leeway in regulating certain subject matters, such as chemicals risks, for instance. It should be borne in mind that regardless of the legal basis, a complete harmonisation curtails the possibility for MSs to adopt stricter national standards than the harmonised ones.[65] Thereby, in the *Toolex* case the Court based its decision on the fact that albeit being classified as a dangerous substance under Directive 76/769/EEC, trichloroethylene was not included in the Annex I setting out the list of restricted substances.

Another relevant point is the possibility for MSs to maintain/introduce stricter national measures than the ones enacted at EU level, once the subject matter has been (partially) harmonised. For maintaining the existing such measures, Article 114(4) stipulates that if an MS deems it necessary to maintain national provisions on grounds of major needs referred to in Article 36, or relating to the *protection of the environment or the working environment*, it shall notify the Commission of these provisions as well as the grounds for maintaining them.

The introduction of more stringent measures, enacted after the harmonisation of the subject matter has taken place, is subject to tighter criteria. For instance, contrary to those listed in Article 36, only the protection of the environment and of the working environment can be invoked as justificatory grounds. In addition, Article 114(5) clarifies that the following conditions should be fulfilled:

- the existence of new scientific evidence;
- the problem shall be specific to the MS invoking the more stringent measures;
- the problem shall arise after the harmonisation has taken place.

The rationale behind the quite distinct procedural and substantial provisions governing MSs' powers to maintain or introduce more strict measures in a (partially) harmonised subject matter is elucidated by the following passage from the CJEU:

> The difference between the two situations [maintaining and introducing] envisaged in Article 95 [Article 114 TFEU] is that, *in the first, the national provisions predate the harmonisation measure. They are thus known to the Community legislature, but the legislature cannot or does not seek to be guided by them for the purpose of harmonisation.* It is therefore considered acceptable for the Member State to request that its own rules remain in force. To that end, the EC Treaty requires that such national provisions must be justified on grounds of the major needs referred to in Article 30 EC [Article 36 TFEU] or relating to the protection of the environment or the working environment. By contrast, *in the second situation, the adoption of new national legislation is more likely to jeopardise harmonisation.* The Community institutions could not, by definition, have taken account of the national text when drawing up the harmonisation measure. In that case, the requirements referred to in Article 30 EC [Article 36 TFEU] are not taken into account, and only grounds relating to protection of the environment or the working environment are accepted, on condition that the Member State provides new scientific evidence and that the need to introduce new national provisions results from a problem specific to the Member State concerned arising after the adoption of the harmonisation measure.[66]

For the sake of clarity, it is relevant to note here that when the legal basis for environmental measures is Article 192 TFEU (environment), MSs are allowed to maintain/introduce more stringent national measures, in accordance with Article 193 TFEU, i.e. respect the Treaty and do not distort the market.[67] An important novelty following the Lisbon Treaty is that standard procedure is now the ordinary one, enshrined in Article 289 TFEU (the previous co-decision procedure). Consequently, the Parliament is now a genuine co-legislator and must be consulted twice on a proposed measure. The Parliament can hence block the adoption of a measure.[68] Given the propensity of the Parliament to advocate for better environmental legislation, this change was a welcomed one.

Article 193 TFEU enshrines the practice of minimum harmonisation as a means for attaining the environmental objectives set out in the Treaty, leaving MSs with the possibility to derogate through the adoption of more protective national measures. However, the national measure adopted pursuant to Article 193 must set forth stricter rules than those of the directive it derogates, and, importantly, the derogated directive must be adopted pursuant to Article 192 TFEU.[69] In other words, the measure must be more stringent and cannot be used to derogate to directives having a basis different from Article 192 TEFU (e.g. Article 114 TFEU).

Further and importantly, the stringent protective measures taken pursuant to Article 193 must be compatible with the Treaty. This means that MSs' measure must observe the Treaty provisions on the free movement of goods, competition, and taxation.[70] Obviously, MSs cannot act in contravention to Article 34–36 TFEU or disregard commitments under secondary legislation. Lastly, provided that all the aforementioned conditions are met, nothing seems to prevent MSs from adopting more stringent derogatory measures, even in the event of a total harmonisation.[71] The measure so adopted must be notified to the Commission.

Against this backdrop, the question arises as to whether REACH harmonises the chemical sectors' regulation also for nanoscale chemicals and how much room for manoeuvre its legal basis leaves to MSs. Before answering this question, the following offers a chronological account of the unprecedented legal and institutional battles leading to the adoption of the most complex piece of legislation ever adopted at EU level and the consideration of nanoscale chemicals in the process culminating in what is today the REACH Regulation.

The regulation of chemicals in the EU before the REACH Regulation

Before 1970, chemical regulation was rather poor. The major gap was the result of the lack of a general duty to test and assess the human and environmental risks of widely produced chemicals, both in Europe and in other Western countries.[72]

Based on a model in which the risk assessment (RA) phase was a pivotal element, decision-making in the EU required a complete RA before any action in regulating chemicals could be brought forward by the competent authorities.[73] Although a proper analysis of the RA procedures will be discussed at length in Chapter 7, a few considerations are of relevance here.

Chemical risk assessment is defined as

> a process to determine the relationship between the predicted exposure [to a chemical] and adverse effects in four steps: hazard identification, dose–response assessment, exposure assessment and risk characterisation.[74]

Such a process is considered fundamentally scientific while the subsequent phase of risk management (RM) represents the policy-making component. Although RA is a science-based process, it has a number of shortcomings connected to the very nature of scientific progress. For instance, *exposure assessment* and *risk characterisation* are particularly affected by data gaps and methodology lacunas, which give way to uncertainty and error.[75]

The sound trust in the scientific nature of RA began to waver during the 1970s when scientific progress on the effects of substances such as *polychlorinated biphenyls* (PCBs) and *dichlorodiphenyltrichloroethane* (DDT) strongly put into question the 'innocent until harm is proven' principle, which governed EU chemical law at the time.[76] A need for precaution and for the reallocation of responsibilities within the sector emerged clearly, given also that the existing chemical laws and directives had failed to address environmental and human health concerns for the great majority of substances commercialised and used in the EU. For instance, only 3 per cent of high production volume chemicals (HPVs) had a full data set (consisting of long-term eco-toxicity, degradation behaviour in environmental media, and mammalian toxicity profiles).[77]

The dichotomy between new and existing chemicals

It should be recalled that the EU chemical law system, in force in the pre-REACH period, was characterised by a highly complex and intertwined cluster of directives and regulations like:

- provision of data was regulated by Directive 67/548/EEC for new substances and Regulation (EEC) 793/93 for existing ones;
- risk assessment requirements were regulated by Directive 67/548/EEC for new substances and Regulation (EC) 1488/94 for existing ones;
- risk management procedures were laid down for both categories in Directive 76/769/EEC.[78]

The backbone of such a system was Directive 67/548/EEC. Adopted in 1967, it represented an important landmark in the EU chemical law since – by approximating the laws, regulations, and administrative provisions of Member States on classification, packaging, and labelling of dangerous substances – it harmonised the subject, transferring regulatory actions on chemicals almost entirely to the European level.[79] However, the several amendments the Directive had undergone, created an ill-functioning system for the chemical area. The inconsistency and the complexity of this system stemmed primarily from the distinction operated between *new* and *existing* substances, a dichotomy introduced with the sixth amendment to Directive 67/548/EEC in 1981. The sixth amendment[80] to Directive 67/548/EEC foresaw that

> in order to control the effects on man and the environment it is advisable that any new substance placed on the market be subjected to a prior study by the manufacturer or importer and a notification to the competent authorities conveying mandatorily certain information; whereas it is, moreover, important to follow closely the evolution and use of new substances placed on the market, and that in order to do this it is necessary to institute a system which allows all new substances to be listed.[81]

The distinction between *new* and *existing* substances is thus an arbitrary one. It is based on sole temporal criterion of the coming into force of such amendment. Consequently, the new provisions applying to the notification of *new* substances, and certain mandatory information and listing requirements, would apply only for substances placed on the market after 1981. However, a positive novelty introduced by the sixth amendment was the inclusion of environmental concerns, alongside those on human health, in the aim of the Directive.[82]

The initial distinction between new and existing substances became more pronounced with the seventh amendment[83] to Directive 67/548/EEC, which established other specific norms and 'uniform principles for risk assessment'.[84]

However, the benefits of the new approach deriving from stricter information requirements on human and environmental health data would apply only to substances entering the market after 1981 and not present in the European Inventory of Existing Commercial Substances (EINECS), considered *new* for regulatory purposes. For *new* substances, Directive 67/548/EEC established a minimum threshold of 10 kg/annum in the volume of production deemed necessary for triggering the obligation on the producer's part to submit a notification dossier. Increasing marketing volumes would determine the extent of testing required, including investigation on physicochemical, toxicological, and ecotoxicological properties. Acute and long-term hazard testing was also dependent on the quantity produced.[85] The obligation to provide a 'base set' of data on human and environmental impact was prefigured only for substances produced in volumes exceeding 1 t/y.[86] Nonetheless, some 2,700 new substances were notified to the EU authorities from 1981 to 2002, with 70 per cent of them classified as dangerous mainly due to their properties such as being 'irritating' and 'dangerous for the environment'.[87]

Greater concerns surrounded *existing* substances present in the EINECS, which in the period preceding REACH, counted more than 100,000 chemicals, making up for 99 per cent of all the chemicals in use.[88] Not contemplated in Directive 67/548/EEC, the law covering the RA of *existing* substances was introduced only in 1993.[89] A reversed tiered approach based on high volumes of production was established for the submission of *available information*, prioritising substances produced in quantities above 1,000tonnes/year (HPV). If the information gathered on HPV substances showed a need for further measures, or if the identified data gap suggested the need for further testing, the substances could be placed on priority lists. Subsequent phases of risk assessment and measures for risk reduction would eventually follow.[90] However, no deadline was set and, as a consequence, in 2002, only 11 of the 140 prioritized HPV substances had a complete RA.[91] It can be argued that the assessment of risk for the *existing* substance was a burdensome and time-consuming activity, performed entirely by the competent authorities on the state or EU level. The complication and slowness of such a process was seriously undermining the communitarian goal of a high level of human and environmental protection as it was allowing for dangerous or untested chemicals to circulate freely in the EU market.

Clearly, the system delineated for existing substances was weak in its legal implications, slow in performing RA, and unable to create any kind of incentive for producers to comply with requirements on human and environmental impacts for chemicals that they were placing quite freely on the EU market. On the contrary, delaying the process of phasing out hazardous chemicals was ' "rewarded" with an extended marketing period'.[92]

As for the *risk management*, for both *new* and *existing* chemicals, it was dealt with by Directive 76/769. Several drawbacks regarding its provisions were soon identified, including the limitations in controlling 'use for certain purposes', limited authority in contemplating bans and restrictions, lack of an automatic link between RA and RM measures, strong emphasis on the cost-benefit analysis, and a general inconsistency deriving from a situation where RA was performed by DG Environment[93] while RM measures were assigned to DG Industry.[94]

According to Dieter Pesendorfer, the pre-REACH chemical policy can be summarised as follows:

1   too complex and too difficult to survey;
2   not supportive enough for innovation and represents a burden on small and medium-sized enterprises (SMEs);
3   lacks an adequate knowledge base;
4   includes institutional blockades;
5   laws at European, national and regional levels are not coherent, consistent and transparent;
6   the precautionary principle, the polluter pays principle and the principle of sustainable development are not respected.[95]

The complexity of the system, as described above, consisted in a fragmented and dense network of legislation, delivering poor control over chemicals risk. Not only did the way the system was designed offer no impetus for innovation, but with a 'softer' regime for existing chemicals, it worked towards the advantage of big companies controlling the chemical market.

Heterogeneity of chemical policy within the EU represented another problem, and chemical laws differed significantly from state to state, with Nordic countries having generally stricter standards.[96] Finally, no precautionary element was embodied in the pre-REACH EU chemical law where obligations for producers (especially those of existing substances) were weak. EU authorities, on the contrary, had to bear the burdensome task of proving negative impacts on human and environmental health on the basis of a detailed risk assessment that would often lead to a 'paralysis by analysis'.[97]

These summarised drawbacks of the pre-REACH chemical policy, emphasising also the waning of the Community top-down approach based on binding and enforceable command-and-control regulations,[98] formed the grounds for a change in the law and in the policy model. The following initiatives, which are considered the immediate predecessors of today's REACH framework, definitively confirmed the need for a radical change and for a new, integrated, and comprehensive approach to chemical regulation at EU level.

From the SLIM initiatives to the White Paper on Chemicals Policy

In 1996, the Commission launched a pilot project with the intent of simplifying the legislation regarding the internal market.[99] Though the focus of this remodelling legislative intervention was placed on the better functionality of the internal market, the Commission argued that this objective should be pursued 'whilst at the same time safeguarding the essential elements of the acquis communautaire and ensuring a high level of health and safety and protection of the environment and of consumers'.[100]

Therefore, in 1998, the Commission stretched the *simpler legislation for the internal market (SLIM) initiative* across other sectors of EU law, including the chemical area, governed by Directive 67/548/EEC. The need to intervene on this Directive was a direct consequence of the complex and entangled net of existing provisions. The Directive had, by the time of SLIM intervention, been amended 8 times and undergone 23 technical updates. Moreover, as shown earlier, the norms governing data submission and RA procedures were laid down in different directives for new and existing substances, creating an inconsistent and non-harmonised system. Hence, a team of experts was entrusted with the task of examining the sector with the intent of identifying common grounds for harmonisation and simplification. In 2000, a report containing some 48 recommendations on Directive 67/548/EEC and the other connected legislation was delivered to the Commission.[101] A structural change of the then existing regulatory system for chemical substances was indicated as necessary. The strictly legal language of the Directive was also to be updated to incorporate the new philosophy and principles that would allow for a holistic chemical management.[102] The work carried out at UN level, in Globally Harmonized System of Classification and Labelling of Chemicals[103] (GHS) and the principles of the Århus Convention[104] established the right for everyone to access environmental information available to public authorities and the right of the public to participate in environmental decision-making. These were highlighted as relevant developments that should be reflected/incorporated in the new EU chemical policy.

Particular attention was devoted to the RA process. Being primarily a duty of EU authorities, it halted the potential of the Directive to deliver environmental benefits. It was suggested that instead producers should be responsible for an initial RA while the authorities should maintain the right to require additional information based on the review of the RA performed by industry. This shift of responsibility within the complicated process of RA should, however, operate in a regime of proportionality in the sense that appropriate triggers such as tonnage bands of production and intrinsic hazards of a given substance should be established by the authorities upfront.[105]

Following the SLIM recommendations, the Commission announced that it would consider specific legislative proposals in the context of the next wider chemical law review.[106]

Before that though, in 2000, the Commission adopted a Communication[107] outlining its position on the subject. Although the PP is explicitly mentioned in the Treaty only once, in addressing environmental protection, the Commission noted that there is no crystallised definition on the EU level. Hence, by outlining the principal features of a precaution-based decision,[108] the Commission endorsed a concept of precaution seen as a 'living principle' in continuous evolution and subject to change and transformation. The Commission operates a differentiation between 'precaution' in decision-making and the 'caution' element that can influence the work of the scientists in their assessment of scientific data.[109] The claim seems to suggest a purely scientific nature of the RA phase where there is no room for genuine precaution. Rather, precaution is clearly seen as a risk management strategy.[110]

The Commission, after a brief overview on the legal basis for the affirmation of the PP on both the EU and international level 'considers that the precautionary principle is a general one which should in particular be taken into consideration in the fields of environmental protection and human, animal and plant health'.[111] Regarding implementation, the Commission suggests that the triggering factor should always be a comprehensive and sound scientific assessment, as complete as possible, capable of identifying and taking into account uncertainties that might arise at each stage of the assessment. Only at the culmination of such a process, can the legislator invoke precaution and implement it in order to manage risks and uncertainties on the basis of the chosen level of protection. The element of the *chosen level of protection* is of particular relevance to the chemical policy. It suggests that before standards, limits, and values of certain regulations are set, the degree of the desirable human and environmental protection should be first determined. There is little doubt on the political nature of this choice. However, the political discretion should be anchored to the level of 'acceptable risk' that the society is willing to tolerate.[112] The reversion of the onus of proof is seen as one expression of the precautionary principle (PP). In some EU legislations, like that on food additives, pesticides, and drugs, which are based on a prior-approval mechanism of a positive list, precaution is contemplated upstream, since it is for industry to generate the scientific evidence on the lack of harmful effects. For other areas of legislation where no safety requirement is established upfront, precaution could be contemplated through the reversion of the onus of proof and the assignment of the duty to produce scientific evidence on the safety of certain substances or products to the manufacturers. However, this shifting should be operated only on a case-by-case basis.[113]

Subsequent to such developments and to the adoption of the Communication on the Precautionary Principle, the much-awaited White Paper (WP) on a new chemical strategy was published in 2001.[114] Although there were some significant modifications, the final text of REACH reflects much of the WP content, so it is useful to examine that briefly here. The WP represented perhaps the most ambitious and far-reaching initiative ever undertaken in the chemical regulation area within the EU and beyond. It announced at the very beginning the key elements that should be embodied in the new law governing chemicals:

- ensuring high levels of protection for both human health and the environment for present and future generations while enabling competitiveness and market functioning;
- applying the precautionary principle when reaching the above-mentioned objectives;[115] and
- fostering innovation by applying the substitution principle.

These ambitious goals faced a significant hurdle in both the 'burden of the past' – constituted by the nearly total gap of data for the majority of existing substances – and the consequent 'burden of the present' – referring to the lack of incentives to develop less hazardous alternatives, a consequence of the grandfathering policy operated in 1981.

A study from the European Commission Joint Research Centre[116] showed that as a result of the grandfathering of existing substances, barely 3 per cent of EU HPV chemicals had a full data set while 15 per cent of HPVs were found to have no data at all. If one considers that only 0.6 per cent of substances were produced and sold in quantities above 1,000 tonnes/year (this was the threshold for being categorised as HPV chemicals), then the data for substances produced in lower tonnage bands were probably almost completely inexistent. The dichotomy between *new* and *existing* substances was considered in the WP to be the major flaw of the existing chemical system. Accordingly, the proposal envisaged the creation of an integrated single system, covering both new and existing substances. It consisted of four separate but interrelated phases, i.e. Registration, Authorisation, Evaluation, and

Restriction. While these phases are analysed in detail in Chapters 3–6 of this book, it is relevant to point out here that there are significant differences between the initial ideation of such phases and the final shape they have been given in the approved text of REACH. Following the WP of 2001, a draft regulation was submitted for comments to stakeholders and the general public in May 2003.[117] Due to strong pressures and lobbying, the draft version was weaker in its provisions than the WP in two fundamental provisions:

• The original provision stipulating the substitution of dangerous substances when a safer alternative already existed was replaced by the possibility for the authorities to simply refuse authorisation without being able to demand the mandatory phasing of the hazardous substance.
• The relevance assigned in the WP to the concept of 'relevant exposure'[118] was substituted by the 1 t/y volume of production and the likelihood of harm, as main criteria triggering the obligation for the producers to provide data and perform pertinent testing.[119]

Disappointing from an environmental and human health perspective, these weakening changes are the result of campaigning and lobbying without precedence in the history of EU legislation.

The chemical industry opposed REACH, as it considered it to be 'unscientific' and capable of putting at risk competitiveness, jobs, and the financial capacity of the EU chemical sector, in particular for SMEs. The European Chemical Industry Council (CEFIC) defined REACH as 'unworkable' and not in line with competitiveness and the Lisbon Strategy.[120] Also, major chemical producers among MSs expressed their strong opposition. In a joint letter to the President of the Commission Romano Prodi, President Jacques Chirac, Prime Minister Tony Blair, and Chancellor Gerhard Schröder expressed their strong opposition to REACH, fearing even a 'risk of de-industrialization'.[121]

This opposition is hardly understandable when bearing in mind that a few months prior to the letter, the authoritative Royal Commission on Environmental Pollution in the UK adopted a Report on the environmental pollution from chemicals, declaring:

> We have little faith that either the present regulatory systems or the proposals coming forward to improve them will provide better answers in the future. We believe that only a substantial paradigm shift will allow a start to be made to rectify this situation, and we believe that such a start needs to be made now.[122]

The Royal Commission (RC) strongly advocated the substitution principle as the only way out of this regulatory deadlock. Moreover, the RC was said to be less certain about its position endorsed in a precedent report,[123] where it held that placing too heavy a burden of proof on the manufacturer regarding the safety of the chemicals they produce might cripple relevant branches of industry and deprive consumers from considerable benefits.[124] An aggressive campaign was also launched by the US and the Bush administration. Interestingly, the main concern, besides trade-related issues, was the fear that REACH might 'export' its model of regulation to the other side of the Atlantic.[125]

Despite the tense political climate, in October 2003 an official proposal was adopted. The final legal proposal was considered to be even more watered down than both the first draft and the WP in terms of ecological and human health protection.[126] Relevant commentators suggested that the new governance models under which REACH was negotiated, allowed business stakeholders to bring the proposal on REACH in line with neo-liberal ideas while a 'radical paradigmatic shift in chemical policy was not reached'.[127]

For the aim of this book, it is relevant to point out that during the REACH ideation process nanosize chemicals were rather marginal in the general discussion, while, for instance, the status of particular chemicals, such as persistent organic pollutants (POPs) and endocrine disrupters whose hazardous nature was (and still is) the object of a complex scientific debate, was widely discussed.

Although it is true that POPs and endocrine disrupters had a more consolidated history of legislative debate, being also incorporated in relevant EU and international directives and Treaties, the argument of this book is that sufficient awareness on nanotechnology to make decisions about its regulatory needs was already available at the time of REACH negotiations.

The proposed nano-specific provisions during the REACH negotiation process

This section aims to illustrate the initial arguments in favour of regulation of nanomaterials under the REACH framework. The following offers an account of how such regulatory suggestions have been ignored while the importance of nanotechnology and the products of its application have been strongly advocated and generously funded by the EU. In other words, an asymmetry can be observed between the priority assigned to the development and commercialisation of nano-enriched products and that for enacting tailored provisions to control their environmental risks. It must be noted that a number of scientific opinions/reports were adopted in the first decade of the 2000s, offering ground-breaking information on the peculiar nature of nano-substances and their unprecedented risk profiles, stressing at the same time the need for regulatory oversight. Based on such information, the importance for an appropriate regulatory coverage of health and environmental risks of nano-substances was emphasised by scientists and some regulators alike. Importantly, the REACH Regulation, at that time still under negotiation, was indicated as one suitable regulatory framework for governing nano-risks. Based on the analysis of such facts, the following tries to make sense of why such facts were overlooked in the regulatory process, leading to the adoption of a final text of REACH that does not incorporate any reference whatsoever to nanoscale chemicals.

The scientific debate and early advocacy for the inclusion of nanosubstances in REACH

It must be noted here that already in 2002, nanotechnology and the products of its application were given high priority within the 6th Framework Programme for Research and Technological Development (FP6).[128] They were listed third in a seven-point prioritised agenda, preceding areas such as 'Food Quality and Safety' and 'Sustainable Development, Global Change and Eco-systems'.[129] This assigned status suggests that the awareness of the EU legislature on the impact and the consequent foreseeable diffusion of nanosubstances and nano-enriched products was supposedly high already at this early stage.

In November 2003, the Commission's Communication on a European initiative on growth, indicated in nanoelectronics a category of crucial relevance for the development and growth of vital sectors of the EU economy.[130] In 2004, the Risk Assessment Unit of the Health and Consumer Protection Directorate-General of the European Commission (DG SANCO, now known as DG SANTE) acknowledged the actual presence of nano-enriched products in the EU market, stating that 'consumers are already being offered products manufactured with nanotechnologies including cosmetics, clothing, and sporting goods'.[131] Holding that unique opportunities might also imply unforeseen risk, the DG called for the establishment of a dialog platform among stakeholders in order to 'set nanotechnologies on a responsible development trajectory, one that will benefit both human and environmental health and global competitiveness'.[132]

On the regulatory level, the DG SANCO called on public authorities to apply, among others, the existing legislative instruments and, when possible, amend them in the light of nano-realities. One suggestion was the application of 'the REACH future European Union regulatory framework being under discussion on chemistry, to manufactured goods including nanoelements'.[133] Given the absence of nano-norms within the REACH proposal, suggestions (like threshold limits criteria) on how to render REACH, nano-compatible already in its embryonic phase, were also given. However, such suggestions fell on deaf ears in the legislature. No nano-specific norms were included in the legislative draft of REACH, which was being debated in Council at the time of the DG SANCO workshop outcomes. During the same period, in May 2004, the Commission adopted 'Towards a European strategy for nano-technology', outlining a number of actions aimed at the strengthening of the European R&D in nanoscience and nanotechnology.[134] Although recognising a general need to address potential human and environmental risks upfront, by generating the necessary data that would enable the performance of a specific risk assessment,[135] the Communication did not indicate any concrete legislative action that might respond to such challenges. However, a greater engagement by the Commission was expressed in the following Communication of March 2005, where the Commission, pending the REACH adoption process, committed to 'examine and, where appropriate, propose adaptations of EU regulations in relevant sectors'[136] with particular (but not exclusive) attention to the following parameters:

> (i) toxicity thresholds, (ii) measurement and emission thresholds, (iii) labelling requirements, (iv) risk assessment and exposure thresholds and (v) production and import thresholds, below which a substance may be exempt from regulation, [given that they] are typically based upon mass quantities.[137]

Later that year, in November 2005, the European Parliament published its first position on the REACH proposal. Despite the prominent importance already assigned to nanotechnology in different Commission documents, none of the norms or the amendments that were discussed in Parliament addressed nanosubstances.[138] During the same period, however, the Commission launched, as part of its emerging policy on nanomaterials, an *Action Plan on Nanotechnology*, consisting of a series of related actions that would allow for rapid, safe, and responsible developments in nanotechnologies and nanoscience research. In line with the Strategy delineated in the previous Communication,[139] the Commission reaffirmed that health and environmental concerns related to nanotechnology and nanoscience applications must be addressed upfront and throughout the entire life-cycle.[140] In pursuing the high level of human health and environmental protection enshrined in the Treaty,[141] also for nanotechnologies and nanoscience applications, the Commission indicated as a possible step forward the need to review relevant legislative acts that might be affected by the innovation in nanoscale. Therefore, the Commission assigned itself the task to review, and if necessary amend, relevant legislations, with particular focus on the elements already mentioned in the Communication from 2005.[142]

Each of the above-mentioned elements mirrors basilar concepts within the REACH framework. The Commission's position would have already suggested an intervention in the draft regulation in order to amend threshold criteria and risk assessment procedures in accordance with nano-specificities. No such intervention was made, but in relation to REACH the assumption was that

> [t]he Commission proposal on REACH may cover some aspects on nanoparticles produced in very high quantities.[143]

This assumption was unlikely to find real recognition in the REACH draft (at the time of the discussion at the Council) given the fact that nanosubstances, due to their particular properties and process of production, were highly unlikely to be produced in very high quantities. The additional lack of any expressed norm on nano-chemicals in the provisions of the draft suggested the lack of any mandatory duty to register nanosubstances under REACH, regardless of their volumes of production. What was later going to represent the main loophole of REACH with regard to nanosize chemicals – namely the lack of a norm clearly considering nanosubstances as *new* for regulatory purposes – was already addressable at this early stage. One can argue that early appropriate regulatory interventions might have eased the following debate on whether and how to regulate nanosubstances under REACH.

It emerges clearly that documents produced at this stage from the EU regulatory and scientific bodies, left little doubt on the awareness that nano-size chemicals deserve and demand tailored legislative intervention. Such intervention did not take place. The high level of environmental protection objective enshrined in the Treaty,[144] would have required the legislature to act, and to act in a timely manner, in order to control risk upfront. It would have also required the legislator to act by targeting those parameters within new and existing laws that would allow risk from nanosize chemicals to be assessed, monitored, and controlled in a life-cycle perspective. Moreover, early scientific evidence already suggested that traditionally used criteria in the field of chemicals regulation were not adequate for dealing with nano-chemicals, and thus were unlikely to deliver reliable risk assessment results. For instance, by the end of July 2004, the highly renowned British Royal Society (RS) had issued a comprehensive Report on nanotechnologies and nanoscience, offering an overview on prospective opportunities and potential risks. Regarding the factors influencing the toxicological behaviour of nano-particles and the correlated health and environmental risks, the Report con-cluded that size alone is not the decisive factor. Of particular relevance is the exposure dose, but contrary to the traditional quantity-exposure correlation, in the case of nanosize particles, two size-related properties influence expo-sure and, thus, toxicity:

- the larger surface rate area of nanosize substances compared to the bulk form ones, given equal mass, and
- surface reactivity and the consequent ability of nanosize chemicals to penetrate deeper in the exposed organisms' cells and sub-cellular tissues.[145]

Neither the adoption of a specific regulatory framework nor the establish-ment of a ban was considered an appropriate and justified measure in light of the existing scientific evidence by the Report in question. Rather, in order to timely address and control societal and environmental risks, the RS called upon legislators to intervene in *existing* regulations and revise them in line with the specific toxicological profiles of nanosubstances, given that they were significantly different from the counterpart bulk material.[146] The RS said that the regulatory review process ought to be an 'evolving' one, based on close monitoring of scientific progress. Specifically, the chemical law area was indicated as the main sector in need for revision given that the REACH proposal – like the old chemical legislation it was aiming to replace – foresaw no additional tests for substances in nanoform. The RS was particularly concerned that the REACH draft implied – incorrectly – that toxicity for humans and environmental organisms is not affected by size. In this regard, the RS suggested a series of amendments on specific triggers and definitions to be incorporated in the latest version of the REACH proposal – and hopefully in the final text of the law – starting with the recommendation to consider nanosubstances as 'new' chemicals under the REACH framework.[147] The Report argued also that the outcome of the REACH negotiation process, which was still ongoing at the time of the Report's adoption, ought to have taken into account such suggestions and other considerations on bioaccumulation and persistency properties of some nanosubstances and nanotubes. By already addressing them in the legal text of the proposal, the result would have been the adoption of a version of REACH 'sufficiently flexible'[148] to take into account those specific properties that determine the different environmental behaviour of nanoparticles.

Despite these clear and specific indications, no amendments was made to the REACH draft. In addition, demonstration of the fact that the awareness of the EU legislature was high and nanotechnology investigation still a priority in the Commission's agenda came in 2005 with the assignment to the newly created Scientific Committee on Emerging and Newly Identified Health Risks (SCENIHR) of the task to assess the appropriateness of existing methodologies of RA also for nanotechnology.[149] The SCENIHR, in line with the conclusions drawn by the RS and after emphasising the need for further data generation, standardisation, and methodological changes to respond to nano-challenges, also addressed the regulatory gaps related to the environmental risks control of nanoparticles. Those gaps were, in the words of the SCENIHR, primarily attributed to the inappropriateness of the existing regulatory triggers to deal with unique properties exhibited by particles when reduced in nanoscale. Hence, the tonnage-based system under the proposed REACH directive and the lack of a separate identification of nanosubstances therein, were criticised as inadequate and in need of revision.[150] Following public consultation, in 2006 the SCENIHR published a modified Opinion based on the 2005 one, confirming its previous position on the need for target intervention on both the technical and normative levels.[151] Specifically with regard to REACH, the Committee's conclusion was

> The regulation of products containing nanoparticles based on tonnage, as proposed for existing chemicals under REACH, needs to be considered further because *there are many more nanoparticles to the tonne than is the case for larger particles, and their behaviour in the body and in the environment may be*

different. If the nanoparticle form of a chemical does have distinctly different properties in biological systems from other physical forms of the same chemical, it will be necessary to readily identify the nanoparticle form of each chemical for the purposes of hazard warning labels etc.[152]

The proposed nano-specific amendments to the REACH draft

The conclusion of the 2005 SCENIHR opinion was taken up by the Parliament during the second reading phase of REACH. The Parliament's draft on the legislative resolution[153] represents a number of relevant amendments, specific to substances in nanoscale, which are entirely justified in light of the SCENIHR's recommendations. For example, Amendment 24 read

> The provisions of this Regulation should ensure an adequate safety evaluation of nanoparticles as a precondition for their manufacture and placing on the market.[154]

Particularly interesting was the proposed Amendment 79, requiring the additional listing of nanoparticles under the letter (f) of what is now Article 57 of REACH, setting out the categories of substances of equivalent concern to substances of very high concern (SVHCs) subject to authorisation.[155] Attention must be paid to the position of the Parliament on this point: given the existing uncertainty on toxicological profiles of nanoparticles, a precautionary approach would have been satisfied only by placing nanosubstances under what was (and still is) REACH's most innovative and revolutionary procedure: the Authorisation phase. Additionally, the Parliament, in Amendment 87, specified that nanoparticles should be automatically prioritised for inclusion in Annex XIV.[156] As we shall see later in this book, the prioritisation process is of vital importance to the successful attainment of Authorisation's scope: phasing out chemicals that can harm the environment and endanger human health through a precautionary process anchored to hazard-based and tonnage-free criteria and to the reversion of the onus of proof. Concerns expressed by the SCENIHR regarding parameters influencing nanosubstances' toxicity led the Parliament to include at Amendment 161 the need to review the minimum tonnage threshold of 1 t/y through

> appropriate legislative proposals to modify the tonnage threshold and the information requirements for nanoparticles to ensure adequate risk assessment, and risk reductions, where necessary, so as to achieve a high level of protection of human health and the environment with regard to nanoparticles.[157]

The last proposed amendment required producers of nanoparticles to comply with the requirements set out in Annex III on the data set to be provided for substances produced in quantities 1–10 t/y.[158]

In spite of such efforts, all the above-mentioned nano-specific amendments did not make it through the legislative procedures, culminating in the adoption of a nano-silent text by the Parliament at the conclusion of the second reading phase. Evidentially, as happened for other innovative provisions, which were negotiated under the co-decision legislative procedure, the political consensus and pressure from different stakeholders representing different and often conflicting interests resulted in legal compromises such as the elimination of nano-provisions from the REACH final text.

On the 12th of December 2006, the final draft was passed and the REACH Regulation was approved. The failure to consider nano-specific norms and eventually embody them in the legal text of REACH, strongly – if not completely – paralysed the capacity of the new law to extend its proclaimed high level of human and environmental protection aim to substances in nanoform. The position of the Commission in this process could be deemed inconsistent and, to some extent, contradictory. On the one hand, the Commission published numerous documents highlighting the increasing importance of nanotechnologies across numerous sectors of the European industry and economy, implying an increase in use and diffusion of substances in nanoscale. On the other hand, the reluctant attitude in introducing nano-tailored norms, especially within one of the most relevant pieces of legislation still under negotiation, is difficult to interpret from an environmental protection perspective. The choice not to act at an early stage is also puzzling considering the nearly exclusive right of legal initiative the Commission held at the time of the REACH proposal.[159] Why the Commission failed to bring nano-chemicals within the REACH proposal appears rather unclear, but one can speculate on the difficulty in bringing together different stakeholders around the need to extend REACH's authority to emerging new substances, which had uncertain status.

A parallel can thus be drawn between the pre-REACH chemical policy based on an artificial distinction between *new* and *existing* substances and the REACH directive, which failed to formulate a distinction between bulk and nanoform chemicals, with the latter category lacking a status of *new substances* for regulatory purposes. It seems that the Commission, in trying to remedy the 'burden of the past' and 'burden of the present' through the adoption of REACH, failed to prevent the emerging 'burden the very small' by not taking a stand of their own on nano-chemicals in REACH. As a consequence of such a burden, under the current REACH framework, the status of nano-substances remains highly uncertain, with huge difficulties (if not total incapacity) to apply current norms to this class of chemicals.

In an attempt to provide some clarity, the salient points of the long and travailed process of REACH adoption and the parallel developments on nanotechnology are summarised in the table contained in the Appendix to this book.

The final text of REACH and the status of nano-chemicals therein

On the 1st of June 2007, the REACH Regulation came into force, repealing and replacing the cluster of directives and regulations that made up for the previous EU chemicals legislation. As already mentioned, REACH was passed under the internal market competence.[160] Under REACH, chemical substances – either on their own or in articles and preparations – are regulated in REACH as *market objects*.[161] Consequently, the mere production and/or placing of chemicals on the EU market, without specific analytic findings on their human and environmental impacts, suffice to bring them under the REACH compass.[162] The REACH is hence a *horizontal* regulation that is product- and technology-neutral.

Technological neutrality can be described as 'a technique of statutory drafting designed to ensure that statutes are able to operate fairly and effectively in diverse technological contexts'.[163] As illustrated by the chronological analysis operated in the previous section, nanosize chemicals are not *explicitly* included in REACH. This is to say that the REACH legal text is completely silent on nanoscale chemicals. While the consequences (in terms of effective risk regulation) of the legislative and political choice to not specifically contemplate nanosubstances will better emerge in Chapters 3-6, it is important to underline here that such a choice was made in a context of relatively high awareness of the need for nano-inclusion in REACH.[164] Lyria B. Moses holds that if technological change was not foreseeable at the time when the law dealing with it was created, then the uncertainty arising as a result of such change may be outside the lawmakers' control.[165] Besides the numerous calls to include nanotechnology in REACH, at the time of REACH negotiation, the food-additive regulation,[166] which is nano-specific, was being discussed at EU level. Therefore, foreseeability can hardly be regarded as one of the factors that contributed to the current legal uncertainty surrounding the status of nanosubstances in REACH. Be this as it may, the kind of legal uncertainty Moses points at must not be confused with the general statutory uncertainty, which is inherent to the language used in legal statutes in general and in the REACH text in particular.

As Friedrich Waismann acknowledged, language has an *open-texture*.[167] He observed that 'even the most precise and carefully delimited empirical terms might nevertheless produce uncertainty in the face of unforeseen and virtually unimaginable instances'.[168] According to Waismann, it would therefore be impossible to have legal rules that are immune to changes in the society and future uncertainty:[169] 'Try as we may, no concept is limited in such a way that there is no room for any doubt.'[170] Applying the open-texture concept to REACH means that the definition of *substance* lying at the heart of REACH cannot be exhaustively comprehensive of all the possible developments in the chemical realm, regardless of the effort put by the legislator into formulating the concept of *substance*. A certain degree of uncertainty will persist, as an intrinsic feature of the language used to express the concept. Therefore, the definitions of *substance* will inevitably lag behind the development in the science of chemical production. The open-texture nature of language not-withstanding, the failure to adopt a specific definition on nano-chemicals, which would have required them to be treated as *new* and *different* substances as compared to their bulk counterparts, has directly contributed to the legal uncertainty on nanosubstances in REACH. In other words, both the ordinary uncertainty owed to the open-texture of language and the legal uncertainty deriving from technological progress, are aggravated in the case of REACH by the negligence to adopt specific provisions on nanosubstances.

With that being said, the REACH framework is *in theory* applicable also to nano-chemicals as an expression of chemical substances. The practice, as Chapters 3–7 will show, is rather different. It is noteworthy here to underline that the current directive of REACH is loaded with ambiguities and uncertainties. As substantiated in Chapter 1, one of the aims of this book is to test the assumption that despite the lack of provisions referring explicitly to nanomaterials in REACH, the general concept of substance still covers this class of chemicals.[171] Further, the Commission appears to be confident enough on the suitability of the regulatory framework of REACH so as to claim that it provides 'the best possible framework' for the risk management of nanomaterials when they occur as substance or mixtures. So high is the trust in REACH's ability to cover nanosubstances that the only successful reform, which took more than one decade to approve, is that to the Annexes and not on the legal provisions of REACH.[172] With REACH currently not containing any definition on nanomaterials and generally silent in its legal text on nanosubstances (a situation that will persist after the nano-specific amend-ments to the Annexes come into force in 2020), it becomes relevant to analyse the possibilities that MSs have under the REACH rule to adopt national measures on nanotechnology. This begs the question: does REACH harmonise the regulation of the entire chemical sector, including chemicals in nanoscale, or does the lack of specific provisions on nanosubstances allow for stricter national provisions? If so, what impact might stricter regulatory actions on the national-level trigger on upper-level legislation?

The legal basis of REACH and the attained degree of harmonisation

At the outset, it is important to recall that the concept of the legal basis is subject to dynamic interpretation. The CJEU jurisprudence has evolved from a position that considered the effect of a measure to determine the effective legal basis of an act, to the 'centre of gravity doctrine'. According to such doctrine, when several objectives are pursued by a measure, it is the predomi-nant aim and component of a measure that determines the correct legal basis of it.[173]

As is known, REACH pursues both a free market objective and a high levels of protection one. Furthermore, REACH is explicitly based on Article

95 TEC[174] (now Article 114 TFEU) and it contains both a free movement clause[175] and a safeguard one.[176] In light of the analysis in the section on EU environmental law above, chemicals (potentially including nano-chemicals) which are considered to be covered by[177] and complying with the REACH system, can be traded freely within the EU.[178] Consequently, at first glance, REACH is about harmonisation of chemicals regulation, pre-empting MSs' powers to enact divergent national measures that could affect the free movement of chemicals.

Nonetheless, as Joanne Scott observes, the novelties introduced through the peculiar hybrid[179] model of governance REACH puts in place, such as information and transparency duties and multi-actor and multi-level decision-making, are responsible for what she calls 'provisional and contestable' harmonisation.[180] In her view, REACH's complex structure encompasses a number of mechanisms that allow 'for the contours of the provisional harmonization bargain to be contested'.[181] More specifically, the REACH model of governance consists, besides the 'traditional regulatory core'[182] relating to obligatory requirements for data submission and substance restrictions, of a number of less traditional governance models including:

- 'mechanisms for public risk communication' allowing for markets, consumers, and the public to react to substances of particular concern;
- 'obligatory self-regulation' for producers with regard to safety management of chemicals along the supply chain; and
- 'cooperative proceduralisation and devolution' given that REACH sets out a framework of basic legal rules and administrative procedures that are going to be fleshed out through implementation guidance documents, standard setting, and further refinement of operational criteria.[183]

As will be explained in some detail in Chapters 3–6, under each of the four phases of REACH and, in particular, under the proper command-and-control procedures of Authorisation and Restriction, MSs (and the Commission) are empowered, on the basis of clearly defined procedural and administrative rules

> to seek to use their local knowledge to persuade the European Union as a whole, of the need to revise applicable norms, in order to ensure effective fulfilment of the Regulation's framework goals (high level of protection of human health and environment in particular).[184]

Hence, notwithstanding Article 114 TFEU as a legal basis, the Commission's regulatory powers in REACH are not absolute. The power monopoly is eroded by the prominent role played by other actors, e.g. MSs, consumers, third parties, and, as we shall see, the European Chemicals Agency (ECHA), especially in the implementation and enforcement phase.

This way, although recourse to treaty-based free movement opt-outs will be pre-empted, the Treaty and, to a greater extent, the nature of REACH as a regulatory hybrid, 'preserve spaces for Member State contestation of the trade/regulation bargain struck'.[185] In sum, as Scott states:

> [REACH] is about product market integration and environmental/health protection. While the former militates in the direction of harmonization, the latter militates against a complacent centre, convinced that it enjoys a monopoly on regulatory wisdom. In keeping with this, REACH is emphatic but tentative in the harmonization which it achieves. It is emphatic in that it leaves little room for unilateral Member State departure from it, as is exemplified by the free movement clause. At the same time, and in a manner which might seem contradictory but is not, REACH is tentative in the harmonization which it achieves.[186]

The question then arises as to whether the harmonisation operated by REACH encompasses also nano-chemicals. Can the Commission and the MSs adopt stringent measures (e.g. subject nanosubstances to authorisation or restriction requirements) on nano-chemicals' risk in order to protect human health and the environment?

As the CJEU has already clarified, a high level of protection 'does not necessarily have to be the highest that is technically possible'.[187] Interestingly, in the Afton case, related to the establishment of levels of metallic additives in fuels, the Court held that 'in an area of evolving and complex technology' the EU legislature has a broad discretion, especially in assessing 'complex scientific and technical facts, in order to determine the nature and scope of the measures which it adopts'.[188] The judgment of the Court was made while the development by the Commission of testing methodologies to assess safe levels on metallic additives in fuel was still pending. The Court found that in a context of difficulties in defining testing methods, the precautionary limits to the level of the methylcyclopentadienyl manganese tricarbonyl (MMT) in fuels, did not infringe the proportionality principle[189] and did not go beyond the objectives laid down in the Directive in question.[190] Therefore, the EU legislature may exercise broad discretion and cannot be precluded

> to achieve a degree of balance between, on the one hand, the protection of health, environmental protection and consumer protection and, on the other hand, the economic interests of traders, while pursuing the objective assigned to it by the Treaty to ensure a high level of protection of health and environmental protection.[191]

It is interesting to question REACH's provisions in the light of the *Afton* case. The similarities are numerous: high and complex uncertainty, equally complex technical and scientific facts to be evaluated for decision-making purposes, lack of appropriate methodologies and testing for nanomaterials. Arguably, the decision enacted on the basis of the REACH rule of law to curtail the risks of chemicals in nanoscale would be justified in the light of the

PP and the discretion that EU institutions and, to a lesser extent the MSs, have in situations of scientific uncertainty.

A few more considerations are warranted here on the MSs' derogation powers concerning nano-chemicals. One peculiarity of the REACH regulatory system is that its four phases set forth rather diversified procedures and could therefore be considered as 'stand-alone, but ostensibly complementary programmes'.[192] It can therefore be argued that stricter national measures might relate differently to different phases of REACH. For instance, an MS might impose an obligation to register, or might decide to restrict or ban nano-chemicals and their application. As Nicolas de Sadeleer has noticed, a problem might arise when MSs want to maintain or introduce stricter measures for chemicals falling within the Authorisation and Restriction phases. MSs can invoke protective measures pursuant to Article 36 TFEU, which allows for 'prohibitions or restrictions on imports, exports or goods in transit justified on grounds of public morality, public policy or public security; the protection of health and life of humans, animals or plants'.

By virtue of the integration principle (enshrined in Article 11 TFEU), Article 36 equally applies to environmental-based measures. However, given the *positive harmonisation* that REACH sets to operate in chemicals law, the subject is deemed to have been completely harmonised by the EU legislature. Therefore, MSs can maintain or introduce stricter national measures for environmental and workers' health protection, when specific conditions exist, only by virtue of Article 114(4)(5). Generally speaking, taking Article 114 TFEU as a legal basis, puts the internal market objective before the political objective of guaranteeing an optimum environmental protection, which remains in the background.[193] Yet, the space for manoeuvring that the harmonisation degree in REACH still leaves to MSs is rather atypical. In other words, although the harmonisation is deemed to be exhaustive, 'the MSs are not silenced'.[194] This means that MSs' multiple tasks and right of initiative (e.g. under substance evaluation and authorisation and restriction proposals) under the REACH system can lead to local knowledge being integrated in 'a bid to provoke regulatory change'.[195] Once this local (i.e. MS-level) knowledge has been presented on the EU level – e.g. by preparing an Authorisation or Restriction dossier – it is then for the EU legislature to justify its decision in relation to it (i.e. accept or reject the initiative); including from the point of the broad objectives that REACH seeks to attain and the precautionary principle that underpins all of its provisions.[196] This view is particularly interesting for the status of nano-chemicals in REACH. To date, several MSs have notified the Commission on mandatory reporting schemes. France passed a national law imposing a mandatory reporting mechanism for companies dealing with nanosubstances.[197] Denmark and Belgium have notified the Commission regarding proposals of registries for nanomaterials.[198] Norway already requires the registration of nanomaterials in the Product Register for quantities $\geq 100\,\text{kg/y}$.[199] So far, none of these national initiatives has raised issues of compatibility with REACH.

It can therefore be envisaged that one way to foster REACH-compatible nano-measures is through MSs' unilateral initiatives on nano-chemicals. If the measure represents an opt-out from Article 114 harmonisation, the MS has to notify it to the Commission, which will then scrutinise the measure under the internal market objective. If such Article 114 opt-out is found to be compatible with REACH and treaty law, it might well act as a 'catalyst for the Commission to consider proposing an adaptation to the regulatory bargain for the Community as a whole'.[200] For example, the French nano decree, which stipulates a mandatory national scheme for the reporting of nanomaterials under very different conditions than those set forth by REACH for chemicals in general (one above all: the minimum threshold of 100 gr), was notified to the Commission[201] which found it compatible with REACH.[202]

Beside the strictly legalistic discourse though, this book's analysis questions whether the REACH legal norms attain a full harmonisation also for nanoscale chemicals, in spite of the lack of clear definition of nano-chemicals as *new and distinct substances*, in need of a specific and separate registration dossier. In other words, does REACH truly harmonise the requirements on manufacture, placing on the market, or use of nanomaterials?[203] The remainder of this book will try to answer this question through a substantial and holistic interpretation of the REACH framework in order to try to address the main research question: does REACH, as it currently stands (i.e. nano-silent) effectively and exhaustively regulate the health and environmental risks of nanoscale chemicals?[204]

The next section offers a brief overview on the role of one of the major actors in the REACH implementation process: the ECHA, which REACH also established. The presentation of the general nature and role of the ECHA within the REACH system is important in order to understand the prerogatives and powers of the Agency, for the successful implementation of the REACH law. In addition, as Chapters 3–7 will better illustrate, the ECHA plays an important role when it comes to the consideration of nanoscale chemicals in REACH.

ECHA decision-making powers beyond the *Meroni* doctrine and implications for nanosubstances in REACH

Even for chemicals that are harmonised by REACH, the centralisation of powers remains still permeable. MSs' degree of participation in the ECHA's organic and administrative structure is responsible for such permeability.[205]

Generally speaking, the EU agencies are divided in two groups: *executive agencies*, 'responsible for performing various executive tasks to assist the Commission in the discharge of its responsibilities'[206]; and *regulatory agencies*, 'actively involved in the executive function by enacting instruments which help to regulate a specific sector'.[207]

Regulatory agencies can be of two types: with or without decision-making powers. Agencies with *decision-making powers* 'may adopt individual decisions but not legislative measures of general application'.[208] Currently there are 41 EU agencies operating in different areas of EU law. As a general rule, EU agencies have to comply with the *non-delegation doctrine* developed in the aftermath of the *Meroni* rulings.[209] Fearing the disturbance of the EU institutional balancing that might derive from broad delegation powers to agencies, the CJEU ruled in the *Meroni case* that only clearly defined executive powers that can be reviewed might be transferred to agencies.[210] The current lack of a legal basis in the Treaty for the creation of the agencies is probably linked to the need to preserve the institutional balance.

The ECHA has been endowed with decision-making powers and its role in the implementation and the clarification on the functioning of the REACH framework is of crucial importance, as the case of nano-chemicals will clearly demonstrate (see Chapter 4). According to Article 75 of REACH, the ECHA is established for the purpose 'of managing and in some cases carrying out the technical, scientific and administrative aspects of this Regulation and to ensure consistency at Community level in relation to these aspects'.

The structure of the ECHA is sophisticated and reflects the intention to remain anchored to the non-delegation tradition, even though, as we shall see, the main facade of the *Meroni* doctrine has started crumbling[211] and the ECHA's powers are quite pervasive. The structure of the Agency encompasses a Management Board, an Executive director, a Committee for Risk Assessment (CRA), a Committee for Socio-economic Analysis (CSA), a Forum for Exchange of Information on Enforcement, a Secretariat, and, finally, a Board of Appeal (BoA).[212] The nature and functions of such formations will be analysed later in this book, in accordance with their specific functions throughout the REACH implementation procedures. Note the fact that MSs' presence dominates each organ and strongly influences ECHA administrative and legal functioning. Article 77 of REACH stipulates that the ECHA provides 'technical and scientific guidance' and tools on the operation of REACH to MSs and the competent authorities (CAs).[213] Although REACH provides for a legal basis for the ECHA Guidance Documents (GDs), this does not mean that the GDs are normative binding acts. To remove all doubt in this sense, GDs contain a legal disclaimer reminding that REACH remains the main text of reference.[214] However, lack of legal binding force does not mean lack of effects on third parties. Lucas Bergkamp and DaeYoung Park argue that the GDs operate an inversion of the onus of proof: it is the regulated entity that shall prove why the guidance is not to be followed (e.g. it conflicts with REACH) rather than the Agency demonstrating why it must be followed.[215] In addition, GDs create legitimate expectance on third parties.

Given the recent modification of some of the REACH Guidance Documents in order to render them nano-specific,[216] it will be interesting to see how the industry will comply with such documents. A decisive input for nano-chemicals' fate might came from a number of cases recently decided by the ECHA Board of Appeal (BoA) concerning the Agency's decision to request additional information on the nanoform of certain chemicals. Such cases and their implications for nanosubstances' regulation in REACH are analysed further in this book. Before moving in that direction, the last part of this chapter tries to situate the massive regulatory shift in chemical regulation that REACH – including not only its new norms and principles but also the new techno-institutional apparatus that sets such norms in motion, e.g. the ECHA and the IT tools the Agency runs – brought about, in the global context. The attention is on the ability of REACH to affect extra-EU jurisdictions, including concerning nanoscale chemicals.

The reach of REACH beyond the EU/EEA

The Brexit example and the Turkish case

A final interesting angle of focus when analysing the impact of REACH, and thus its 'reach' in terms of broad applicability, is that from the perspective of two countries which are in a peculiar position in relation to the EU: the UK, as a MS soon-to-be third party on the one hand; and Turkey, as a third country currently working its way towards ascension to EU membership. Both countries share the characteristic of having a prosperous chemical sector that yields high turnovers and enables other strategic sectors of the respective national economies to operate successfully.

Out of REACH: the Brexit example

As the UK prepares to give up its EU membership, questions arise as to the terms pursuant to which the two entities will regulate their relationship, once the legal and institutional divorce is finalised. One pressing question concerns the applicability of a massive law like REACH in a post-Brexit reality. In the UK, the chemical industry represents the second biggest manufacturing industry overall. In 2017, the UK exported chemicals and chemical products to the value of £28.3 billion.[217] The chemical sector is a profitable activity not only because of the significant quantities of production and commercialisation of 'raw' chemicals, but also due to the feeding of such chemicals into other neuralgic sectors of the British industry like the aviation, pharmaceutical, and agriculture ones. At the same time, the British chemical sector is closely intertwined with the EU market: 60 per cent (to the value of £17.0 billion) of chemical exports in 2017 went to EU MSs, and 75 per cent of chemical imports came from the EU. It is no surprise thus that REACH compliance is of primary concern in a post-EU British economy. In fact, UK companies hold a total of 12,000 registrations in REACH, which make for 13 per cent of the total registrations under REACH.[218] In addition to the undeniable relevance of the chemical sector for British industry and trade, what these numbers clearly demonstrate is the fact that it would be arduous for the British economy to thrive without access to the EU chemical market, once Brexit is finalised. There are two possible scenarios for the post-Brexit period and it is worth analysing to some extent the implications of each of them in relation to the REACH status in general and the question of nano-scale chemicals therein in the specific.

The first scenario is that of an exit made with a deal secured. In this case the UK could adopt the Norwegian model, i.e. be a non-EU country that is part of the EEA, or alternatively, like Switzerland become a country that is outside of the single market but has secured free trade agreements with the EU.[219] The difference being that while Norway has adopted REACH and regularly implements the regulation, Swiss companies trading chemicals with the EU must ensure that the importers or only representatives (ORs) register the substances pursuant to REACH. In either case, the UK will lose its vote not only in Council and Parliament, but also in the many committees REACH operates through, thus losing its voice on chemical regulation matters for good. Further, the registrations currently held by the UK will be invalid, if not agreed otherwise. The UK Government has stated in a *White Paper* that it will seek active participation in EU agencies, in particular 'those EU agencies that provide authorisations for goods in highly regulated sectors – namely the European Chemicals Agency',[220] in order to make it possible for UK companies to register directly with the ECHA instead of appointing ORs.

Also, the UK claims to want to seek access to the IT system the ECHA uses to operationalise REACH, so that the transfer of data between the UK and the EU authorities is done in a prompt and efficient manner.[221] This, the White Paper continues, would be part of the broader proposal for securing 'an economic partnership' with the EU. Such partnership will be ideally premised on a *common rulebook for goods* 'covering only those rules necessary to provide for frictionless trade at the border – meaning that the UK would make an upfront choice to commit by treaty to ongoing harmonisation with the relevant EU rules [...]'.[222]

If a trade agreement is to be concluded, UK products would need to comply with EU standards pertaining to the manufacturing of certain goods. The REACH Regulation, as a standard setter *par excellence* (as demonstrated by the fact that it is being 'copied' also by extra-EU jurisdictions like Japan, Korea, and China, among others), would certainly impose the adoption of a good part of its rules and standards on the UK companies, if the frictionless trade in question is to be secured also for the chemical sector. Although no final decision has been reached yet on a potential exit deal, it has been observed that even in the event of such a deal, one thing is obvious: the UK will not remain in REACH because fully submitting to the regulation means, among other things, crossing the clearly marked red line of Brexit, i.e. accepting the jurisdiction of the CJEU, which is the ultimate entity that settles disputes pertaining to REACH.[223]

However, the EU for its part is unlikely to allow the UK to cherry-pick on laws and institutions while exiting, particularly for what concerns the jurisdiction of the CJEU. It is therefore rather unclear what a potential deal would look like and what it will stipulate in terms of REACH compliance and its applicability to the UK.

The second scenario, the '*no deal scenario*', prospects the exit of the UK without a deal with the EU being reached. The UK would consequently become a third country. In this case, it would still make sense for the UK to seek participation in REACH, and in its *Registration* system as a minimum, even if this comes at a price, which the UK will need to pay in fees (while losing any decisional power within the REACH system). Retaining full participation in and application of REACH has been already ruled out for this second scenario, since for the UK, REACH fully embodies the single market mechanisms Brexit is aiming to extricate the country from. Hence, although the UK is likely to seek access to the single market, it will do so by submitting to the strict minimum required rather than remaining fully involved in laws like REACH.[224] However, as a rule, once the UK becomes a third country, UK REACH registrations will, also in this second option, become invalid. In order for UK companies to retain their registrations and generally be able to sell chemicals or chemical-based products in the EEA, they would need to either transfer their registrations to an EU-based entity 'as part of a business transfer to that entity of the assets relating to the registration';[225] or transfer them to an OR based in the EU. The second option will be available only to UK *manufacturers* but not to UK *importers*, which would presumably need to register their substances directly with the ECHA.[226]

Alternatively, in a no-deal scenario, the choice for the UK could be that of enacting a national chemicals legislation and the necessary infrastructure and institutions for administering and implementing it, so as to fill the void created as a result of abandoning REACH. In practice though, this REACH-like model would be a very expensive undertaking. It has been estimated that replacing ECHA functions with national law across the EU, would entail administrative costs above 224 million. What the exact share of that would be for a post-Brexit UK remains unclear. What is certain is that the costs would be in the range of tens of millions of pounds.[227]

What is more, adopting a legal text emulating REACH will not suffice. Rather, the UK will need to build a supporting IT system like the one ECHA uses to administer REACH (the IUCLID 6), and, importantly, appoint an entity that performs the ECHA's tasks and functions. So far, the UK Department for Environment, Food and Rural Affairs (DEFRA) has been working to develop an IT tool that should 'replicate the EU's REACH IT system as closely as possible',[228] which was planned to be in place by March 2019. The costs of such a tool are estimated at £32.8 million for the 2018–2020 period.[229] The UK government has also claimed that it would maintain the current standards of human health and environmental protection and that the Health and Safety Executive (HSE) would act as the lead UK regulatory authority, given the experience it already has with REACH compliance procedures. Still, UK companies will need to transfer their *registrations* to EU-based organisations (ORs). Likewise, UK importers and downstream users of authorised substances would need to take the necessary steps in order to register and obtain authorisation, respectively, so as to be able to keep commercialising with EEA-based companies. Further, starting from 2019, such companies would be required to provide specific notifications to the HSE. For new chemicals to be placed in the EEA (and UK) market after Brexit, the burden for UK companies will be double as they will need to register the new substances twice: first with the ECHA (through the ORs) and then with the national appointed authority, the HSE for instance, with the data provided being the same in both cases.

In such a situation, providing 'specialist capacity to evaluate the impact of chemicals on health and the environment'[230] will become necessary, as the UK will not be able to partake in the knowledge-generation process, nor share the cutting-edge information circulating between EU MSs due to the REACH obligations. How this is to be attained without accessing the valuable ECHA database and the rich information that has been produced on chemicals risk since the enactment of REACH, remains a critical point.

Clearly, leaving REACH, and eventually, the replication of its legal text, its supporting institutions, and its implementing mechanisms, best exemplifies that complicated 'process of disentangling both legislative standards and governance structures' that Brexit will entail for the UK, particularly in the area of environmental law.[231]

But Brexit will most likely be finalised by the end of 2019. The last deadline for registration in REACH was May 2018 and UK companies had to comply with it. What will happen to the costly and valuable registrations already completed by UK companies? It must be noted that the possibility of a *buffer period* to facilitate the UK's transition to its post-Brexit reality will only be possible if a final *Withdrawal Agreement* is reached.[232] During this period and in order not to cause burdensome interruption to the economic activities involving commercialisation of chemicals, the UK government foresees a general carry-across and grandfathering of registrations and authorisations already held by UK companies complying with REACH.[233] The general idea is to keep all the approvals, certifications, and goods authorisations under EU law valid for the entire transition period.[234]

However, whether this would be possible and, if so, under which terms and conditions, will depend on the terms of the agreement that the EU and UK might ultimately manage to strike.

REACHing out to EU: KKDIK and the Turkish case

Beyond the EU, REACH is becoming a world standard for chemicals regulation. Korea, Japan, China, and recently Turkey, have adopted REACH-like regulations without having any direct legal obligation to do so. The case of Turkey is an interesting counter-example to the prospected scenario(s) in the post-Brexit UK.

Before 2008, the chemical sector in Turkey operated under a very light regulatory regime with few rules and constraints in place. After REACH was enacted, and in light of Turkey's advanced membership request, Turkey began to adopt a number of *by-laws* to implement EU chemicals legislation. Examples of such laws include the SAE (CLP By-law), i.e. *Regulation on Restrictions for the Manufacture, Marketing and Use of Certain Dangerous Substances and Preparations* (26.12.2008/27092) and the SDS, i.e. *Safety Data Sheets Regulation* (26.12.2008/27092) by-law.[235] However, both laws represented only late transposition of old repealed EU legislation, i.e. Directive 67/548/EC and Directive 99/45/EC in the case of the SAE; Directive 76/769/EC (now REACH Annex XVII) and Directive 91/155/EC (now REACH Annex II) in the case of the SDS. Although such by-laws were significant in that they helped Turkey to shape a chemical legislation in line with the EU procedures and standards on chemicals regulation, they were not the equivalents of the REACH reform. However, the Turkish by-law that most closely mirrored the REACH framework was the so-called KEK/CICR or *Kimyasalların Envanteri ve Kontrolü Hakkında Yönetmelik/Chemicals Inventory and Control* by-law (28.12. 2008/27092).

Pursuant to Article 1 of the KEK the aim of this by-law was to

> set out administrative and technical procedures and principles related to inventory creation and control to *provide effective protection against the adverse effects that chemicals may have on human health and the environment.*[236]

What is more, the KEK, at Article 6(2), stipulated for the first time that it was essential to provide *adequate protection* for human health and the environment by reducing risks of dangerous chemicals. This is a close transposition of the EU concept of high levels of protection that REACH has at its basis. The KEK also operated on the basis of a tiered approach, setting forth data requirements for producers of chemicals on the basis of a two-pronged system: small quantities i.e. 1–1,000 t/y and higher volumes i.e. > 1,000 t/y. Still, the KEK was more a transcription of the Council Regulation (EEC) No. 793/93 of 23 March 1993 on the evaluation and control of the risks of existing substances, than of the complex and massive REACH Regulation. The KEK had nonetheless a positive impact on the oversight of chemicals produced and commercialised in Turkey given that by 2011, some 2,888 substances manufactured or imported in quantities ≥ 1 t/y and < 1,000 t/y and 597 substances manufactured or imported at 1,000 t/y (considered HPV substances) were registered with the Turkish Ministry of Environment and Urban Planning (MoEUP) under the KEK inventory.[237] The result is significant also when considering that for the first time, registrants had to provide data on (eco)toxicity and the physicochemical properties of some of the most common chemicals on the Turkish market, which, just like in the pre-REACH EU situation, had been used and commercialised completely unchecked until then. Of these, 131 were prioritised for evaluation.

Turkey did not stop there. In 2013, this official candidate for membership in the EU launched an overhaul of its young EU-like chemicals legislation, with the aim of bringing it more in line with the ultimate system of rules and procedures brought about by EU REACH and the CLP Regulations. Recent laws adopted in such an intent include:

- The SEA, i.e. the new by-law on the Classification, Labelling and Packaging of Substances and Mixtures (11.12.2013/28848);
- The SDS, i.e. the new by-law on Safety Data Sheets on Hazardous Substances and Mixtures, known also by its Turkish acronym as GBF Regulation (13.12.2014/29204);
- Kimyasalların Kaydı, Değerlendirmesi, İzni ve Kısıtlanması Yönetmelik or KKDIK (23.12.2017/30105), translated as Regulation on the Registration, Evaluation, Permission and Restriction of Chemicals.

The merit of such by-laws has been to introduce a progressive set of duties and obligations for the producers and importers of chemicals in Turkey, triggering that process of data generation on chemical risk so crucial to the adoption of measures that can ensure a control of risk deriving from chemical exposure, in line with the now fully-flagged principle of high levels of protection of human health and environmental protection inspired by the EU environmental policy. And nowhere is this more visible in the Turkish EU-like chemical legislation than in the KKDIK.

The KKDIK was adopted with significant delay on 23 June 2017 and entered into force on 31 December 2017. This is the actual much-awaited Turkish-REACH which closely follows its EU prototype. Like its EU counterpart, the KKDIK has been referred to as 'the most comprehensive and stringent Turkish chemical legislation to date'.[238]

The aim of the KKDIK is:

> to ensure a *high level of protection of human health and the environment*, including the promotion of alternative methods for assessment of hazards of substances while enhancing competitiveness and innovation.[239]

Clearly this is almost a transposition of REACH's Article 1 into Turkish national law. It is significant that in the time span of less than one decade, Turkey has tried to catch up with the latest developments taking place in EU chemicals legislation – with notable results. The KKDIK will replace by 2023 the SEA, SDS/GBF, and the KEK, bringing the provisions of these separate pieces of legislation under a unified law. This Turkish-REACH sets also two general deadlines: the 2020 deadline for the pre-registration of all chemicals produced in quantities ³ 1 t/y in order to give Turkish businesses a way to adjust to the new requirements of the law, and the final deadline of 2023, when all chemicals subject to the regulation are required to be registered. The KKDIK adopts many of the REACH milestones, including the four tonnage bands and the relative incremental data requirement criterion, the authorisation procedure (including the Candidate Substance List and the Annex of Substances Subject to Authorisation), the restriction procedure, the registration of monomers used to produce a polymer (but not the polymer itself), etc.[240] Interestingly, in order to help companies comply with the REACH-like requirements, the Turkish Ministry of Environment and Urban Planning (MoEUP) has delegated the task of training of chemical safety experts to another institution. The criteria for being certified as such an institution are set out in a specific annex to the KKDIK.[241] It is relevant to point out here that only trained and qualified experts, known as Certified Chemical Safety Assessors (CCSAs) can sign off registrations to be submitted to the MoEUP under the new KKDIK, compile dossiers on Chemical Safety Assessments (CSAs) and on Chemical Safety Reports (CSRs), procedures that KKDIK has also borrowed from REACH.[242]

Importantly for the focus of this book and the question of nanosubstances in REACH, the Turkish-REACH copies, almost verbatim, the Authorisation procedure, including concerning the identification of SVHCs and the use of such chemicals in articles (as well as the 0.1 per cent weight by weight (w/w) threshold thereof). Similarly, the Restriction phase of REACH is faithfully transposed in the KKDIK although the number of entries (66 to date) is lower if compared to the restricted substances included in REACH's Annex VII.[243] Yet, if the legal void characterising Turkish chemicals law in the pre-REACH period is considered, the recent developments are clearly a positive achievement under the profile of human health and environmental protection.

It is important to underline that the KKDIK does not incorporate any specific provision referring to nanomaterials. However, just like with REACH, the assumption is that such chemicals are covered by the KKDIK definition of substance. Notwithstanding the debate on whether this is actually the case, it can be hypothesised here that given the close and rather prompt transposition of REACH and its milestones in the KKDIK, it is very likely that Turkey will soon update its KKDIK Annexes so as to accommodate at least some of the amendments made to the EU REACH Annexes concerning nanotechnology.

One final remark needs to be made on the fact that the KKDIK, just like REACH, will apply to all companies trading chemicals on the Turkish market. Hence, chemical companies operating outside Turkey will need to appoint a local OR in Turkey in order to register their chemicals under the KKDIK. In this regard, it might be interesting to point out that the major import countries for the Turkish chemical sector are China (12%), Germany (10.3%), Russia (9.8%), and USA (5.4%), whereas the main export markets are Germany (9.3%), UK (7.3%), Iraq (5.9%), Italy (4.8%), and USA (4.4%).[244] Such numbers suggest that the new requirements of the REACH-like KKDIK are likely to resonate far across the Bosporus,[245] with the probable consequence of 'exporting' the REACH model – or at least, some elements of it – to trade partners as diverse as Russia and Iraq.

This far-reaching reach of REACH can be seen as a sort of double *California Effect*:[246] on the one side, Turkey saw it necessary to align its national chemical legislation to the REACH model so as to secure a stable trade with the EU/EEA area, especially in light of its future membership, while on the other, countries which might have a strong interest in commercialising chemicals with Turkey might feel compelled to enact REACH-like norms similar to those of the KKDIK, so as to remove obstacles to the trade flow with Turkey. It remains to be seen how things will develop in the next four years, when the final deadline of the KKDIK would make it mandatory to comply with REACH-like norms for all *new* and *existing* chemicals circulating in Turkey. In particular, it will be interesting to follow the way Turkey will choose to incorporate into its new REACH-like statute the approved nano-specific amendments to REACH, which are to come into force in 2020, when the pre-registration/notification deadline of the KKDIK is also due. Ideally, a modification to the KKDIK Annexes so as to reflect the REACH nano-amendments could be enacted before the final 2023 deadline expires, so as to prompt specific registrations for nanoscale substances under the KKDIK.

Conclusions on Brexit and the Turkish-REACH

From the contraposition of the UK potential approaches to REACH in the aftermath of Brexit, and that of Turkey which, while it awaits to join the EU, has adopted its own REACH-like regulation, the KKDIK, a few preliminary conclusions can be drawn on the far-reaching effect of REACH as the new global-setter in chemicals regulation.

First, concerning the general area of EU environmental law, which is unprecedented in its scope, breadth, and level of innovation, the UK move appears – at least, as far as REACH is considered – to be a sinister attempt to bring the wheel of integration back in time: the country will need to go back to the standardisation rules, undoing that long and strenuous process of progressive harmonisation that has finally granted a specific legal basis to the environmental protection aim, elevating it to (primary) Treaty law level. Brexit, which appears at best awkward for its government and at worst catastrophic for its citizens, will send the UK back to square one, where, before all the elaborated case law and treaty reforms, it was common to use rudimental and often improvised legal tools, e.g. product standard harmonisation rules, for protecting the environment. It is unclear how the UK will be able to use such outdated tools and the now-obsolete thinking they represent, to operate in a landscape, like that of modern EU environmental law, which is now highly sophisticated and completely transformed since those tools were last used to such purpose.

No other EU environmental statute puts this problem in such stark relief as REACH. The Regulation, as shown at the beginning of this chapter and as will be further demonstrated in the next ones, is the fruit of long-fought battles for securing, first, a better knowledge of chemicals' nature and their risks, and second, a better control of such risks on an EU-wide basis, in line with the Union's high level of protection objective. Disruptive, expensive (the UK companies have spent as much as £250 million for registration purposes as of May 2018, which will become invalid after Brexit), burdensome, and hardly innovative, the post-Brexit substitute for REACH seems like a clumsy attempt at redoing alone a collective endeavour in which the UK had invested significant resources and expertise, and from which it was finally harvesting bountiful fruits in terms of human health and environmental protection and gains in knowledge. Further, the REACH framework operates through duties and rules that are premised on cooperation, mutual obligations, and reciprocal oversights and controls. This is because the EU legislator enacted REACH in the full realisation that knowledge generation – especially in the complex realm of chemicals, where risks can be highly uncertain while being at the same time diffused and often irreversible – is best done through a collaborative, coordinated, and transparent process. Moreover, the free circulation of chemicals thrives better if such functions and the data generation demanded by REACH are done in a shared and concordant process. Lastly, the communal fulfilment of REACH tasks allows for cost-sharing while maximising knowledge gains. By leaving the EU, the UK will lose access to all this while being at the same time required to pay substantial fees in case some access to REACH will be granted.

One might ask what will then be the gain if a country is willing to face such burdensome consequences so far into the REACH implementation process. Some see a potential in the new possibility that a post-Brexit UK will allow for use of chemicals that are banned or otherwise restricted elsewhere in the EU. Hence, this argument goes, freeing UK enterprises from the burden of REACH would constitute a silver lining of opportunities,[247] since costly compliance procedures would be avoided. However, the prospect of the UK searching for economic opportunities by bringing back dangerous chemicals that it took the EU decades to restrict or phase out, would represent a betrayal to its own citizens and ecosystems, which would be exposed again to chemicals proven to pose unacceptable risks. Furthermore, the time and resources already invested by the UK in REACH are so high, and the process of REACH implementation so advanced, that it appears difficult to envisage any positive gain from an out-of-REACH situation. All the considerations above tend to be even more acute when nano-chemicals are considered. The choice of the UK to leave REACH now that the nano-specific amendments to the Annexes are finally approved will certainly render the regulation of such chemicals by means of national laws only an arduous one. The UK is likely to lag behind in terms of information-generation and risk-understanding for this class of chemicals.

Moreover, the fact that other countries, like Turkey prominently, are voluntarily embracing the strict rules of authorisation and restriction in REACH, invites reflection. What is more, Turkey, aware of the complexity of the tasks REACH compliance entails, is devoting special attention to the training of experts that can sign off/certify properly prepared chemical safety sheets/dossiers, whereas the UK, renouncing the possibility to exchange valuable information in the pertinent fora, will probably lose also technical expertise. Finally, while in the case of Turkey and its extra-EU partners, the adoption of a REACH-like chemicals legislation is thought to prompt a positive race to the top, in the fashion of a double California Effect, Brexit risks exposing the UK to the danger of dumping policies[248] and a race to the bottom. Such consequences would be particularly worrisome for the case of nano-pollutants if we consider that their risks are thought to be of potentially infinite impacts.[249]

In sum

In general, REACH is a critically important piece of legislation for reducing the introduction of toxic pollutants into the environment. As it applies to chemical substances, the control, prevention, and reduction of risks posed by hazardous chemicals is operated upfront, without considering the specificities related to the dispersion in different environmental compartments. Perhaps because of this generalised application, which attributes an over-arching nature to its set of legal provisions, REACH will contribute and benefit also other single-media regulations' objectives in terms of reduction and/or phasing out of hazardous chemicals.

REACH's impact is certainly felt beyond the EU area, as demonstrated by the fact that third countries are embracing some of its core elements, elevating the regulation to the rank of global standard-setter. This is certainly one strong point of REACH. At the same time though, the failed attempts to bring nanoscale chemicals under the REACH rule in general and its Authorisation process in the specific, represent a weakness that, as will be shown, is proven difficult to remedy now that the Regulation is fully operative. It is regrettable that scientific development on nanotechnology and nanotechnology's legal status in REACH followed parallel tracks, leading to a statute that is currently not nano-specific in its legal text. Yet, as this chapter demonstrated, negotiating REACH and securing the necessary consensus for passing a law of such proportions was not an easy one. It is perhaps therefore not surprising that in the attempt to have such a law in place, the aim to include the then-emerging issue of nanoscale chemicals had to be postponed. As will be shown, this choice turned out to be a huge and perhaps irremediable missed opportunity in terms of attaining a high level of human health and environmental protection also for nanoscale substances – more so, if it is considered that the only nano-specific changes to REACH will be contained only in its Annexes, but not in the legal text of its Articles.

Notes

1 The first Directive on chemicals regulation dates back to 1967 and REACH came into force in 2007.
2 See Tanja Ehnert, *The EU and Nanotechnologies: A Critical Analysis* (Hart Publishing 2017) 145–147.
3 Stokes refers to the Commission in this regard as the 'gatekeeper' of the existing status quo. See Elen Stokes, 'Nanotechnology and the Products of Inherited Regulation' (2012) 39 *Journal of Law and Society* 93, 98.
4 Ibid. 94.
5 Charlotte Burns and Neil Carter, 'The Environmental Policy' in Erik Jones, Anand Menon, and Stephen Weatherill (eds) *The Oxford Handbook of the European Union* (Oxford 2012) 512.
6 Treaty establishing the European Economic Community, EEC Treaty (Treaty of Rome) [1957].
7 Jan H. Jans and Hans H.B.Vedder (eds) *European Environmental Law: After Lisbon* (4th edn, Europa Law Publishing 2012) 3. The phases of EU environmental law development elucidated in this chapter are based mainly on and draw significantly upon this book.
8 Council Directive 67/548/EEC of 27 June 1967 on the approximation of laws, regulations and administrative provisions relating to the classification, packaging and labelling of dangerous substances [1967] OJ 196/1.
9 Directive 67/548/EEC, Article 1.
10 Directive 67/548/EEC, recital (1).
11 Council Declaration of 22 November 1973 on the programme of action of the European Communities on the environment [1973] OJ C112/1.
12 Council Directive 85/210/EEC of 20 March 1985 on the approximation of the laws of the Member States concerning the lead content of petrol [1985] OJ L96/25.
13 Council Directive 78/319/EEC of 20 March 1978 on toxic and dangerous waste [1978] OJ L84/43.
14 Article 235 EEC read:

> If any action by the Community appears necessary to achieve, in the functioning of the Common Market, one of the aims of the Community in cases where this Treaty has not provided for the requisite powers of action, the Council, acting by means of a unanimous vote on a proposal of the Commission and after the Assembly has been consulted, shall enact the appropriate provisions.

15 Jans and Vedder (n 7) 5.
16 Case 240/83 *Procureur de la République v ADBHU* [1985] ECLI:EU:C:1985:59.
17 Ibid. para 13; The Court reaffirmed the status of the environmental protection as 'one of the Community's essential objectives' also in the Danish Bottle case, Case-302/86 *Commission v Denmark* [1988] ECLI:EU:C:1988:421, para 8.
18 See Maria Lee, *EU Environmental Law: Challenges, Change and Decision-Making* (2nd edn, Hart Publishing 2014) 3.
19 *ADBHU* (n 16) para 15.
20 Council Directive 79/409/EEC of 2 April 1979 on the conservation of wild birds [1979] OJ L103/1.
21 Council Directive 82/884/EEC of 3 December 1982 on a limit value for lead in the air [1982] OJ L378/15.
22 See Jans and Vedder (n 7) 6.
23 Ingmar von Homeyer, 'The Evolution of EU Environmental Governance' in Joanne Scott (ed.), *Environmental Protection: European Law and Governance* (OUP 2009) 8–9.

24 Ibid. 10–11.
25 Single European Act [1986] OJ L169/1.
26 Christian Zacker, 'Environmental Law of the European Economic Community: New Powers Under the Single European Act' (1991) 14 B.C. Int'l & Comp. L. Rev. 249, 250.
27 Ibid. 250.
28 Ibid. 250.
29 von Homeyer (n 23) 12.
30 Ibid. 13.
31 Treaty on European Union [1992] OJ C191/1.
32 Jans and Vedder (n 7) 7.
33 Lee (n 18) 3.
34 von Homeyer (n 23) 15.
35 Ibid. 18.
36 Treaty of Amsterdam amending the Treaty on European Union, the Treaties establishing the European Communities and certain related acts – Final Act [1997] OJ C340/115.
37 Article 2 EC, see also Jans and Vedder (n 7) 9.
38 Roger J. Goebel, 'The Treaty of Amsterdam in Historical Perspective: Introduction to the Symposium' (1998) 22 Fordham International Law Journal S7, S20.
39 von Homeyer (n 23) 18–19.
40 The challenge of invisibility and uncertainty persist for some of the most pressing environmental problems. See on this point Hans Christian Bugge, 'Twelve Fundamental Challenges in Environmental Law' in Christina Voigt (ed.), *Rule of Law for Nature: New Dimensions and Ideas in Environmental Law* (CUP 2013) 10–11.
41 von Homeyer (n 23) 22.
42 Ibid. 22–23.
43 Treaty of Nice amending the Treaty on European Union, the Treaties establishing the European Communities and certain related acts [2001] OJ C80/1.
44 Consolidated version of the Treaty on European Union [2012] OJ C326/13.
45 Consolidated version of the Treaty on the Functioning of the European Union [2012] OJ C326/47.
46 Article 3(1), TEU.
47 Articles 11, 13, and 194 (2) TFEU. See also Eléonore Maitre-Ekern, 'Towards an Integrated Product Regulatory Framework Based on Life Cycle Thinking' in Beate Sjåfjell and Anja Wiesbrock (eds), *The Greening of European Business under EU Law: Taking Article 11 TFEU Seriously* (Routledge 2015).
48 See M. Setälä and Th. Schiller (eds) *Citizens' Initiatives in Europe: Procedures and Consequences of Agenda-Setting by Citizens* (Palgrave Macmillan 2012).
49 See Case C-64/09 *Commission v France* [2010] ECLI:EU:C:2010:197, para 30.
50 Article 13(2) TFEU.
51 Jans and Vedder (n 7) 13.
52 Opinion 2/00 of the Court [2001] ECLI:EU:C:2001:664, para 5; See also Nicolas de Sadeleer, 'Environmental Governance and the Legal Bases Conundrum' (2012) 31 Yearbook of European Law 373.
53 Nicolas de Sadeleer, *EU Environmental Law and the Internal Market* (OUP 2014) 1.
54 Ludwig Krämer, *EU Environmental Law* (7th edn, Sweet & Maxwell 2011) 5–6.
55 Krämer (n 54) 72 explains that this is owed to the fact that the residual powers that Articles 114, 192, and 193 provide for MSs, are very different and, therefore, a double basis would create legal uncertainty.
56 See Nicolas de Sadeleer 'The Impact of Registration, Evaluation and Authorisation (REACH) of Chemicals Regulation on the Regulatory Powers of the Nordic Countries' in Nicolas de Sadeleer (ed.), *Implementing the Precautionary*

Principle: Approaches from the Nordic Countries, EU and USA (Earthscan 2007) 339–341.

57 The permitted grounds for derogation are set out in Article 36(1) TFEU and include 'public morality, public policy or public security; the protection of health and life of humans, animals or plants; the protection of national treasures possessing artistic, historic or archaeological value; or the protection of industrial and commercial property'.

58 de Sadeleer 2007 (n 56) 340.

59 Ibid. 339.

60 Case C-473/98 *Toolex* [2000] ECLI:EU:C:2000:379.

61 Council Directive 76/769/EEC of 27 July 1976 on the approximation of the laws, regulations and administrative provisions of the Member States relating to restrictions on the marketing and use of certain dangerous substances and preparations [1976] OJ L262/201.

62 *Toolex* (n 60) para 35.

63 Ibid. para 49.

64 Ibid. para 38.

65 de Sadeleer 2007 (n 56) 341.

66 Case C-3/00 *Denmark v Commissions* [2003] ECLI:EU:C:2003:167, para 58, emphasis added; see also de Sadeleer 2007 (n 56) 347.

67 ClientEarth, 'The Impact of the Lisbon Treaty – An Environmental Perspective' (2010) 18, available at: www.clientearth.org/reports/clientearth-briefing-lisbon-treaty-march-2010.pdf accessed 24.10.2016.

68 Jans and Vedder (n 7) 59.

69 See Case C-6/03 *Deponiezweckverband Eiterköpfe* [2005] ECLI:EU:C:2005:222.

70 Jans and Vedder (n 7) 115.

71 For a good discussion on this point, see Jans and Vedder (n 7) 113–122.

72 Gunnar Lind, 'The Only Planet Guide to the Secrets of Chemicals Policy in the EU: REACH – What Happened and Why?' (Inger Schörling 2004).

73 Ibid. 50.

74 Commission, 'Strategy for a Future Chemicals Policy' (White Paper) COM (2001) 88 final, 30.

75 Kathleen Cooper et al., 'Environmental Standard Setting and Children's Health' (CELA 2000) 128.

76 Ibid.

77 Lind (n 72) 52.

78 See Ralf Nordbeck and Michael Faust, 'European Chemicals Regulation and Its Effect on Innovation: An Assessment of the EU's White Paper on the Strategy for a Future Chemicals Policy' (2003) 13 European Environment 79.

79 Ibid. 80.

80 Council Directive 79/831/EEC of 18 September 1979 amending for the sixth time Directive 67/548/EEC on the approximation of the laws, regulations and administrative provisions relating to the classification, packaging and labelling of dangerous substances [1979] OJ L259/10.

81 Ibid. 10.

82 Nordbeck and Faust (n 78) 82.

83 Council Directive 92/32/EEC of 30 April 1992 amending for the seventh time Directive 67/548/EEC on the approximation of the laws, regulations and administrative provisions relating to the classification, packaging and labelling of dangerous substances [1992] OJ L154/1.

84 Ibid. 1.

85 Nordbeck and Faust (n 78) 81.

86 Ibid. 84.

87 Ibid. 82.

88 COM (2001) 88 final.
89 Council Regulation (EEC) 793/93 of 23 March 1993 on the evaluation and control of the risks of existing substances [1993] OJ L84/1.
90 Nordbeck and Faust (n 78) 82.
91 Ibid. 83.
92 COM (2001) 88 final, 19 and Nordbeck and Faust (n 78) 84.
93 The EU Commission is divided into several departments and services. The departments are known as Directorate-Generals (DGs) which are classified according to the policy they deal with.
94 See Nordbeck and Faust (n 78) 95–97.
95 Dieter Pesendorfer, 'EU Environmental Policy under Pressure: Chemicals Policy Change between Antagonistic Goals?' (2006) 15 Environmental Politics 95, 96.
96 See in general: de Sadeleer 2007 (n 56).
97 Christian Hey, Klaus Jacob, and Axel Volkery, 'Better Regulation by New Governance Hybrids? Governance Models and the Reform of European Chemicals Policy' (2007) 15 Journal of Cleaner Production 1859, 1860.
98 Ibid. 1861.
99 Commission, 'Simpler Legislation for the Internal Market (SLIM): A Pilot Project' (Communication) COM (96) 204 final.
100 Ibid.
101 Commission, 'Result on the Fourth Phase of SLIM' (Report) COM (2000) 56 final.
102 COM (2000) 56 final, recommendation 1, 15.
103 United Nations, *Globally Harmonized System of Classification and Labelling of Chemicals (GHS)* (4th edn, UN 2011).
104 Convention on Access to Information, Public Participation in Decision-Making and Access to Justice in Environmental Matters Alternative (Aarhus Convention), 28 June 1998, (1999) 38 ILM 517.
105 COM (2000) 56 final, recommendations 39–40, 19.
106 COM (2000) 56 final, 8.
107 Commission, 'Communication on the Precautionary Principle' (Communication) COM(2000) 1 final.
108 According to the Commission, precautionary-based measures should be:

> proportional, non-discriminatory; consistent with similar measures already taken; based on an examination of the potential benefits and costs of action or lack of action (including, where appropriate and feasible, an economic cost/benefit analysis); subject to review, capable of assigning responsibility for producing the scientific evidence necessary for a more comprehensive risk assessment.
>
> COM (2000) 1 final, 4

109 COM (2000) 1 final, 3.
110 COM (2000) 1final, 9.
111 COM (2000) 1 final, 10.
112 COM (2000) 1 final, 16.
113 COM (2000) 1 final, 21.
114 COM (2001) 88 final.
115 Of note here is that the definition of precaution endorsed in the White Paper is weaker than the one contained in the Rio Declaration. It reads:

> Whenever reliable scientific evidence is available that a substance may have an adverse impact on human health and the environment but there is still scientific uncertainty about the precise nature or the magnitude of the potential damage, decision-making must be based on precaution in order to prevent damage to human health and the environment.

116 Remi Allanou, Bjørn G. Hansen, and Yvonne van der Bilt, 'Public Availability of Data on EU High Production Volume Chemicals' (EUR 18996, European Commission JRC 1999).

117 Pesendorfer (n 95) 109.

118 COM (2001) 88 final, 8 reads:

> Given the vast number of existing substances on the market, the Commission proposes that first priority is given to substances that lead to a high exposure or cause concern by their known or suspected dangerous properties – physical, chemical, toxicological or ecotoxicological,

suggesting the intention of making exposure, not necessarily linked to the volume of production, a criterion valid per se when requiring data from industry.

119 Lind (n 72) 83.

120 Pesendorfer (n 95) 108.

121 Lind (n 72) 86; the letter can be found here: www.ambafrance-uk.org/Risks-of-de-industrialization accessed 03.04.2017.

122 Royal Commission on Environmental Pollution, *Twenty-fourth Report: Chemicals in Products, Safeguarding the Environment and Human Health* (HMSO 2003) 10.

123 Royal Commission on Environmental Pollution, *Second Report – Three Issues in Industrial Pollution* (HMSO 1972).

124 Royal Commission 2003 (n 122) 3.

125 Lind (n 72) 85.

126 Lind (n 72).

127 Pesendorfer (n 95) 111.

128 Council Decision 1513/2002/EC of 27 June 2002 concerning the sixth framework programme of the European Community for research, technological development and demonstration activities, contributing to the creation of the European Research Area and to innovation (2002 to 2006) [2002] OJ L 232/1.

129 Ibid. 5.

130 Commission, 'A European Initiative for Growth – Investing in Networks and Knowledge for Growth and Jobs – Final Report to the European Council' (Communication), COM (2003) 690 final/2, 35.

131 European Commission, Community Health and Consumer Protection, 'Nanotechnologies, a preliminary risk analysis on the basis of a workshop organized in Brussels on 1-March 2004 from the Health and Consumer Protection Directorate General of the European Commission' (2004).

132 Ibid. 3.

133 Ibid. 132.

134 Commission, 'Towards a European Strategy for Nanotechnology' (Communication) COM (2004) 338 final, 3.

135 Ibid. 4.

136 Commission, 'Nanosciences and Nanotechnologies: An Action Plan for Europe 2005–2009' (Communication) COM (2005) 243 final, 11.

137 Ibid.

138 ★★★I Position of the European Parliament, adopted at first reading on 17 November 2005 with a view to the adoption of Regulation (EC) No …/2006 of the European Parliament and of the Council concerning the Registration, Evaluation, Authorisation and Restriction of Chemicals (REACH), establishing a European Chemicals Agency and amending Directive 1999/45/EC (EP-PE_TC1-COD(2003)0256) P6_TA(2005)0434.

139 COM (2004) 338 final, 4.

140 COM (2005) 243 final, 2.

141 Respectively Articles 152 and 174 TEC.

142 COM (2005) 243 final, 11.

143 COM (2005) 243 final, 10.
144 Article 3(3) TEU stipulates: 'The Union shall work for sustainable development of Europe based on balanced economic growth and price stability ... *and a high level of protection and improvement of the quality of the environment*'; emphasis added.
145 The Royal Society and The Royal Academy of Engineering, *Nanoscience and Nanotechnologies: Opportunities and Uncertainties* (The Royal Society 2004) 45–50.
146 Ibid. 76.
147 Ibid. 71.
148 Ibid. 72.
149 See Scientific Committee on Emerging and Newly Identified Health Risks (SCENIHR), 'Opinion on the Appropriateness of Existing Methodologies to Assess the Potential Risks Associated with Engineered and Adventitious Products of Nanotechnologies' (28–29 September 2005).
150 Ibid. 55.
151 SCENIHR 'Modified Opinion (after public consultation) on The Appropriateness of Existing Methodologies to Assess the Potential Risks Associated with Engineered and Adventitious Products of Nanotechnologies' (10 March 2006).
152 Ibid. 55.
153 ***II RECOMMENDATION FOR SECOND READING on the Council common position for adopting a regulation of the European Parliament and of the Council concerning the Registration, Evaluation, Authorisation and Restriction of Chemicals (REACH), establishing a European Chemicals Agency, amending Directive 1999/45/EC of the European Parliament and of the Council and repealing Council Regulation (EEC) No. 793/93 and Commission Regulation (EC) No. 1488/94 as well as Council Directive 76/769/EEC and Commission Directives 91/155/EEC, 93/67/EEC, 93/105/EC, and 2000/21/EC (7524 /8/2006–C6–0267/2006–2003/0256(COD)), FINAL A6–0352/2006.
154 Ibid., Amendment 24, 17.
155 Such choice is based on the fact that:

> According to 'Science', the very small size of nanomaterials can modify the physico-chemical properties and create the opportunity for increased uptake and interaction with biological tissues. This combination can generate adverse biological effects in living cells that would not otherwise be possible with the same material in larger form. According to SCENIHR, information about the biological fate of nanoparticles (e.g. distribution, accumulation, metabolism and organ specific toxicity) is still minimal. Nanoparticles should therefore fall under authorisation.
>
> Ibid., Amendment 79, 51

156 This is because:

> According to SCENIHR, a wide variety of nanoscale materials and functional nanoscale surfaces are in use in consumer products, including cosmetics and sunscreens, fibres and textiles, dyes, fillers, paints, emulsions and colloids. Given the combination of a) very worrying adverse effects by nanoparticles, b) their widespread use in consumer products and c) the minimal knowledge about the biological fate of nanoparticles, they should be prioritised within the authorisation system of REACH.
>
> Ibid., Amendment 87, 55

157 Ibid., Amendment 161, 94.
158 The justification for such a provision was the following:

> So far, nanoparticles are often only produced in very low quantities. But given their major potential to create adverse biological effects, as a very minimum,

nanoparticles between 1 and 10 tonnes should be considered to be priority substances for which at least the whole base set information of Annex VII should be provided in the absence of nanoparticle-specific tests.

Ibid., Amendment 165, 97

159 Paolo Ponzano, Costanza Hermanin, and Daniela Corona, 'The Power of Initiative of the European Commission: A Progressive Erosion?' (*Notre Europe*, 2012) http://providus.lv/article_files/2324/original/Commission_Power_of_Initiative_NE_Feb2012_01.pdf?1355306495 accessed 01.03.2019.

160 Article 114 TFEU, previous Article 95 TEC.

161 For a broader discussion on chemicals as regulatory objects and the approaches of different regimes see Elisabeth Fisher, 'Chemicals as Regulatory Objects' (2014) 23 RECIEL 163, 167.

162 Fisher (n 161) 168 explains also that the American Toxic Substances Control Act takes another view on chemicals as regulatory objects, treating them as 'risky objects', where the EPA must meet a number of analytic requirements in terms of demonstration of unacceptable risk, before being able to regulate chemicals under the Toxic Substances Control Act (TSCA).

163 Lyria Bennett Moses, 'Recurring Dilemmas: The Law's Race to Keep Up with Technological Change' (2007) UNSW Law Research Paper 21/2007, 1.

164 As early as 2005, there was a clear indication from the SCENIHR that REACH parameters and triggers, at the time under negotiation by EU institution, were inappropriate for nano-chemicals and that a reconsideration was needed before the law was passed. See the Appendix on the REACH history of adoption.

165 Moses (n 163) 36.

166 Council Regulation (EC) 1333/2008 of the European Parliament and of the Council of 16 December 2008 on food additives [2008] OJ L354/16.

167 Friedrich Waismann, 'Verifiability' in Antony Flew (ed.) *Logic and Language, the First Series* (1951), available at: www.ditext.com/waismann/verifiability.html accessed 18.02.2019.

168 Frederick Schauer, 'On the Open Texture of Law' (2011) University of Virginia School of Law http://ssrn.com/abstract=1926855 accessed 18.02.2019.

169 Moses (n 163) 35.

170 Waismann (n 167).

171 Commission, 'Regulatory Aspects of Nanomaterials' (Communication) COM (2008) 366 final 4.

172 Commission, 'Second Regulatory Review on Nanomaterials' (Communication) COM (2012) 572 final 13.

173 Pål Wennerås, 'Towards an Ever Greener Union? Competence in the Field of the Environment and Beyond' (2008) 45 Common Market Law Review Environment 1645, 1669.

174 REACH, recital (1).

175 REACH, Article 128.

176 REACH, Article 129.

177 The Commission has taken the view that nano-chemicals are covered by the definition of substance in REACH and that therefore REACH's provisions apply. See: COM (2008) 366 final, 4; COM (2012) 572 final, 13.

178 REACH, Article 128.

179 On the hybrid nature of REACH see in general Hey, Jacob, and Volkery (n 97).

180 Joanne Scott, 'REACH: Combining Harmonization and Dynamism in the Regulation of Chemicals' in Joanne Scott (ed.), *Environmental Protection: European Law and Governance* (OUP 2009) 58.

181 Ibid.

182 Hey, Jacob, and Volkery (n 97) 1864.

183 Ibid.
184 Scott (n 180) 58.
185 Ibid. 68.
186 Ibid. 91.
187 Case C-341/95 *Bettati v Safety Hi-Tech* [1998] ECLI:EU:C:1998:353, para 47.
188 Case C-343/09 *Afton Chemical* [2010] ECLI:EU:C:2010:419, para 28.
189 Ibid. para 55.
190 Council Directive 2009/30/EC of 23 April 2009 amending Directive 98/70/EC as regards the specification of petrol, diesel and gas-oil and introducing a mechanism to monitor and reduce greenhouse gas emissions and amending Council Directive 1999/32/EC as regards the specification of fuel used by inland waterway vessels and repealing Directive 93/12/EEC [1999] OJ L 140/88.
191 *Afton* (n 188) para 56.
192 Lucas Bergkamp and Nicolas Herbatschek, 'Regulating Chemical Substances under REACH: The Choice between Authorization and Restriction and the Case of Dipolar Aprotic Solvents' (2014) 23 RECIEL 221, 221.
193 de Sadeleer 2014 (n 53) 160.
194 Scott (n 180) 68.
195 Ibid.
196 Ibid. 68–69.
197 See Nadia Kaddour, 'No Laws in Nanoland: How to Reverse the Trend? The French Example' (2013) 30 Pace Envtl. L. Rev. 486.
198 'Nanomaterials – the Current State of Play' (*CW*, October 2015) https://chemical watch.com/43068/nanomaterials-the-current-state-of-play accessed 22.02.2019.
199 'Guide to Completing the Form' (*Norwegian Environment Agency*, 12 February 2015) www.miljodirektoratet.no/en/Areas-of-activity1/Chemicals/The-Product-Register/Guide-to-Completing-the-Form/ accessed 22.02.2019.
200 Scott (n 180) 73.
201 Journal Officiel de la République Française, 'Arrêté du 6 août 2012 relatif au contenu et aux conditions de présentation de la declaration annuelle des substances à l'état nanoparticulaire, pris en application des articles R. 523–12 et R. 523–13 du code de l'environnement' (10 August 2012) www.legifrance.gouv.fr/affichTexte.do?cidTexte=JORFTEXT000026278450&categorieLien=id accessed 22.02.2019.
202 Commission, 'Order relating to the content and submission conditions of annual declarations of nanoparticle substances, adopted pursuant to Articles R. 523–12 and R. 523–13 of the Environment Code' 2011/673/F, available at http://ec.europa. eu/growth/tools-databases/tris/en/index.cfm/search/?trisaction=search.detail&year=2011&num=673&mLang=EN accessed 22.02.2019.
203 Jean-Philippe Montfort et al., 'Nanomaterials under REACH: Legal Aspects' (2010) 1 EJRR 51, 58.
204 It must be noted that the specific nano-amendments to the REACH Annexes, approved as this book was being finalised and coming into force in 2020, most likely will not, due to their nature and the location (in the Annexes) in REACH, automatically provide answers on issues of harmonisation or the coverage of nanosubstances under each stage of REACH.
205 Lee (n 18) 214.
206 Commission 'The Operating Framework for the European Regulatory Agencies' (Communication) COM (2002) 718 final, 11.
207 Tanja Ehnert, 'The European Chemicals Agency – Beyond the Scope of the Meroni Doctrine?' (University of Maastricht 2008) 13.
208 COM (2002) 718 final, 11.
209 Case 9–56 *Meroni v High Authority* [1958] ECLI:EU:C:1958:7 and Case 10–56 *Meroni v High Authority* [1958] ECLI:EU:C:1958:8.

210 Ehnert 2008 (n 207) 7.
211 Ibid. 67.
212 REACH, Article 76.
213 REACH, Article 77(g)–(h).
214 Such notice reads:

> This document contains guidance on REACH explaining the REACH obliga-
> tions and how to fulfil them. However, users are reminded that the text of the
> REACH Regulation is the only authentic legal reference and that the informa-
> tion in this document does not constitute legal advice. The European Chem-
> icals Agency does not accept any liability with regard to the contents of this
> document.

215 Lucas Bergkamp and DaeYoung Park, 'The Organizational and Administrative
     Structures' in Lucas Bergkamp (ed.) *The European Union REACH Regulation for
     Chemicals: Law and Practice* (OUP 2013) 28.
216 The GDs are accessible at: https://echa.europa.eu/guidance-documents/guidance-
     on-information-requirements-and-chemical-safety-assessment accessed 01.03.2019.
217 NAO/DEFRA, *Progress in Implementing EU Exit* (Report, HC 2017–2019, 1498) 11.
218 House of Commons, *Brexit and Chemicals Regulation (REACH)* (CBP 840,
     2018) 3.
219 'Will Brexit Mean Avoiding the Burden of REACH?' (*CW*, 2016) https://
     chemicalwatch.com/47567/will-brexit-mean-avoiding-the-burden-of-reach
     accessed 18.02.2019.
220 HM Government, *The Future Relationship between the United Kingdom and the
     European Union* (White Paper, Cm 9593, 2018) 8.
221 Ibid. 22.
222 Ibid. 8, emphasis added.
223 (CBP 840, 2018) 4.
224 Environmental Audit Committee, *The Future of Chemicals Regulation after the EU
     Referendum* (HC 2016–17, 912) para 12.
225 (CBP 840, 2018) 1.
226 Ibid. 19.
227 (HC 2016–17, 912) para. 13.
228 (Report, HC 2017–2019, 1498) 28.
229 Ibid. 24.
230 DEFRA, *Guidance Regulating Chemicals (REACH) if There's No Brexit Deal*
     (Updated 19 December 2018) available at: www.gov.uk/government/publications/
     regulating-chemicals-reach-if-theres-no-brexit-deal/regulating-chemicals-reach-if-
     theres-no-brexit-deal accessed 19.12.2018.
231 European Union Committee, *Brexit: Environment and Climate Change*, (HL
     2016–17, 109) para 21.
232 (CBP 840, 2018) 15.
233 (White Paper, Cm 9593, 2018) 22.
234 Ibid.
235 See Ahu Çekim, 'Overview of current Turkish legal framework for chemical
     control legislation. Including Turkey's classification and labelling regulation
     (SEA(CLP By-Law))', [PowerPoint Presentation, 2014] slide 3, available at:
     http://kimyasallar.csb.gov.tr/uploads/file/Presentation.pdf accessed 18.02.2019.
     Note: the acronyms refer to the names of regulations in Turkish, which have
     been translated when referring to them in full length.
236 KEK, Article 1.
237 'Turkish Chemical Substance Inventory' (ChemSafetyPRO 2016–01–26) www.
     chemsafetypro.com/Topics/Turkey/Turkish_Chemical_Substance_Inventory.
     html accessed 23.01.2019.

238 'Turkish Regulation on Registration, Evaluation, Authorisation and Restriction of Chemical Substances' (*Doruksistem*) www.doruksistem.com.tr/Default. asp?P=0&L=2&K=0&K1=136 accessed 18.02.2019.
239 KKDIK, Article 1.
240 'Introduction to Turkish KKDIK Regulation 2017' (*ChemSafetyPRO*, 2019–03–10) www.chemsafetypro.com/Topics/Turkey/Turkey_REACH_KKDIK_ regulation.html accessed 18.02.2019.
241 'Turkish Ministry Appoints New Head of Chemicals' (*CW*, 12 September 2018) https://chemicalwatch.com/70171/turkish-ministry-appoints-new-head-of-chemicals accessed 18.02.2019.
242 Selcuk Bilgin, 'TURKREACH (abbreviated as) KKDIK: The new Turkish by-law on registration, evaluation, authorization & restriction of chemicals', [PowerPoint Presentation, 2018] slide 42, available at: https://chemspain. org/wp-content/uploads/2018/01/2.-TURKREACH-Doruksistem.pdf accessed 19.02.2018.
243 Ibid., slide 53.
244 See Timur Erk and Caner Zanbak, 'Turkish Chemical Industry 2015–2016', (*Chemical News*, August 2016) 35 http://tksd.org.tr/doc/2016_TKSD_Indian_ Chemical_News.pdf accessed 18.02.2019.
245 Nertila Kuraj, 'REACHing across the Bosphorus. The transposition of the EU chemicals law reform into Turkish national legislation; fostering innovation, sustainability and high levels of protection for human health and the environment', [PowerPoint Presentation, Boğaziçi University, 2017], Boğaziçi University.
246 For a definition of the term, see David Vogel, 'Environmental Regulation and Economic Integration' (1999), Yale Center for Environmental Law and Policy October www.iatp.org/sites/default/files/Environmental_Regulation_and_ Economic_Integrat.pdf accessed 18.02.2019.
247 'Will Brexit Mean Avoiding the Burden of REACH?' (*CW*, 7 June 2018) https://chemicalwatch.com/47567/will-brexit-mean-avoiding-the-burden-of-reach accessed 23.01.2019.
248 See Céline Charveriat and Andrew Farmer, 'The Implications of Brexit for Future EU Environmental Law and Policy' (2017) (1) Elni Review, 11–16, www.elni.org/fileadmin/elni/dokumente/Archiv/2017/Heft_1/elni2017-1_ Charveriat-Farmer.pdf accessed 18.02.2019.
249 See Dennis Pamlin et al., *Twelve Risks that Threaten Human Civilisation: The Case for a New Risk Category* (Global Challenges Foundation 2015).

3   Registration

Introduction

Based on the principle that manufacturers, importers, and downstream users are to prove that chemicals placed on the market and used as such do not adversely affect human health and the environment, the REACH Regulation[1] sets up a system of four phases: Registration, Evaluation, Authorisation, and Restriction. Core elements of the legislation include: detailed technical and scientific provisions; re-thinking of the role of different actors along the entire supply chain of chemicals; and implementation of relevant environmental principles such as the precautionary principle,[2] the substitution principle,[3] and the (implied) polluter pays principle. The aim of the legislation is

> to ensure a high level of protection of human health and the environment, including the promotion of alternative methods for assessment of hazards of substances, as well as the free circulation of substances on the internal market while enhancing competitiveness and innovation.[4]

In contrast to the previous chemical law, the human and environmental protection aim precedes, in the text of Article 1(1), that of free circulation of chemicals and marked functioning. This subordination of aims is not only the result of the wording formulation Article 1 adopts, but has already been consolidated in early case law.[5] Regarding the primary law level, REACH's legal basis is constituted by Article 114 TFEU. Article 114(3)[6] calls upon the Commission to take as a base 'a high level of protection' when drafting a legislative proposal, which, pursuant to Article 114(1), concerns 'health, safety, environmental protection and consumer protection'.

Starting from this consideration and taking into account the position of the Commission that nanosubstances are covered in REACH by the general concept of 'substance'[7] and that REACH, overall, 'sets the best possible framework for the risk management of nanomaterials',[8] the present chapter embarks on an analysis of whether the concrete provisions of REACH truly provide the legal and conceptual elements in favour of such a claim. In other words, the ability of REACH to deliver high levels of human and environmental protection also for nanosize chemicals is questioned in an attempt to identify the drawbacks requiring revision and to eventually suggest how to improve the current framework. The necessary starting point of such analysis is what can be considered as the gateway to the REACH system, i.e. the Registration phase.

No data, no market

REACH registration deadlines and implications for nanosubstances

The 'no data, no market'[9] principle represents the backbone of the REACH framework. The general reversion of the onus of proof stated in Article 1(3) and based on the precautionary principle[10] that underpins REACH's provisions requires all substances, on their own, in articles, and in preparations, to be registered before being commercialised and placed in the EU market.[11] The rationale behind the registration requirement is that producers shall bear the responsibility (and the relative costs) of developing and providing scientific data supporting the safety of the chemicals they intend to put on the market.

This choice of REACH to subordinate the possibility of using and trading chemicals to the prior assessment of their safety, represents a shift forward in the producers' responsibility concept, new to the EU chemical policy. In addition, requiring producers to bear the costs of such an operation also represents an anticipation of the polluter pays principle at the very source of potential chemical pollution.

In its attempt to remedy the inconsistency of the previous EU chemical law, REACH foresees an obligation to register for both *new* and *existing* substances, produced or imported in quantities of 1 tonne or more per producer/importer per year (1 t/y).[12] However, REACH maintains a connection to the old classification, distinguishing, in terms of registration deadline, between *phase-in* and *non-phase-in chemicals*.

Phase-in substances encompass:

• the category of existing substances holding an EINECS[13] number;
• substances that have been manufactured in the EU (including the countries that joined on 1 January 2007) but have not been placed on the EU market after 1 June 1992;
• substances that qualify as no-longer polymers.[14]

As shown in Chapter 2, EINECS substances represent nearly 30,000 chemicals in use as a result of the grandfathering system of 1981, with little or no data on their environmental hazards. However, given the practical impossibility of assessing and registering this enormous quantity of substances at once, the REACH system foresees transitional measures that, based on the hazardous properties of a chemical and the volumes of production, seek to ensure a smooth and reasonably feasible registration transition under the REACH framework. According to Article 23 of REACH, the deadlines for registration were as follows:

- *30 November 2010*
  For phase-in substances that, according to Directive 67/548/EEC, are classified as:

  a   carcinogenic, mutagenic, or toxic to reproduction category (CMR) 1 and 2, produced/imported in quantities above 1 t/y;
  b   very toxic to aquatic organisms which may cause long-term adverse effects in the aquatic environment, produced/imported in quantities above 100 t/y.

- *31 May 2013*
  For phase-in substances produced/imported in quantities 100–1,000 t/y;
- *31 May 2018*
  For phase-in substances produced/imported in quantities 10–100 t/y.

In establishing such an approach, the EU legislature's intention seems to be that of 'alleviating' the burden of the past by prioritising for registration substances that, because of hazardous properties and/or high production volumes, might determine relevant exposure for humans and the environment. A general prerequisite for benefiting from transitional measures and time dilations was that of pre-registration of these categories by 1 December 2008, providing, when possible, the substances' EINECS and Chemical Abstracts Service (CAS) numbers.[15]

While transitional measures are pretty common in legislative practice, it can be argued that in the case of REACH, the extended deadlines for phase-in substances might in principle represent a loophole regarding registration of phase-in nano-chemicals. Given the current absence of a legal requirement to consider nanosubstances 'new for regulatory purposes', a producer/importer might have chosen to observe this timeline instead of registering *existing* nanosize chemicals right away. And yet, this eventuality would represent a best-case scenario, as the producer might be 'exempt' from registering a nanosubstance at all due to a lack of legal norms within REACH that would explicitly impose enforceable duties for a separate identification and registration of nanosize substances. Until the nano-specific amendments to the Annexes come into force in 2020, this situation is likely to persist.

By exclusion, the *non-phase-in* category of substances encompasses those chemicals not produced and used in the EU prior to 1 June 2008, unless they have been notified in accordance with Directive 67/548/EEC. These are considered *new* substances and have to comply with REACH from the very first stage of their production/importation and prior to commercialisation.[16] As a matter of course, phase-in substances for which the producer/importer failed to comply with the pre-registration requirements cannot benefit from the transitional deadlines and consequently must be registered forthwith.

Conversely, substances notified under Directive 67/548/EEC and listed in the European List of Notified Chemical Substances (ELINCS) are deemed registered under REACH. The almost automatic transposition of the registered status of chemicals that were considered *new* according to the system operated in 1981 may well conceal chemicals in nanoform holding an ELINCS number. No provision under Directive 67/548/EEC refers to the shape and scale of chemicals.[17] Thus, it is possible for nanosize chemicals to have entered REACH without a proper assessment based on their nanoscale properties and without the legislator being aware of the nanoscale.

These preliminary observations on nanosubstances under REACH only begin to scratch the surface of what this book refers to as the '*burden of the very small*', i.e. the inability of the current REACH framework to properly and exhaustively deal with nanosize chemicals. We argue that there are two main legislative and conceptual shortcomings that prevent ensuring a high level of environmental and human health protection for nanosubstances: the definition of substance and the incremental tonnage mechanism. These are objectionable already at the very first phase of REACH (Registration). In the following part, the importance of such elements in general and their relevance for nanosize chemicals in particular is discussed. Further, this book advances the claim that the REACH Annexes now modified so as to contain nano-specific provisions notwithstanding, such loopholes are likely to remain problematic as long as the legal text of REACH, and in particular the definition of 'substance' therein, remains nano-silent.

The centrality of the 'substance' definition under REACH and its ability to cover nanosubstances

The entire REACH framework is built on the concept and definition of 'substance' as its provisions apply to the manufacture, placing on the market or use of such chemical substances on their own, in preparations, or in articles.[18] Hence, determining what categories are encompassed under this definition identifies which chemicals are and are not subject to the legal requirements of REACH. Article 3(1) defines 'substance' as

> a chemical element and its compounds in the natural state or obtained by any manufacturing process, including any additive necessary to preserve its stability and any impurity deriving from the process used, but excluding any solvent which may be separated without affecting the stability of the substance or changing its composition.

In order to ensure effective management of different aspects[19] of REACH on a Community level, the European Chemicals Agency (ECHA) was established by REACH. Although the wording of Article 75[20] of REACH clearly invests the ECHA with managerial tasks, that same wording does not prevent the ECHA from exercising regulatory powers with binding effects on third parties.[21] Overall, the ECHA's task is to provide 'the best possible scientific and technical advice on questions relating to chemicals'.[22] In this regard, the guidance documents (GDs) prepared by the ECHA pursuant to Article 76(1) (g) of REACH are of particular interest for the clarification and interpretation of REACH's provisions and the technical requirements therein. Are these documents of any assistance in identifying nano-chemicals? While the structure and the main tasks of the ECHA were elucidated in Chapter 2, the remaining part of the current chapter engages with the detailed obligations imposed by the REACH text and the pertinent ECHA GDs, and their applicability for *substances* in nanoscale.

Substances on their own

A key GD is that on substance identification, which sets forth criteria for identifying chemicals subject to REACH's rule of law. According to the ECHA, 'to ensure that the REACH processes are working properly, correct and unambiguous substance identification is essential'.[23] Hence, it is crucial to question the suitability of the criteria that REACH indicates (and the ECHA clarifies) for identifying chemicals in general, and also for nanosubstances specifically.

Generally, substance identification is dealt with in Section 2, Annex VI of REACH. In case the substance holds a European and/or international identification,[24] the number/name/code shall be stated in the registration dossier.[25] In addition, other physical and chemical characterisers shall be provided when registering a substance. The ECHA GD on substance identification specifies that the following information is to be provided:

- Information related to the molecular and structural formula of each substance such as:

    - molecular and structural formula;
    - information on optical activity and typical ratio of (stereo) isomer;
    - molecular weight or molecular weight range.[26]

- Composition of each substance such as

    - degree of purity (%);
    - nature and degree of impurities;
    - spectral data (ultra-violet, infra-red, nuclear magnetic resonance, or mass spectrum);
    - description of the analytical methods or the appropriate bibliographical references for the identification of the substance and, where appropriate, for the identification of impurities and additives.[27]

These criteria mirror those specified in REACH's Annex VI – Sections 2.1, 2.2, 2.3. The ECHA requires substance identification to be based on a combination of the above-mentioned parameters.[28] But while some parameters, like a CAS or IUPAC number might be relatively easy to identify, others, like the chemical composition for instance, might require further consideration.

Indeed, the ECHA establishes a main distinction between 'well-defined substances', whose composition might be identified qualitatively and quantitatively according to the criteria endorsed in Section 2 of Annex VI of REACH, and 'substances of Unknown or Variable composition, Complex reaction products, and Biological materials (UVCB)', the variability of which is large and/or poorly predictable.[29] Well-defined substances can be divided into two further subcategories: *mono-constituent*[30] and *multi-constituent*[31] substances.

Although it is beyond the scope of this book to provide a full and complete analysis of the chemical specificities and the relative scientific debate, it is important to notice how the definition of mono- and multi-constituent chemicals is mass-related given that the determination of the 'chemical composition' is based on the mass-fraction concept and expressed as the ratio of a chemical constituent to the mass of the total substance, i.e. weight by weight (w/w). In other words, the 'abundance' of an element within a chemical formulation is determined by its weight within that formulation. The ECHA's guidance explains further that, beside the main constituent(s) a chemical substance may be composed of impurities and additives. Logically, mono-constituent substances have one main constituent (as a 'rule of thumb' this shall be present in quantities ≥ 80 per cent (w/w)) while the multi-constituent substances have several main constituents (present in the substance in a concentration ≥ 10 per cent (w/w) and < 80 per cent (w/w)).[32] Impurities present in the chemical substance should be indicated in the registration dossier. Hazardous impurities might also impact the classification of the substance under the Classification, Labelling, and Packaging Regulation (CLP) and, as a consequence, must be reported in the safety data sheets (SDSs).[33]

A question then naturally arises: are these specific parameters capable of capturing nano-chemicals? Given that nanomaterials are not explicitly tackled within the REACH legal norms (and when the currently approved Annex modifications come into force in 2020, only certain Annexes will be equipped with nano-specific provisions), to what extent (if at all) do the ECHA specificities enable a successful registration of nanosize chemicals?

As already mentioned, in 2008 the Commission stated that nanosubstances fall within the definition of 'substances' and are therefore covered (in principle) by REACH.[34] The Parliament, in a Resolution in 2009, called for explicitly labelling nanomaterials *new* chemicals under REACH.[35] From the Parliament's point of view, parameters such as size, solubility/persistence, and other specific and new intrinsic properties arising from the nanoscale represent some of the most important characterisers for identifying risks posed by nanomaterials. As a result, the resolution called for:

> the introduction of a comprehensive science-based definition of nanomaterials in Community legislation as part of nano-specific amendments to relevant horizontal and sectoral legislation.[36]

The Parliament also solicited the Commission to promote the adoption of a harmonised definition of the term *nanomaterial* on an international level and update the European one accordingly.[37] On these premises, in 2011 the Commission endorsed a Recommendation on the definition of the term nanomaterial.[38] The aim of such a document is, in the Commission's words, to provide a definition of 'nanomaterial' which can be used for legislative and policy purposes within the EU.[39]

Based on the Scientific Committee on Emerging and Newly Identified Health Risks (SCENIHR),[40] Joint Research Centre (JRC),[41] and International Organization for Standardization (ISO)[42] previous definitions, the Commission adopted the following formulation:

> 'Nanomaterial' means a natural, incidental or manufactured material containing particles, in an unbound state or as an aggregate or as an agglomerate and where, for 50% or more of the particles in the number size distribution, one or more external dimensions is in the size range 1 nm–100 nm.[43]

This far-reaching definition embraces not only manufactured nanomaterials, intentionally created as such, but also nanosize materials that occur as a result of natural processes or as by-products of industrial activities. According to this definition, certain categories of nanomaterials such as fullerenes, graphene flakes, and single-walled carbon nanotubes (SWCNTs) shall be considered nanomaterials even when they have one external dimension below 1 nm.[44] The derogation from the general formulation appears to relate to the intrinsic hazardous properties of these carbon-based nanomaterials. SWCNTs, for example, have been proved to cause asbestos-like pathogenicity in lung tissues.[45] Hence, the implication would be that these materials should be treated as nanomaterials, not only based on size-related considerations but also other size-dependent factors, such as toxicity and dangerousness. In this case, the lower-limit of 1 nm in size can be derogated because of the known dangerousness of the nanoform. Indeed, the acknowledged toxicity of certain carbon-based nanoparticles led the Commission to modify the status of carbon and graphite within REACH. Pursuant to Article 2(7)(a), substances listed in Annex IV shall be exempted from Title II (Registration)[46] on the premise that for those substances, sufficient available information shows a minimum risk related to their intrinsic properties. However, Article 138(4) of REACH required the Commission to carry out a review of Annex IV by June 2008. As the result of such a review, the Commission adopted a Regulation amending Annex XIV by removing carbon and graphite from the Annex: 'due to the fact that the concerned Einecs and/or CAS numbers are used to identify forms of carbon or graphite at the nano-scale, which do not meet the criteria for inclusion in this Annex'.[47]

In the Commission's view, too little is known about these substances to maintain that they pose a minimum risk and are, therefore, subject to the

Annex XIV exemptions. The Commission did not have to prove the risk of such substances, but in the light of uncertainty and lack of information opted for a precautionary approach, subjecting them to Registration duties and further REACH provisions. Articles 131 and 133(4) of REACH indicate, in Article 5a(1) to (4) and Article 7 of Decision 1999/468/EC, the procedures through which such an amendment is carried out. The consequence is that today, carbon and graphite in nano-scale must be registered.

In 2018, as this book was being finalised, the first registration of SWCNTs was successfully submitted to the ECHA. The registration dossier[48] in question concerns TUBALL single-wall carbon nanotubes produced and commercialised in Europe by the Luxembourg-based OCSiAl in quantities of 10 t/y, and was the fruit of a collaboration between OCSiAl, UK research firm Envigo, and the Intertek Pittsfield.[49] Note that no chemical safety assessment was performed due to the tonnage band of production but OCSiAl states that in the coming years it might increase its volumes of production to 60 t/y, a quantity that would trigger the duty to perform a chemical safety assessment (CSA). Although the registration in question concluded that there is no risk to aquatic toxicity, the methods used to reach that conclusion are being questioned since they contrast with recent scientific studies on the same point.[50] It remains to be seen how this dossier will impact the fate of carbon nanotubes in REACH. It certainly represents a first step from industry in the direction of trying to bring nanoscale chemicals under the REACH framework. Note that the toxicity of multi-walled carbon nanotubes (MWCNTs) has also been observed[51] and MWCNTs are currently on the Community Rolling Action Plan (CoRAP) for evaluation by Germany, expected in 2019 (see Chapter 5).

Further, in its 2011 Recommendation, the Commission's definition refers also to *aggregates* and *agglomerates* as possible expressions of nanomaterials, which may exhibit the same behaviour of unbound substances. Therefore, in case the constituents of such chemical bounds are in the range of 1–100 nm, aggregates and agglomerates should fall under the definition of nanomaterial, in spite of the fact that their compressive size may exceed the upper limit of 100 nm.[52] Although it is the agglomerate/aggregate size that is usually responsible for the diffusion and transportation fate,[53] it is possible that from the life-cycle perspective, smaller nanoparticles might be released from the compound.[54] Taking into account this eventuality, the Commission, not without a note of precaution, opts for the inclusion of 'larger' forms of nanomaterials expressed in aggregates and agglomerates, in the definition of nanomaterial.

The last part of the definition suggests that 'when technically possible and requested by specific legislation', the *volume-specific surface area or VSSA* (which should be greater than $60 \, m^2/cm^3$) parameter, *in addition to size* and *number size distribution*, can be used in defining a nanomaterial. However, the size and number-size-distribution can still define a nanomaterial even though its specific surface area by volume might be smaller than $60 \, m^2/cm^3$.[55]

Hence, in addition to size, the core element of the definition in question is the number–size–distribution threshold.[56]

A general revision of the definition was set for December 2014, and the Commission stated that the review should be primarily focused on the number–size–distribution criteria threshold of 50 per cent and decide whether to increase or decrease it.[57] As mentioned in Chapter 1, said revision is currently ongoing. Although the Commission claims that no major modifications are to be made to the general definition of the term 'nanomaterial' contained in the Recommendation, disagreement has emerged with regard to the use of the VSSA parameter thereof. The VSSA criterion has been categorised as 'overprotective' by a recent study which holds that the use of such parameter 'identifies more nanomaterials than in reality'.[58] However, the JRC defended the criterion, pointing out the flawed methodology used in the study by André J. Lecloux et al. and reaffirming that, as substantiated in its 2015 Report, the opposite is in fact true: a VSSA of over $60\,m^2/cm^3$ indicates a nanomaterial but a lower value does not lead to the classification as a non-nanomaterial. In fact, in certain cases the JRC noticed, the VSSA might even be more reliable than other parameters in identifying nanomaterials.[59] However, the JRC specifies, the VSSA should be used together with the other screening methods but not as the sole identifier of the nanoform.[60] Beyond the outcome on this point, the other point of concern regarding definition, is that the revision in question is yet to be adopted, meaning that it was not approved in time for the last REACH registration deadline, which was 31 May 2018. Any nano-registration dossiers submitted by this deadline would have used a definition that will soon become outdated.

Another point to be considered on the definition of nanomaterials, concerns the non-binding nature of the Recommendation, which does not oblige regulators to observe the exact formulation endorsed by the Commission. In fact, the Recommendation itself allows for derogations and adaptations of the definition it endorsed in line with specific aims and purposes of sectoral legislation. By way of example, the definition contained in Regulation (EU) No. 1169/2011 on the provision of food information to consumers overall reflects some of the elements indicated in the Commission's Recommendation above. However, such Regulation contemplates only 'engineered' nanomaterials (ENMs), introducing the element of 'intentionality' of the nanoscale, given that ENMs are 'created' as such. In addition, size consideration is based on a '100 nm or less' criteria, while Recommendation 2011/696/EU establishes a size range between 1 and 100 nm, derogating to the lower limit of 1 nm only for some carbon-based nanosubstances.

Another example in this direction is represented by the EU cosmetics Regulation.[61] For the purpose of the Regulation, 'nanomaterial' means:

> an insoluble or biopersistent and intentionally manufactured material with one or more external dimensions, or an internal structure, on the scale from 1 to 100 nm.[62]

The different parameters underlined here can be attributed to the fact that the Regulation text was adopted before the Recommendation. The inclusion of the need for the nanomaterials to be of a specific hazard (biopersistent) and of intentional nature in order to trigger the application of the cosmetics Regulation in question seems questionable from an environmental and human health perspective. Very little is known in general about the nature of nano-chemicals, and limiting the new set of rules to a very small portion of the entire category, i.e. nanomaterials manufactured as such, means placing the burden for regulating other nano-chemicals – which may not be biopersistent or intentionally produced, but might nonetheless pose significant risks – entirely on the authorities. However, the cosmetics Regulation contains a specific clause which requires the Commission to update the definition of the term 'nanomaterial', in line with possible scientific and technical progress and having regard for potential internationally agreed definitions.[63]

It is clear that the legal debate on definition is a crucial one, since the way a definition is formulated determines the object of a regulation, tracing a line between what is legal and what is not. Definitions are also essential to the principle of legal certainty. However, how legislators tackle the issue of definition depends on a range of legal, political, and scientific considerations and policy choices. Nanomaterials and the scientific uncertainty surrounding their nature and effects on human and environmental health pose a considerable challenge for legislators. In this regard, the American Food and Drug Administration (FDA) recommended in 2007 'not to adopt' a fixed and detailed definition,[64] whereas the EU legislator has constantly engaged in the process of definition that culminated in the 2011 Recommendation and its ongoing revision mentioned above. Such definition relies considerably on different scientific opinions prepared by SCENIHR and European Food Safety Authority (EFSA).[65] The nature of the definition of 'nanomaterial' endorsed in such documents has been labelled policy-driven rather than scientifically and evidence-based. In this direction, influential commentators like Andrew D. Maynard have questioned the scientific soundness of the 2010 SCENIHR's opinion outcomes on the definition of the term 'nanomaterial'.[66] Maynard argues that 'no-one it seems is prepared to challenge the base-assumption that a regulatory definition of nanomaterials is needed'.[67] Rather than focusing on definition, Maynard suggests identifying other factors that would permit decisions on nanomaterials to be taken 'on a science-based approach that links dose to response'.[68] As we shall see, in Chapter 7, this suggestion remains at the core of the current debate on nano-risk regulation. In a recent article Maynard et al. adopt the view that, instead of a clear-cut definition, three principles might be best employed for identifying risk associated with current nanomaterials and future sophisticated materials: *the emergent risk, the plausibility of such a risk, and the impact of it.*[69] The suggested identifying criteria of *plausibility and impact of emergent risk* would however need to rely on the recognition of the status of nano-chemicals as 'new material', and that is not currently the case. One plausible option for operationalising such criteria would be the use of the precautionary principle which can enable regulators to take action in the face of uncertain risk.[70]

While initial legal norms on definition might suffer the shortcomings deriving from a limited understanding of the specific physicochemical properties emerging at nanoscale and a constant need to be updated in accordance with rapid scientific developments in nanotoxicology, the necessity of addressing in a timely manner the environmental and health concerns posed by these unique intrinsic properties emerging in nanoscale, urges legal action. Although the Commission indicates that legal intervention can range from legally binding norms to research project and recommendation,[71] this book argues that the introduction of a clear status of nanosubstances as 'new for regulatory purposes' is necessary and should be embodied in legal provisions. More so, in the case of REACH, conceptualised and enacted as an overarching legislative platform, the introduction of a legally valid definition is essential. The current definition of substance endorsed by REACH[72] lacks any reference to *size, number-size distribution,* or *surface area by volume.*

This lacuna is likely to be remedied, albeit only partially, by the inclusion of a nano-definition in the amended Annex VI (a) to REACH together with a set of nano-specific requirements to be provided for the characterisation of the 'nanoform'. Starting from 2020, *particle number size distribution* with the indication of the number fraction of constituent particles in the size range 1–100 nm; description of *surface functionalisation* or *treatment;* shape, aspect ratio, and other *morphological characterisation;* and importantly, *surface area, either as VSSA or as specific surface area by mass, or both* will have to be provided for the nanoforms *covered by registration.*[73]

As to the definition of substance contained in the legal text of REACH, which will not be affected by the nano-specific changes in the Annexes, doubts remain as to its ability to cover nano-chemicals. Given that the definitions of 'main constituent', 'impurities', and 'additive' – themselves part of the definition of 'substance' – are to date size-neutral and mass-related (being expressed in w/w per cent), they fail as such to address the correlation between nano-properties and environmental and health hazards. As an example, scientific studies have already demonstrated in the case of nano silver that the coating of the surface area can either increase or decrease toxicity.[74] How would the coating be treated under REACH? As an impurity (hazardous) or additive? Can the nanosubstance formulated as such be considered a mixture?[75] The same questions can be raised for other categories of substances identified under REACH such as *intermediates*[76] and *catalysts.* In the light of these considerations, it can be concluded that the definition issue under REACH remains an open one.

Substances in articles

REACH's legal provisions apply also to chemical substances in articles, imposing upon producers a duty to register.[77] Considering that 'article' means nearly any product other than the chemical bulk substance – including electronics, textiles, furniture, and separate parts of unfinished products[78] – their regulation under REACH is of genuine environmental relevance, especially since certain categories of articles contribute significantly to diffuse pollution. In addition, nano-chemicals are being increasingly[79] applied to a wide array of consumers' products including batteries, automotive components, electronics and computers, children's toys, clothing, sporting goods, cosmetics, etc.[80] Hence, the legal status of nanomaterials under REACH inevitably affects the legal requirements that would apply to nano-enriched products categorised as 'articles' in accordance with the provision laid down in Article 3(2) of REACH and further elaborated by the specific ECHA GDs on this point.[81]

According to Article 7 of REACH, a producer/importer shall register chemicals contained in articles if a substance is present in those articles in quantities totalling more than 1 t/y per producer/importer *and* if such substance is 'intended to be released under normal and foreseeable conditions of use'. A preliminary observation here is that the 1 t/y minimum threshold, though capable of potentially capturing high-volume produced nanosubstances, is unlikely to cover other nanomaterials that are being manufactured in smaller quantities and incorporated in consumers' goods.[82]

Additionally, in case a substance present in articles in concentrations greater than 0.1 per cent (w/w) belongs to the Candidate List for Authorisation, it shall be *notified* to the ECHA, unless the producer/importer can exclude human and environment exposure under normal or reasonably foreseeable conditions of use, including the disposal phase.[83] However, given the hazardous nature of the substance in question, Article 33(1) of REACH requires suppliers of articles to provide 'recipients' of such articles with information on the safety uses of the article, including disposal, and as a minimum, provide the name of the substance. Nevertheless, contrary to what would seem logical, the term 'recipient' does *not* include the ordinary consumer. The ECHA specifies[84] that the term refers only to industrial and professional users. Consumers can separately file a request in order to obtain from the supplier the same information that is provided by default to industrial recipients, with the name of the substance as a minimum requirement.

Considering that the provisions of Article 33 apply regardless of the quantity produced, they could be in principle applicable to smaller quantities of nanosubstances classified as SVHCs. However, these provisions suffer a number of limitations such as the 0.1 per cent (w/w) threshold and the impossibility for consumers to obtain information on the presence of such substances in articles without an explicit request. The necessity for the consumers' activation in this case becomes particularly burdensome in the eventuality of nanosubstances of very high concern present in articles under the conditions referred to in Article 33(2). Given that consumers' awareness on nanotechnology remains low,[85] it is hard to imagine an extensive exercising of the right to know enshrined in Article 33(2). What is more, the reference to the 0.1 per cent threshold in Article 7(2)(b) has led to different and conflicting interpretations between Member States (MSs), which in turn might lead to different views on the duty to inform, according to Article 33. Controversies on interpretation emerge with regard to complex articles, which contain several components, each of them satisfying the 'article' definition in REACH. Should the threshold refer to each component as such, or to the finished final article? The ECHA initially suggests a calculation of the threshold on the article as such, and not with regard to the concentration in each component of the article.[86] Hence, in case of a garment, for example a coat, containing different decoration elements and buttons, the SVHCs contained in a plastic button would have needed to be calculated in relation to the entire mass of the coat. However, settled case law indicates that guiding documents cannot establish binding interpretation of EU law.[87] And the perspective changes completely, if, as some MSs with dissenting views suggested, each component of the garment is independently considered an article in the sense of REACH. In this last case, it would be much easier for the SVHCs used in a button to reach the 0.1 per cent w/w threshold, if the base for such computation is the button weight. Germany, France, Austria, Belgium, Sweden, Denmark, and Norway held that there was no legal basis in REACH (especially in Article 3, where the definition of 'article' is laid down) to suggest that: 'an article will "cease to be an article" when it is joined together with other articles to form a larger more complex article'.[88]

With the motto '*Once an Article, always an Article*', these MSs held that both complex articles and parts of articles independently satisfy the REACH definition of 'article'. Therefore, both the coat as such and the single elements therein, i.e. the plastic button, have to comply with Article 33 notification requirements, in case SVHCs are used in producing them. Obviously, the interpretation of 'article' and the obligation to inform are crucial to the free movement of goods in the EU market because different interpretations might result in different legal regimes for articles containing SVHCs.

The case brought before the Court concerned a preliminary ruling by the French Conseil d'État, and it concerned the interpretation of Articles 7(2) and 33 of REACH.[89] The referred question asked:

> Where an 'article' within the meaning of [the REACH Regulation] is composed of several elements which themselves meet the definition of 'article' given by the regulation, are the obligations resulting from Article 7(2) and Article 33 of the regulation to apply only with regard to the assembled article or with regard to each of the elements which meets the definition of 'article'?[90]

In its Opinion, the Advocate General (AG) took the view that a component of an article does not cease to be an article once it is integrated into a bigger, complex article but rather, as Norway and Belgium held on the basis of Article 2(2) of REACH, an article is no longer considered as such, only when it becomes waste for the purpose of EU law.[91] Put it differently, only when an article loses those features that define it as such under REACH – shape, surface, or design which determines its function to a greater degree than does its chemical composition – does it cease to be considered an article for REACH purposes.[92] The AG held thus that when calculating the threshold, the component article rather than the entire complex one should be taken as the base for such calculation.[93] The Court, disregarding the position of the Commission and the ECHA's technical guidance on the subject, aligned its interpretation with that of the five MSs and ruled that the 0.1 per cent w/w threshold must be calculated in relation to each component of the complex article. Also, following the AG Opinion on this point, the Court ruled that the duty to notify of the presence of SVHCs in articles pursuant to Article 7(2) of REACH, applies to both producers and importers. However, in the case of *composed articles*, the duty to notify covers only those articles that the *producer* has herself made or assembled. If the article is manufactured by a third party, the duty to notify does not apply for the producer that uses it as an input in a composed article. Nonetheless, the third party is subject to the notification duty for the article it makes or assembles.[94] The importer of the composed article, on the other hand, should be considered also the importer of the component articles and comply with the notification obligation accordingly. As the AG noted in her Opinion, the obligation to notify to ECHA the presence of SVHCs in articles stems directly from the objective of a high level of protection that REACH pursues. There is a need to close the information gap on such substances in order to address the significant risks they represent. In this, the obligation to register is in line with the spirit of the PP concerning the part about burdening the risk-creating entities, i.e. producers/importers.

However, neither the AG not the Court made any considerations on the fact that, because of their hazardous properties and deleterious effects for human health and the environment, the use of SVHCs should be limited to the greatest extent possible. Therefore, the 1 per cent rule might be in the future challenged for its effectiveness in ensuring high levels of protection from risks of complex chemicals like endocrine disrupting chemicals (EDCs) or nanoscale chemicals, for which mass is not the right dose identifier.

The outcome of this case is nonetheless a positive development concerning the risks of SVHCs in articles, especially in light of the aim to protect consumers and the right to know pursuant to Article 169(1) TFEU and Article 38 of the Charter of Fundamental Rights of the European Union (CFREU).[95] The right of consumers to know is also consecrated in the REACH preamble (recitals 56 and 117), and the transparency in the supply chain that REACH enables is thought to constitute one of the new regulatory tools of REACH.[96] In addition, the new ECHA GD on substances in articles now states that the concentration threshold limit 'applies to each article of an object made up of more than one article, which were joined or assembled together (complex objects)'.[97] Yet the mass-related 0.1 per cent w/w threshold remains deeply problematic for the case of potential nano-SVHCs used in articles.

It can be concluded that the definition of substance (both on its own and in articles and preparation) as articulated in the current legal text of REACH, does not reflect the physicochemical properties that render nano-chemicals different from their macro-scale counterparts. Indeed, according to authoritative scientific bodies, these very properties, responsible for the environmental fate and the health implications of such substances, represent better identifiers than mass-related criteria, currently employed for registration (among others) purposes under REACH.[98] It can therefore be argued that the current normative provisions, triggering registration obligations, do not reflect the real nature of nanosubstances, rendering their status under REACH rather uncertain. This assumption seriously undermines the ability of the legal framework of REACH, to which registration represents the 'access point' to ensure the declared aim of high level of human and environmental protection, also for this category of substances.

The paramount procedural and legal importance of the registration phase was clearly stated in the first case law on REACH brought before the CJEU. A reference for a preliminary ruling on the interpretation and validity of Article 6(3) of REACH was made in the course of proceedings between different companies operating in the chemical sector and polymers production,[99] and the Secretary of State for the Environment, Food, and Rural Affairs in front of the English High Court. Article 2(9) of REACH exempts polymers from the requirements of Title II and Title VI of REACH, with the consequence that registration requirements and evaluation procedures do not apply for this category of substances. However, by virtue of Article 6(3), monomers and other substances composing the polymer must be registered when certain concentrations and weight thresholds are met.[100] REACH establishes that 'a 'monomer unit' means the reacted form of a monomer substance in a polymer.[101] However, Article 6(3) refers generally to monomers without defining them as 'reacting'. The claimant companies' argument was that if the interpretation of 'polymer' referred to in Article 6(3) was also to encompass reacted monomers, it would make no sense to require such monomers (but not the polymers they form) to be registered because, once monomers have reacted in polymerisation, the final polymers are generally stable and safe.[102] Hence, the CJEU was requested to rule on Article 6(3) of REACH under a threefold profile: with regard to the *clarification of the term monomer*, the *proportionality* of the requirement to register monomers in relation to the objective of protecting human health and the environment and the *principle of equal treatment* given the obligation to register monomers also for importers.[103]

The Court ruled that the concept of monomer in Article 6(3) 'relates only to *reacted monomers* which are incorporated in polymers'[104] and that the duty on both producer and importers to register such substances does not infringe on the principle of equal treatment (and is, thus, not invalid on these grounds) because 'the obligation to register is identical for Community manufacturers and for importers'.[105] It is interesting to point out that when ruling on such matters, the Court stated that Article 6 'sets out a general principle of registration, not of exemption'.[106] The implication on the legal plan would be that all chemical substances produced/imported in quantities above 1 t/y must be registered under REACH, unless subject to specific and expressed exemption. Hence, it would appear that the global obligation to register derived from the interpretation of Article 6, would also apply for nano-chemicals. However, as shown earlier in this section, the technicalities involved in the case of nano-substances seem to subordinate their effective registration to an amendment of the legal text of REACH *and* the pertinent Annexes. However, the modification of the sole Annexes is likely to allow many of the above problems to linger as long as the legal text of REACH is not in turn rendered nano-specific.

Relevant to the fate of nanosubstances is also what the Court held on the principle of proportionality. Although the Court avoided expressing an opinion on the justification, under the scientific profile, of the choice operated by REACH to register monomers (but not polymers), the Court stated that the exemption to register polymers is a temporary exemption, in accordance with the previsions laid down in Article 138(2) and Recital 41 of REACH. However, such provisions maintain the right for the Commission to enact specific legislation for polymer registration, once effective methods are in place.[107] Until then, the duty to register monomers 'satisfies the *precautionary principle* as referred to in Article 3(1) of REACH'.[108] As a consequence of this ruling, the status of precautionary principle is, for the first time, consolidated in the CJEU case law regarding REACH as a principle that can determine and guide the legislator's choice to act (register monomers) or not to act (exempt polymers) until scientific progress enabling better legislative provisions takes place.

Against this background, it could be argued that a universal registration duty stemming from the text of Article 6, together with a precautionary approach in presence of scientific uncertainty, could constitute the legal grounds for the delineation of a general obligation to register nano-chemicals. And yet, contrary to what can be observed for monomers, the general silence of REACH's legal provision on nanosize substance contributes to a sort of legal leeway for this category of chemicals.

Regarding the scope of REACH, the CJEU also stated in its judgment that

> the Community legislature established, as *the main purpose* of the obligation *to register* laid down in Article 6(3) thereof, the first of those three objectives [ensure a high level of human health and environmental protection; ensure the free circulation of substances in the internal market; enhance competitiveness and innovation], namely to ensure a high level of protection of human health and the environment.[109]

For the first time[110] since the entry into force of REACH, the priority of the objective of protection of human health and environment (over the free circulation of substances on the internal market) is consolidated with regard to Registration. Interestingly, the Court, recalling Recital 19 of REACH[111] noted that

> the means by which to achieve such an objective is … the registration obligation imposed on producers and importers.[112]

Registration is hence the quintessence of REACH not only because once initiated, it triggers the application of specific provision foreseen in the subsequent phases, but also because the existence of an obligation to register implies the fulfilment of complementary tasks that are of particular relevance from an environmental standpoint. The tasks in question include: the generation of data for registration purposes, the preliminary assessment of risks based on such data, and the indication of risk reduction/management measures. In line with the precautionary principle, it is for industry to provide such data. In the present moment of scientific uncertainty and overall data paucity on nano-chemicals, registration would foster data generation and precautionary ruling over nanosubstances.

Despite the holding of the Court – that Article 6 of REACH establishes a universal duty to register substances, either on their own or in articles and preparation, and the holding of the Commission – that nanosubstances fall within the general concept of 'substance,' the legal status of nanosubstances in REACH remains uncertain. The major hurdle to Registration remains the lack of an explicit mention of chemicals in nanoscale in REACH, defined after those very special properties that relate to their toxicity for humans and the environment. In addition, the lack of acknowledgement of their status as 'new for regulatory and legal purposes' represents an important shortcoming.[113] At least until the amended REACH Annexes become applicable to registrants of nanosubstances (early 2020), the registration of nano-chemicals relies heavily (if not completely) on producers' discretion.

In the last version of the guidance on substance identification, the ECHA concluded that

> The current developments in nano-technology and insights in related hazard effects may cause the need for additional information on size of the substances in the future. The *current state of development is not mature enough to include guidance on the identification of substances* in the nanoform in this guidance document.[114]

However, regardless of the legal fate of the definition of nanosubstances within REACH, another structural-conceptual element of REACH – the incremental tonnage bands – is of peculiar relevance for the legal status of nanosize chemicals. The next section demonstrates why the system of the tonnage bands through which REACH operates is problematic for nano-chemicals, representing thus a second major hindrance to their regulation in REACH, after that of substance definition.

The incremental tonnage system: is it effective in ensuring high levels of environmental protection?

Another pivotal element of REACH's policy and of its legal provision is the incremental tonnage system. The overall[115] idea is that greater volumes of production correspond to greater exposure for humans and the environment. Hence, greater volumes of production trigger greater data sets to be provided to the ECHA by producers and other actors along the supply chain.

Pursuant to Article 10 of REACH, producers of substances in quantities of at least 1 t/y must submit a *technical dossier* for registration purposes. Of particular relevance for the case of substances in nanoform, is the indication given in the GD applicable in this phase,[116] which states 'Under REACH, registrants are obliged to collect all relevant and available information on the intrinsic properties of a substance, regardless of the quantity manufactured or imported.' This would suggest the existence of a legal obligation for producers of nanosubstances to 'collect' and/or generate data on chemical substances' intrinsic physicochemical properties. However, despite the fact that GDs might bear some legal effects, such a provision is not contained in the main legal body of REACH. Also, its general and loose formulation can hardly suggest its enforcement for nanosubstances.

The actual legal obligations on data generation spring from Article 12 of REACH,[117] and in this case they are tonnage-dependent. In seeking to ensure a high level of environmental and human health protection, REACH adopts a stepwise approach; the set of data that must be provided increases with the increase of tonnage bands. Annexes VI to XI describe the information to be submitted for registration and evaluation purposes. Once a higher tonnage band is reached, the additional data foreseen in the next Annex must be provided.[118] The data submission process is articulated in the following steps:

- gather and share existing information;
- consider information needs;
- identify information gaps;
- generate new data propose testing strategies.[119]

According to this provision, producers of nanosubstances would be required to gather and share the information, and given the current difficulties in testing nano-chemicals, a joint submission pursuant to Articles 11 and 19 of REACH could help mitigating costs while defining better testing strategies. Pursuant to Article 10 of REACH and Annex VI, the technical dossier to be submitted for registration purposes should contain the following information:

- general registrant information on registrants such as contact, location, etc.;
- identification of the substance with reference to all the parameters analysed in detail above, such as any international or European identification number (e.g. EINECS, ELINCs, or CAS number), molecular weight, degree of purity, etc.;[120]

- information on the manufacture and uses of the substance;[121]
- classification and labelling;[122]
- guidance on the safe uses of the substance.[123]

The approved amendments pertaining to the Annex VI requirements include a reference to the nanoform specifying now that substances, as identified in Article 3(1), can occur in more than one form. The new provisions in the Annex stipulate that when the substance *being registered* is *also* manufactured or imported in nanoform, certain specific information related to the nanosize must be provided. To this end, nanoforms shall be characterised pursuant to the '*Guidance note on nanoforms*' to be included in Annex VI, and particularly in line with the new Section 2.4 thereof on the characterisation of nanoforms.[124]

Beside this general information, in REACH, the tonnage band determines the data the producer must generate and present to the ECHA, in accordance with the pertinent Annex:

- Annex VII requires the following data to be provided for substances produced in quantities <u>1–10 t/y</u>:[125]

  - Information on the physicochemical properties such as boiling point and density. Of note here is that size or other nano-relevant criteria such as a number-size distribution threshold are to date not contemplated;[126]
  - Toxicological information including skin irritation (*in vitro*) and skin corrosion, skin sensitisation, eye irritation, mutagenicity, and acute toxicity;[127]
  - Ecotoxicological information including aquatic toxicity, short-term toxicity on invertebrates, degradation, and ready biodegradability.[128]

Currently, the newly approved amendment to the text of Annex VII states that 'any relevant physicochemical, toxicological and ecotoxicological information shall include characterisation of the nanoform tested and test conditions'.[129] In line with such provision, specific references to the nanoform are included in some of the existing parameters and testing methodologies laid down in the Annex in question. For each of these categories, REACH foresees the possibility to adapt, omit, and replace the required information, stating the reasons for making such a choice.[130]

- Annex VIII sets forth the *additional* information to be provided for substances produced in volumes <u>10–100 t/y</u>:[131]

  - Toxicological information such as *in vivo* skin and eye irritation, *in vitro* gene mutation study in mammalian cells, acute dermal toxicity, reproductive toxicity, and toxicokinetics;
  - Ecotoxicological information such as short-term (or long-term if the producers consider it relevant to conduct such a test) toxicity testing in fish, degradation, fate, and behaviour in the environment.

It can be argued that some information like toxicokinetics,[132] environmental fate, and degradation would be particularly relevant for nanosubstances' coverage under REACH, considering that numerous authoritative opinions from SCENIHR and EFSA stress the crucial importance of parameters such as solubility/persistency and toxicokinetics in determining nanosubstances' risk.[133] In an ideal scenario, REACH would need to take into account such parameters; both legal provisions and GDs should emphasise nano-specific criteria since doing so would help to understand and, hence, efficiently define the object of regulation. Yet, the language of the Annexes has been so far silent on nano-specific properties and on tests and methodologies to be employed in order to obtain data on specific endpoints, relevant for the toxicological profiles of nanosubstances.[134] The same applies to the language of Article 12, from which the obligation to comply with the provision of the Annexes derives.

However, the approved amendments to Annexes VII and VIII include a specific reference to the nano-specific information to be provided in accordance with the testing methodologies and parameters put forth by the Annexes' sections thus far discussed. Many of these sections have been modified so as to explicitly include indications on how to perform a required test study when the substance is in nanoform.[135] Moreover, the waiving of certain studies to be performed for the scope of obtaining the necessary toxicity information (provided scientific justification for doing so is supplied) for specific endpoints, which represented considerable perplexities for nanosubstances, has now been also modified. According to the new subsections to Annex VIII–IX, certain characteristics that would justify waiving in the case of bulk substances cannot alone be used to justify waiving of a study required to be performed also for the nanoform. For instance, the new Section 9.1.1 in Annex VII stipulates that the *Short-term toxicity testing on invertebrates (preferred species Daphnia)* cannot be waived on the mere justification of insolubility for substances in nanoform.[136] Likewise, for the nanoform, high insolubility in water, the new Section 9.2.2 to Annex VIII states, cannot serve as a justification for waiving the *Abiotic* study that would normally not be required for substances which are readily biodegradable or highly insoluble in water.[137]

According to Article 12(1)(d) of REACH, Annex IX specifies information to be provided for substances produced in quantities <u>100–1,000 t/y</u>, which include the following:

- Information on the physicochemical intrinsic properties (e.g. stability in organic solvents), identification of relevant degradation products, viscosity, etc.;
- Toxicological information such as short-term repeated dose toxicity study (28 days), one species, male and female, sub-chronic toxicity study (90 days) and reproductive toxicity;
- Ecotoxicological information such as aquatic toxicity including short- and long-term toxicity on fish, bioaccumulation in aquatic species,

preferably fish, effects on terrestrial organisms such as invertebrates, micro-organisms, and plants (short-term).[138]

For this Annex too, the Draft Regulation foresees the introduction of specific requirements regarding the information to be provided for the nanoform of substances produced in these quantities. Importantly in this regard, further testing shall be considered by the registrant or *may be required by ECHA*, if there is an indication that nano-specific properties influence *hazard of* or *exposure* to those nanoforms.[139] Additional exceptions from and/or justifications for waiving the requirement for certain information are now put in place by the amending Draft Regulation in REACH's Annex IX.

Finally, pursuant to Article 12(1)(e), Annex X sets forth what can be considered the widest set of information foreseen under the REACH framework to be provided for substances produced in very high quantities, concretely ≥ 1,000 t/y:

- Toxicological information such as long-term repeated dose toxicity (if deemed necessary under certain conditions explained in column II of the Annex in question), developmental toxicity, two-generation reproductive toxicity and carcinogenicity;
- Ecotoxicological information, including long-term toxicity to terrestrial organisms, plants, sediment organisms, and long-term or reproductive toxicity on birds.[140]

Two considerations can be underlined here. Generally speaking, from an environmental and human health prospective, it is striking that certain data and testing, like long-term toxicity and carcinogenicity, are required only for substances of very high volume of production. Starting from 1990, the number of new substances reported each year was nearly 300.[141] Of these, only 0.6 per cent was being produced in volumes exceeding 1,000 t/y. About 30 per cent of new chemicals was being produced in quantities less than 1 t/y.[142] While under the pre-REACH chemical law, there was an obligation to at least notify this last category of substances (given the previous threshold of 10 kg/y), with the adoption of REACH, paradoxically, this great portion of chemicals will be left out of the new testing and regulatory regime – given the new minimum threshold of 1 t/y – and nano-chemicals make no exception.

In particular for nano-chemicals, the great scientific uncertainty on their nature and the intrinsic properties combined with an increasing scientific literature on the ability of certain nanoparticles to cause oxidative stress and DNA damage[143] would suggest a need for data on their carcinogenic properties. Eventually, only producers of nanosubstances of quantities greater or equal to 1,000 t/y would be required to submit data on carcinogenicity.

Annex X has also been amended to include nano-specific requirements with regard to the possibility of conducting long-term toxicity testing when certain conditions are met.[144]

Important and ground-breaking as they are, such new provisions and the specific requirements on the nanoform they put forth, apply for 'nanoforms covered by registration'.[145] Therefore the minimum volume of production of 1 t/y, which constitutes one of the major loopholes of REACH with respect to nanomaterials and other non-threshold chemicals (like EDCs), will remain. Even in light of the current approved amendments, this threshold will allow for a broad range of low-volume nanosubstances to go unregulated under REACH. Considering that the toxicity of nano-chemicals is correlated to their intrinsic properties that transcend mass-related exposure, low-volume chemicals would be likely to 'evade' the REACH framework for as long as the minimum threshold remained unchanged.

Concerning the studies to be conducted for each specific endpoint mentioned in the Annexes VI–XI, the ECHA has issued specific guidance documents (GDs).[146] The GDs describe information requirements under REACH with regard to substance properties, exposure, uses, chemical safety assessment, and risk management. In addition, they include specific testing methods that need to be employed by industry when complying with REACH requirements. Interestingly, although REACH is nano-neutral (and until 2020 this is the case for both its legal body of legal Articles and its Annexes), as a result of the RIP-oN projects,[147] since 2012, several GDs have an Appendix containing 'recommendations for nanomaterials', which set forth advice for producers of nanomaterials on how to comply with the data and testing requirements for each specific endpoint foreseen in Annexes VI–XI in the case of nanoscale substances. Of note here is also the fact that the ECHA has recently adopted a number of *new* nano-specific Appendixes to some of its GDs and/or *updated* some of the existing ones. The ECHA states that the updates will help registrants meet the specific information requirements for the nanoform, as required by the approved amendments to the REACH Annexes.[148] The role of such GDs' Appendixes and their limitations are further analysed in Chapter 7.

Summing up

As this chapter showed, the whole architecture of REACH rests on two key elements – the concept of substance as defined by Article 3 of REACH, and minimum threshold of 1 t/y of production or import of substances thus defined – in order for the rules and obligations of the complex REACH framework to be triggered, starting with the Registration phase. However, this book has so far shown that both elements are problematic when it comes to their validity for chemicals in nanoscale. Not only is the definition of substance at Article 3 not nano-specific, but, the minimum threshold for entering REACH uses a metric, which as will be shown in the subsequent chapters of this book, is not suitable to the specific mode of toxic action through which nanoscale chemicals act.

The recently approved amendments to the REACH Annexes, including for Annexes that set out data to be provided for registration purposes, contain now a few relevant nano-specific provisions. This way, the inclusion of a specific reference to the separate registration of nanoforms in Annex I and VI and, most importantly, of the nano-specific characterisers of the 'nanoform', are a welcome effort as, for the first time, they impose a clear requirement for assessing and documenting separately the hazardous profiles of the nanoform (as compared to the bulk form) in terms of humans and the environmental impacts.[149] This would provide some degree of clarity on the status of nanomaterials in REACH. However, such amendments allow for the two main nanomaterials loopholes of REACH to persist. First, with regard to substance definition, not only do such amendments to the Annexes make use of the term 'nanoform' (instead of, for instance, 'nanomaterial' or 'nanosubstance') but they leave the definition of 'substance' in the legal body of REACH unaltered, i.e. non-nano-specific. Second, the clear indication in the amendments' text that the new requirements 'apply only to nanoforms when they are covered by the registration' reiterates the second identified loophole of REACH with regard to nanomaterials, i.e. the minimum threshold of 1 t/y. This will continue to allow for low-volume nanosubstances which, due to the mechanisms described in Chapter 1, might still pose unacceptable risks for humans and the environment, to fall out of registration obligations. Such loopholes notwithstanding, the adoption of the nano-specific provision to the REACH Annexes will arguably 'ensure further clarity on how nanomaterials are addressed and safety demonstrated in registration dossiers'.[150]

However, until such amendments come into force in early 2020 and, importantly, with the legal text of REACH remaining nano-silent even after that date, it is relevant to understand to what extent the other three programmes of REACH – Evaluation, Authorisation, and Restriction – remedy or perhaps even add to the existing loopholes in the Registration process.

The next chapter therefore deals with the status of nanomaterials under the Evaluation phase of REACH.

Notes

1 Council Regulation (EC) 1907/2006 of 18 December 2006 concerning the Registration, Evaluation, Authorisation and Restriction of Chemicals (REACH) [2006] OJ L 396/1.
2 REACH, Article 1(3).
3 REACH, recitals (73) and (74) and specifically Title VII on Authorization.
4 REACH, Article 1(1).
5 See C-558/07 *S.P.C.M. and Others* [2009] ECLI:EU:C:2009:430.

6   The Commission, in its proposals envisaged in paragraph 1 concerning health, safety, environmental protection and consumer protection, will take as a base a high level of protection, taking account in particular of any new development based on scientific facts. Within their respective powers, the European Parliament and the Council will also seek to achieve this objective.

7 Commission, 'Regulatory Aspects of Nanomaterials' (Communication) COM (2008) 366 final, 4.

8 Commission, 'Second Regulatory Review on Nanomaterials' (Communication) COM(2012) 572 final, 11.
9 REACH, Article 5(1).
10 Article 1(3) and recitals (9) and (69) of REACH clearly refer to the precautionary principle.
11 Ibid.
12 The 1 t/y minimum registration requirement is established at Article 6(1) of REACH.
13 European Inventory of Existing Commercial Chemical Substances.
14 REACH, Article 3(20)(a)(b)(c) REACH.
15 REACH, Article 28.1 (a).
16 'Registration Process' (*ECHA*) http://echa.europa.eu/web/guest/support/dossier-submission-tools/reach-it/nons accessed 19.02.2019.
17 Article 2.1(a) of the Directive refers generally to chemical substances as 'chemical elements and their compounds as they occur in the natural state or as produced by industry'.
18 REACH, Article 1(2) and Article 5(1).
19 Recital 15 of REACH refers precisely to technical, scientific, and administrative aspects of REACH Regulation.
20 Article 75(1) of REACH, which establishes the creation of the ECHA, reads 'A European Chemicals Agency is established for the purposes of managing and in some cases carrying out the technical, scientific and administrative aspects of this Regulation and to ensure consistency at Community level in relation to these aspects.'
21 See Lucas Bergkamp and DaeYoung Park, 'The Organizational and Administrative Structures' in Lucas Bergkamp (ed.), *The European Union REACH Regulation for Chemicals Law and Practice* (OUP 2013) 25–26. According to Article 75(1) ECHA can also 'carry out' technical, scientific, and administrative aspects which it usually manages, indicating a regulatory power deriving directly from REACH.
22 REACH, Article 76(1).
23 ECHA, 'Guidance for the Identification and Naming of Substances under REACH and CLP' (ECHA-16-B-37.1-EN, May 2017) 9.
24 Such as substances holding an EIECS (European Inventory of Existing Commercial Chemical Substances), ELNCS (European List of Notified Chemical Substances), and an NLP (No Longer Polymer) – number; substances holding a CAS (Chemical Abstracts Service), IUPAC (International Union of Pure and Applied Chemistry), or other trade name or abbreviations. ECHA (n 23) 22 and REACH Section 2, Annex VI.
25 ECHA-16-B-37.1-EN (n 23) 22.
26 Ibid.
27 Ibid. 23.
28 Ibid. 24.
29 Ibid.
30 'A mono-constituent substance is a substance in which one constituent is present at a concentration of at least 80% (w/w) and which contains up to 20% (w/w) of impurities.' Ibid. 25.
31 'A multi-constituent substance is a substance consisting of several main constituents present at concentrations generally ≥ 10% and < 80% (w/w).' Ibid.
32 Ibid. 32.
33 See Lucas Bergkamp and Nicolas Herbatschek, 'Key Concepts and Scope' in Lucas Bergkamp (ed.), *The European Union REACH Regulation for Chemicals Law and Practice* (OUP 2013) 42–44.
34 See COM (2008) 366 final.

35 Parliament resolution of 24 April 2009 on regulatory aspects of nanomaterials (2008/2208(INI)), P6_TA(2009)0328 [2009] OJ C184E/82.
36 Ibid. 7.
37 Ibid. 8.
38 Commission Recommendation 2011/696/EU of 18 October 2011 on the definition of nanomaterial [2011] OJ L275/38.
39 Ibid., recital (4).
40 SCENIHR, 'Scientific Basis for the Definition of the Term "Nanomaterial"' (6 July 2010).
41 Göran Lövestam et al., 'Considerations on a Definition of Nanomaterial for Regulatory Purposes' (European Commission JRC 2010).
42 ISO, 'Nanotechnologies – Terminology and definitions for nano-objects – Nanoparticle, nanofibre and nanoplate' (ISO/TS 27687:2008).
43 Recommendation 2011/696/EU, point 2.
44 Ibid., point 3.
45 See Chiu-Wing Lam, John T. James, Richard McCluskey, and Robert L. Hunter, 'Pulmonary Toxicity of Single-Wall Carbon Nanotubes in Mice 7 and 90 Days after Intratracheal Instillation' (2004) 77 Toxicol. Sci. 126; Anna A. Shvedova et al., 'Unusual Inflammatory and Fibrogenic Pulmonary Responses to Single-Walled Carbon Nanotubes in Mice' (2005) 289 Am. J. Physiol. Lung Cell Mol. Physiol. 698; Craig A. Poland et al., 'Carbon Nanotubes Introduced into the Abdominal Cavity of Mice Show Asbestos-Like Pathogenicity in a Pilot Study' (2008) 3 Nature Nanotechnology 423.
46 Article 2(7)(a) exempts substances included in Annex IV not only from Title II (Registration) but also from Title V (Downstream users) and Title VI (Evaluation) on the basis that 'sufficient information is known about these substances that they are considered to cause minimum risk because of their intrinsic properties'.
47 Commission Regulation (EC) 987/2008 of 8 October 2008 amending Regulation (EC) No 1907/2006 of the European Parliament and of the Council on the Registration, Evaluation, Authorisation and Restriction of Chemicals (REACH) as regards Annexes IV and V [2008] OJ L268/14, recital (3).
48 'Registration Dossier SWCTs' (*ECHA*, 2018) https://echa.europa.eu/registration-dossier/-/registered-dossier/18023 accessed 14.01.2019.
49 'Single-Wall Carbon Nanotubes Complete REACH Registration' (*CW*, 2016) www.compositesworld.com/news/single-wall-carbon-nanotubes-complete-reach-registration accessed 09.01.2019.
50 See 'REACH Registrant Finds No Aquatic Toxicity for SWCNTs' (*CW*, 2018) https://chemicalwatch.com/71515/reach-registrant-finds-no-aquatic-toxicity-for-swcnts accessed 09.01.2019.
51 Lan Ma-Hock et al., 'Inhalation Toxicity of Multiwall Carbon Nanotubes in Rats Exposed for 3 Months' (2009) 112 Toxicol. Sci. 468; Julie Muller et al., 'Respiratory Toxicity of Multi-Wall Carbon Nanotubes' (2005) 207 Toxicology and Applied Pharmacology 221.
52 Recommendation 2011/696/EU, recital (12).
53 'Useful Terminology' (*NanoComposix*) http://nanocomposix.com/pages/useful-terminology accessed 19.02.2019.
54 Recommendation 2011/696/EU, recital (12).
55 Ibid., point 5.
56 The centrality of this parameter was strongly advocated by SCENIHR's 2010 Opinion (n 40).
57 Recommendation 2011/696/EU, point 6.
58 See André J. Lecloux et al., 'Discussion about the Use of the Volume Specific Surface Area (VSSA) as a Criterion to Identify Nanomaterials According to the

EU Definition. Part Two: Experimental Approach' (2017) 9 *Nanoscale* 14952, 14960.

59 Hubert Rauscher et al., 'Towards a Review of the EC Recommendation for a Definition of the Term "Nanomaterial": Part 3: Scientific-Technical Evaluation of Options to Clarify the Definition and to Facilitate its Implementation' (European Commission JRC 2015) 18.

60 Ibid.

61 Council Regulation (EC) 1223/2009 of 30 November 2009 on cosmetic products [2009] OJ L342/59.

62 Regulation 1223/2009, Article 2(1)(k).

63 Regulation 1223/2009, Article 2(3).

64 FDA, 'Nanotechnology: A Report of the U.S. Food and Drug Administration Nanotechnology Task Force' (25 July 2007), 6–7.

65 As documented above, this refers to SCENIHR, 'The Existing and Proposed Definitions Relating to Products of Nanotechnologies' (29 November 2007); SCENIHR 'Risk Assessment of Products of Nanotechnologies' (19 January 2009); SCENIHR, 'Scientific Basis for the Definition of the Term "Nanomaterial"' (6 July 2010), and EFSA, 'The Potential Risks Arising from Nanoscience and Nanotechnologies on Food and Feed Safety' (2009) 958 The EFSA Journal 1; EFSA, 'Guidance on the Risk Assessment of the Application of Nanoscience and Nanotechnologies in the Food and Feed Chain' (2011) 9 EFSA Journal 2140. The latest opinion to have been adopted is the SCENIHR 'Nanosilver: Safety, Health and Environmental Effects and Role in Antimicrobial Resistance' (10–11 June 2014).

66 Andrew D. Maynard, 'Don't Define Nanomaterials' (2011) 475 Nature 31.

67 Ibid.

68 Andrew D. Maynard, David B. Warheit, and Martin A. Philbert, 'The New Toxicology of Sophisticated Materials: Nanotoxicology and Beyond' (2011) 120 (suppl 1) Toxicol. Sci. 109, 125.

69 Ibid. 119–120.

70 Commission, 'On the precautionary principle' (Communication) COM (2000) 1 final, 22.

71 COM (2000) 1, 4.

72 REACH, Article 3(2).

73 Commission (Draft Regulation) (EU) .../... of XXX amending Regulation (EC) No. 1907/2006 of the European Parliament and of the Council on the Registration, Evaluation, Authorisation and Restriction of Chemicals (REACH) as regards Annexes I, III,VI, VII, VIII, IX, X, XI, and XII to address nanoforms of substances, XXX [...] (2017) XXX draft, Annex Ares(2017) 4925011–09/10/2017 (Hereafter, Ares(2017)4925011) 9.

74 Anil K. Suresh et al., 'Silver Nanocrystallites: Biofabrication using Shewanella Oneidensis, and an Evaluation of Their Comparative Toxicity on Gram-Negative and Gram-Positive Bacteria' (2010) 44 Environ. Sci. Technol. 5210.

75 The definition of 'mixture' under REACH is based on the lack of chemical reaction between the (two or more) mixed substances, which shall as a result be registered separately. See Bergkamp and Herbatschek (n 33) 46.

76 REACH, Article 3(15). The different categories of intermediates will be analysed under the section dealing with exceptions from REACH.

77 Article 3(3) defines the term *article* as 'an object which during production is given a special shape, surface or design which determines its function to a greater degree than does its chemical composition'.

78 Bergkamp and Herbatschek (n 33) 50.

79 In 2013, the PEN Nanotechnology Consumer Products Inventory listed 1,628 nano-related products introduced on the market since 2005. The number of

products registered in 2013 represented a 24 per cent increase compared to the number registered in 2010. See 'Inventory Finds Increase in Consumer Products Containing Nanoscale Materials' (*PEN*, 13 October 2013) www.nanotech project.org/news/archive/9242/ accessed 19.01.2019.

80 For an overview of the categories see 'Categories' (*PEN*) www.nanotechproject. org/cpi/browse/categories/ accessed 19.02.2019.

81 ECHA, 'Guidance on Requirements for Substances in Articles' (ECHA-17-G-19-EN, June 2017).

82 The Commission holds that some nanomaterials already authorised by EFSA in FCMs, like synthetic amorphous silica and carbon black, were being produced in quantities of 1.5 and 9.5 million t respectively. However, the data refer to the global market and do not provide specificities on individual manufacturers. See in this regard: Commission, 'Types and Uses of Nanomaterials, Including Safety Aspects Accompanying the Communication from the Commission to the European Parliament, the Council and the European Economic and Social Committee on the Second Regulatory Review on Nanomaterials' (Staff Working Document) SWD (2012) 288 final, 10.

83 REACH, Article 7(2)(3).

84 ECHA-17-G-19-EN (n 81) 26.

85 See in general David Bennet, 'Public Perceptions of Nanotechnologies: Lessons from GM Foods' in Q. Chaudhry, L. Castle, and R. Watkins (eds), *RSC Nanoscience & Nanotechnology: Nanotechnologies in Food* (Royal Society of Chemistry 2010).

86 ECHA, 'Guidance in Nutshell, Requirements for Substances in Articles' (ECHA-11-B-05-EN June 2011) 6.

87 Case C-279/12 *Fish Legal and Shirley* [2013] ECLI:EU:C:2013:853, para 38.

88 'Once an article – Always an article' [PowerPoint common presentation], available at: http://echa.europa.eu/documents/10162/13636/presentation_dissenting_ms_caracal_en.pdf accessed 22.02.2019.

89 Case C-106/14 *FCD and FMB* [2014] ECLI:EU:C:2015:576.

90 Ibid. para 20.

91 Case C-106/14 *FCD and FMB* [2014] ECLI:EU:C:2015:93, Opinion AG Kokott, paras 31–33.

92 Ibid. para 35.

93 Ibid. para 36.

94 Ibid. para 55.

95 On consumers' protection and the right to know under the TFEU and the CFREU see M. Jagielska and M. Jagielski, 'Are Consumer Rights Human Rights?' in J. Devenney and M. Kenny (eds) *European Consumer Protection, Theory and Practice* (CUP 2012).

96 Joanne Scott, 'REACH: Combining Harmonization and Dynamism in the Regulation of Chemicals' in Joanne Scott (ed.) *Environmental Protection: European Law and Governance* (OUP 2009) 3.

97 ECHA, 'Guidance in a Nutshell on Requirements for Substances in Articles' (ECHA-17-G-26-EN, December 2017) 8.

98 The Royal Society and The Royal Academy of Engineering, *Nanoscience and Nanotechnologies: Opportunities and Uncertainties* (The Royal Society 2004); SCENIHR 2010 (n 40).

99 The claimant companies included: S.P.C.M. SA. (France), C.H. Erbslöh KG (Germany), Lake Chemicals and Minerals Ltd (UK), and Hercules Inc. (USA).

100 According to Article 6(3)(a)(b) the registration of monomer units is required when 'the polymer consists of 2% weight by weight (w/w) or more of such monomer substance(s) or other substance(s) in the form of monomeric units and

chemically bound substance(s)' and 'the total quantity of such monomer substance(s) or other substance(s) makes up 1 tonne or more per year'.

101 REACH, Article 3(5)(b).

102 Jean-Luc Laffineur, 'Analysis First ECJ Ruling on REACH: Choosing Registration over Exemption. Case C-558/07, R (on the application of SPCM SA, CH Erbsloh KG, Lake Chemicals and Minerals Ltd, Hercules Inc.) v Secretary of States for the Environment, Food and Rural Affairs' (2010) 22 Journal of Environmental Law 135, 140.

103 Ibid.

104 *S.P.C.M. and Others* (n 5) para 27.

105 Ibid. para 75. The Court asserted also that while it might require importers an additional effort to acquire information on monomers used in the polymers they aim to place on the EU market, exempting them for registering such monomers would in practice determine a favourable treatment, de facto distorting completion rules applicable to the internal market. See also paragraphs 77–81.

106 Ibid. para 31.

107 Laffineur (n 102) 9.

108 *S.P.C.M. and Others* (n 5) para 54.

109 Ibid. para 44.

110 A similar view was also endorsed in a recent decision from ECHA's Board of Appeal, stating

> although the protection of human health is, together with protection of the environment, the most important of the objectives of the REACH Regulation it must be weighed against the other objectives of the REACH Regulation and EU law more widely.

See Decision of the Board of Appeal of ECHA, Case A-005-2011 *Honeywell v ECHA* [2013] para 122.

111 Recital 19 of REACH reads:

> Therefore, the registration provisions should require manufacturers and importers to generate data on the substances they manufacture or import, to use these data to assess the risks related to these substances and to develop and recommend appropriate risk management measures. To ensure that they actually meet these obligations, as well as for transparency reasons, registration should require them to submit a dossier containing all this information to the Agency. Registered substances should be allowed to circulate on the internal market.

112 *S.P.C.M. and Others* (n 5) para 46.

113 See Michael R. Taylor, 'Regulating the Products of Nanotechnology: Does the FDA Have the Tools it Needs?' (PEN5 2006). Taylor suggested also that nanoscale materials should be considered new 'for safety evaluation purposes'.

114 ECHA-16-B-37.1-EN (n 23) 36, emphasis added.

115 However, for certain categories of substances, like those delineated in Article 57 of REACH and considered of 'very high concern', the *main* criterion used for assessing risks to humans and the environment is not that of the volume of production (thus exposure) but rather the intrinsic hazardousness of the substances in question, regardless of exposure.

116 ECHA, 'Guidance on information requirements and chemical safety assessment Chapter R.2: Framework for generation of information on intrinsic properties' (ECHA-2011-G-11-EN, December 2011) 2.

117 REACH, Article 12 is entitled '*Information to be submitted depending on tonnage*'.

118 REACH, Annex VI.

119 REACH, Annex VI.

120 See REACH, Annex VI.

121 REACH, Annex VI, section 3. Interestingly, information on the technological process of production is required for producers of articles but not for producers of substances.

122 REACH, Annex VI, section 4.

123 REACH, Annex VI, section 5.

124 Ares(2017)4925011, Annex VI, 6–9.

125 REACH, Article 12(1)(a)(b).

126 REACH, Annex VII, section 7.

127 REACH, Annex VII, section 8.

128 REACH, Annex VII, section 9.

129 Ares(2017)4925011, Annex VII (a), 11.

130 See Column II of each table belonging to sections 7–9 of Annex VII.

131 REACH, Article 12(1)(c).

132 Toxicokinetics consisting in 'the science dealing with absorption, distribution, metabolism and excretion (ADME) of substances in the body' is of primary importance for understanding and evaluating risks associated with nanoparticles. Toxicokinetics studies have always accompanied the Opinions delivered by SCENIHR and EFSA. The main concerns identified so far through such studies are related to the possible accumulation of insoluble nanoparticles in secondary target organs and their possible migration, form exposure routes, to the brain and unborn foetus. See SCENIHR, 'Risk Assessment of Products of Nanotechnologies' (19 January 2009) 24, 29.

133 Ibid. SCENIHR (2009) 7, reaffirmed that 'free and low solubility nanoparticles (nanomaterials) are a priority concern in the context of human and environmental risk.' at p. 7 Also, EFSA lists solubility/persistency and bioaccumulation among the main factors influencing a potential high exposure to nanoparticles. See EFSA 2011(n 65) 10.

134 An endpoint is an observable or measurable inherent property of a chemical substance. It can for example refer to a physical-chemical property like vapour pressure or to degradability or to a biological effect that a given substance has on human health or the environment, e.g. carcinogenicity, irritation, aquatic toxicity.

135 Ares(2017)4925011, 11–14.

136 Ares(2017)4925011, Annex VII (g) point 9.1.1, 11.

137 Ares(2017)4925011, Annex VIII (h) section 9.2.2, 16.

138 See REACH Annex IX, sections 7–9.

139 Ares(2017)4925011, Annex IX (b), 17.

140 See REACH Annex X, sections 8–9.

141 Ralf Nordbeck and Michael Faust, 'European Chemicals Regulation and its Effect on Innovation: An Assessment of the EU's White Paper on the Strategy for a Future Chemicals Policy' (2003) 13 European Environment 79, 82.

142 Ibid.

143 See for example Kyung-Taek Rim, Se-Wook Song, and Hyeon-Yeong Kim, 'Oxidative DNA Damage from Nanoparticle Exposure and Its Application to Workers' Health: A Literature Review' (2013) 4 Safety and Health at Work 177.

144 Ares(2017)4925011, (b) point 8.6.3, 21.

145 Ares(2017)4925011, 3/8/17/19/24.

146 'Guidance on Information Requirements and Chemical Safety Assessment' (*ECHA*) http://echa.europa.eu/guidance-documents/guidance-on-information-requirements-and-chemical-safety-assessment accessed 19.02.2019.

147 'RIPoN' (*European Commission*) http://ec.europa.eu/environment/chemicals/nanotech/reach-clp/ripon_en.htm accessed 18.02.2019.

148 Lynn L. Bergeson and Carla N. Hutton, 'ECHA Publishes REACH Guidance for Nanomaterials' (May 2017) https://nanotech.lawbc.com/2017/05/echa-publishes-reach-guidance-for-nanomaterials/ accessed 18.02.2019.
149 CIEL, 'Revision of REACH Annexes for Nanomaterials – Position Paper' (2015) www.ciel.org/wp-content/uploads/2015/10/Position-Paper-REACH-Annexes-Final.pdf accessed 18.02.2019.
150 'Consultation' (*European Commission*) http://ec.europa.eu/environment/consultations/nanomaterials_2013_en.htm accessed 18.02.2019.

4   Evaluation

Introduction

If the Registration were to deliver the high levels of human and environmental protections it aspires to, it is reasonable to expect that the broad spectrum of information, data, and testing requirements it triggers will be carefully scrutinised in order to establish the accuracy and compliance of such data with the normative provisions under REACH. As it is virtually impossible for the ECHA to evaluate every single dossier submitted, REACH foresees different procedures that enable the ECHA's performance of an overall check of compliance under the procedure of Evaluation.

REACH foresees three types of Evaluation: dossier evaluation,[1] substance evaluation,[2] and evaluation of intermediates.[3] For the purpose of this chapter, the first two categories will be analysed.

Dossier evaluation

Under dossier evaluation (DE), the ECHA performs both the *examination of testing proposals* in accordance with Annexes IX and X of REACH and the *compliance check* of the registration dossiers.[4] The ECHA's Board of Appeal (BoA) acknowledged the importance of dossier compliance check pursuant to Article 41, stating that its aim is that of ensuring that the dossiers under examination comply with '*all* relevant information requirements set out in REACH regulation'.[5] It is in principle a valid tool that the ECHA can employ in ensuring that the registration dossiers of chemicals in nano-form do effectively comply with *all* the requirements REACH imposes on the producers/importers/downstream users.

However, the different types of examination the ECHA can conduct under the general Evaluation programme, envisaged under Title VI of REACH, are based on a set of criteria which might hinder the performance of such examinations on chemicals in nanoscale.

DE's two subprogrammes, namely the examination of testing proposals and the compliance check, are analysed in the following.

Testing proposals

Article 10(ix) of REACH specifies that among other standard information to be included in the technical dossier (TD) for registration, for substances produced in quantities ≥ 100 and ≥ 1,000 t/y, proposals for testing in accordance with Annexes IX and X of REACH should also be included. Particular relevance is given to SVHCs since the ECHA is required to prioritise substances that show persistent, bioaccumulative, and toxic (PBT), very persistent and very bioaccumulative (vPvB), and carcinogenic, mutagenic, or toxic to reproduction (CMR) properties and other substances classified as 'dangerous' according to the criteria of Directive 67/548/EEC.[6] While for substances of very high concern (SVHCs) the ECHA screening is a hazard-driven process, for the existing dangerous substance, Article 40(1) requires, besides the minimum threshold of production of 100 t/y, the existence of '*uses resulting in widespread and diffuse exposure*'. Hence, in the case of SVHCs, the mere concern arising from their intrinsic properties is sufficient to trigger the ECHA's examination on testing proposals. Whereas for substances classified as 'dangerous' under the pre-REACH regime, the actual *risk*, estimated on exposure basis, is the regulatory driver instead. Arguably, the burden on the ECHA is greater in this latter case, as it determines that relevant exposure must occur before assessing testing proposals for such substances. However, in both cases, the minimum[7] threshold of 100 t/y makes the application of this provision difficult for nano-chemicals in low volumes despite their potential categorisation as SVHCs.

An important aim of the ECHA's check-up on the testing proposals on TDs submitted for Registration is safeguarding animal welfare by avoiding unnecessary testing and encouraging data sharing.[8] In this regard, REACH's approach to animal testing is represented by the Three Rs concept, as follows: '*Replacement* of animals in experiments, *Reduction* of the numbers used, and *Refinement* of husbandry and procedures to reduce suffering and improve welfare'.[9]

The testing methods for obtaining the information on the intrinsic properties of chemicals for different endpoints identified and required by the REACH Annexes are set out in the Annex to Council Regulation (EC) No. 440/2008.[10] Articulated in over 700 pages, the Regulation in question brings together validated test methods approved and adopted on Community level, in accordance with REACH requirements. The principle of *replacement, reduction, and refinement* is at the core of the design and adoption of testing strategies[11] and the Commission is entrusted with the duty to review testing methods in order to reduce the use of vertebrate animals.[12] The mere existence of validated non-testing methods[13] seems to be sufficient to trigger reviewing (and perhaps replacement) of existing animal testing methodologies.

Non-testing methods under the REACH framework and their applicability to chemicals in nanoscale

At the time of the REACH negotiations, a study from the Joint Research Centre (JRC) foresaw that nearly 3.9 million additional test animals could potentially be used as a result of the introduction of REACH, in case alternative methods were not accepted by the authorities. And this only during the implementation period of REACH (11 years).[14] The study in question notes, however, that 'for some of the most test animal intensive endpoints, no alternative tests are currently available'. Therefore, contributions from different actors like the EU, OECD, academia, and industry for the development of no-testing methods, such as Q(SAR) and *in vitro* studies, are seen as a principal goal for the future of the chemical policy in REACH and the reduction of animal testing therein.[15] It ought to be recalled here that animal welfare is listed among the key principles the EU should respect in policy formulation and implementation, as substantiated in Article 13 of TFEU:

> In formulating and implementing the Union's agriculture, fisheries, transport, internal market, research and technological development and space policies, the Union and the Member States shall, since animals are sentient beings, pay full regard to the welfare requirements of animals, while respecting the legislative or administrative provisions and customs of the Member States relating in particular to religious rites, cultural traditions and regional heritage.

Considering how many animals are used in the safety testing of chemicals, it is evident that reducing the number of animals used and/or the unnecessary suffering of laboratory animals, lies at the heart of animal welfare related measures. For animals used for scientific purposes, welfare issues are addressed through Directive 2010/63/EU.[16] As a consequence, Member States (MSs) have some discretion and flexibility for translating the norms of the directive in national law. In the case of REACH, as it is a regulation, the provisions referring to use of vertebrate animals in experimenting and testing are immediately and directly binding upon MSs. It is thereby quite understandable that the promotion of the use of non-testing methods represents an essential element of the normative framework delineated by REACH. Such alternative non-testing methods are aimed at allowing the registrant to meet information requirements, while minimising or avoiding unnecessary testing on animals.

In fact, REACH permits the testing on vertebrate animals only as a 'last resort' rule.[17] This view has been confirmed by the ECHA's BoA, which ruled that in case of an identified information gap[18] presented to the ECHA, the Agency 'must ensure that testing on vertebrate animals is undertaken only as a last resort'.[19] Instead, comparison and grouping of structurally similar substances, specialised computer modelling like (Q)SARs, Weight of Evidence approach, and *in vitro* studies using cells rather than live animals are encouraged to be used by the registrant for obtaining data on chemicals' toxicity.[20] Scientifically speaking, all non-testing methods (excluded the *in vitro* ones) are based on the *similarity principle* which implies that chemicals having similar structures are expected to exhibit similar biological activities.[21] The possibility to use alternative test methods also for chemicals in nanoscale represents a prerequisite for the application of the Three Rs to this group of chemicals. In addition, such validity affects the burden placed on the registrant/ECHA when considering the necessity for vertebrate animal testing. In case these non-testing methods were unreliable or not technically possible for nano-chemicals, animal testing, which according to REACH must be used only as a last resort, would become the normal procedure. Therefore, a short analysis of the existing non-testing methods and their applicability to nano-chemicals becomes relevant for understanding the ECHA's range of discretion and enforcement powers when evaluating potential dossiers on nanosubstances in the light of Article 40 of REACH.

i (Q)SAR

Structure–activity relationships (SAR) are qualitative relationships that relate a (sub)structure to the presence or absence of a property or activity of interest.[22] Quantitative structure–activity relationships, (Q)SARs, are mathematical models (often statistical correlations) relating one or more quantitative parameters derived from chemical structure to a quantitative measure of a property or activity of a chemical substance (e.g. a (eco)toxicological endpoint).[23] In other words, the (Q)SARs are *theoretical models* that can be used to predict in a qualitative or quantitative manner the toxicity of chemical compounds from a knowledge of their chemicals structure.[24] In REACH, (Q)SARs methods are encouraged to be used for data generation, either in concomitance with other methods (including testing) – like in the case of Article 13(1) – or as an alternative to *experimental* data, provided that certain criteria are meet, as foreseen by Annex XI of REACH.[25] Thus, in case (Q)SARs applications generate relevant, reliable, adequate, and appropriately documented results, these results could, in principle, be used on their own for regulatory purposes. In other cases, especially in presence of scientific uncertainty, (Q)SAR results can be combined with other information that compensates for such uncertainty – for example in the context of the *Weight of Evidence approach*.[26] The ECHA explains that for the purposes of REACH, the validation of (Q)SAR models shall be performed in reference to the OECD internationally agreed principles for validation of (Q)SAR, suggesting a certain degree of interdependence between the OECD principles that govern the validity of the model[27] and the use of that model under REACH. From an analysis of the OECD principles,[28] it becomes clear that a thorough understanding of the structural descriptors of a substance is crucial to the predictability of its biological activity through (Q)SAR algorithms.

Given the great scientific uncertainty surrounding the physicochemical properties of nanosubstances, it is unlikely that such a model can be successfully applied for assessing the hazardous properties of chemicals in nanoscale. Indeed, already in 2007, SCENIHR concluded that

> [i]t is also premature to apply the QSARs approach to nanoparticles since current knowledge on the main characteristics determining the environmental fate and effects of nanoparticles is too limited to enable a simple classification of nanoparticles to be developed for environmental risk assessment purposes.[29]

In SCENIHR's opinion, the challenge in applying (Q)SARs for nanosubstances is owed to the 'general lack of knowledge of which physicochemical properties of nanoparticles are responsible for any specific toxicity'[30] and the fact that 'the bulk chemical still provides the ultimate structure activity relationship for the same basic chemical composition; even though difference in toxicity between the larger bulk and nanosized forms have been demonstrated in some cases'.[31] To date, (Q)SAR studies for predicting the toxicity of nanochemicals have been rarely reported and, although useful in the case of bulk chemicals, the concept of nano-(Q)SAR remains underdeveloped.[32]

ii Structural similarity: grouping and read-across

Chemicals that share a similar structure are also likely to display similar physicochemical and (eco)toxicological properties. Thus, they can be grouped and assessed following a 'category' approach. Instead of assessing the properties of every single chemical belonging to the group, such properties are assessed on the evaluation of the group of chemicals as a whole. The benefits of this approach include consideration for animal welfare, resources and time reduction, and the possibility to fill possible gaps on certain properties and endpoints without the need to conduct new testing. In case there is a lack of data for one or more members of the same group, read-across from other chemicals within the same category can be performed to fill such a gap.[33]

Considering the scope of REACH – ensuring a high level of human health and environmental protection – it is relevant to point out that the category approach might in certain cases be applicable and justified only for human health endpoints or for environmental ones only.[34] The ECHA distinguishes between *category approach* and *analogue approach* on one hand, used to group together structurally similar chemicals; and *read-across*[35] on the other, which can be used to fill in data gaps within the groups identified through the category and the analogue approach.[36]

Against this background, it is important to recall the fact that a case-by-case approach has been repetitively recalled and 'encouraged' by several EU scientific bodies[37] and backed up by several legislative documents with regard to the assessment and the consequent management of potential risks deriving from nanosubstances.[38] It therefore seems logical to assume that grouping and read-across is unlikely to find practical application when regulating nano-chemicals in REACH. In addition, the peculiarities that nanosubstances exhibit due to their size, surface shape, surface reactivity, coating, biodegradation, accumulation, and aggregation, etc., are still pretty unclear and form the object of broad scientific research, which aims to mitigate uncertainties and generate reliable data, essential to effective regulatory measures.

Given these shortcomings, the OECD considers it premature to develop guidance on grouping specifically for nanomaterials.[39] Therefore, until more data becomes available, grouping and read-across for nanosubstances do not seem feasible, and the usage of such non-testing methods for regulatory purposes in general, and specifically under REACH, is highly improbable.

A final relevant observation is that the step-wise approaches that the ECHA advocates when it comes to non-testing methodologies are heavily dependent not only on basic data on the characterisation of nano-chemicals, but also, to a certain extent, on the possibility of some valid non-testing methods, already applicable to nano-chemicals. The existence of valid non-testing methodologies can 'feed' data to the performance of other non-testing in a progressive process for data generation.

In the *Nickel Institute* case, the CJEU, while recognising the validity of the read-across method for classification and labelling purpose, held that while

> the method based on structure-activity relationships displays certain differences from the read-across method, the fact remains that those two methods are not to be regarded as independent since they are both founded on the principle of extrapolation from existing data on certain substances in order to assess and classify other substances which have a similar structure and on which there are very limited or no data.[40]

The Court's position suggests an interconnection (not exclusivity) between (Q)SAR and read-across, based on the necessity for both models to rely on existing data. Given the paucity of such data for chemicals in nanoscale, it is unlikely that in the near future a read-across method will be employed for the classification of nanosubstances under REACH and CLP. In this regard, the Appendix to Chapter R.8 *Characterisation of dose [concentration] – response for human health* to the ECHA's Guidance on Information Requirements and Chemical Safety Assessment, states:

> it should be noted that the use of non-testing data such as read-across, grouping or (Q)SAR approaches in addressing data gaps for nanomaterials is very limited at this time. In addition to this the use of such *in-silico* models for nanomaterials has also yet to be established. Therefore the potential use of non-testing approaches for nanomaterials in deriving an assessment of hazard for humans must be scientifically justified on a case by case basis.[41]

The GD adds:

> Regarding nanomaterials, the use of a read across approach in addressing data gaps for nanomaterials may not be considered suitable at this time as the use of such approaches for nanomaterials has yet to be established. Therefore the potential use of read-across and other non-testing approaches for nanomaterials in deriving an assessment of hazard for humans must be scientifically justified on a case by case basis.[42]

A similar approach is taken by the ECHA when it comes to environmental effects of nanomaterials, holding that

> the use of read-across from available data on bulk or other forms of the material in place of specific data for the nanomaterials being assessed must be scientifically justified and may be associated with additional uncertainty.[43]

The overall conclusion is that of a current impossibility to employ read-across and *in silico* models – in alternative to animal testing – for generating data on different endpoints on human and environmental toxicity, required under REACH. Moreover, trying to extrapolate such data from the bulk form must be backed by strong scientific facts (unlikely in a moment of scientific uncertainty). It is relevant to point out here that a read-across from the bulk to the nanoform of a chemical substance must be discouraged as it might add to the existing uncertainty and possibly lead to distorted outcomes.

iii Weight of the evidence

When a complete study on a specific endpoint is lacking but fragmented scientific information on that endpoint can be derived from other studies such as (Q)SAR, invalidated *in vitro* studies, literature review, and independent other sources, no additional testing might be needed.[44] This fragmented information must then be evaluated for accuracy, quality, consistency, and consequences in case it leads to a wrong decision, in what is called the *Weight of Evidence* method.

In principle, this method could be used for assessing the toxicity of nanochemicals for a given endpoint. However, as this method is heavily dependent on the accuracy of already performed tests and previously generated data 'weighted' in the process, it seems unlikely that the Weight of Evidence is going to be successfully employed in the assessment of human and environmental toxicity of chemicals in nanoscale under the REACH and CLP regime.[45]

Therefore, for nanosubstances under REACH, it can be held that to date, limitations and consequent lack of plausible *in vitro*[46] and *in silico*[47] models make it difficult to apply and enforce the Three Rs concept for this group of chemicals. Consequently, it can be speculated that the 'last resort' rule evoked by REACH on animal testing is actually the only available practice for testing (eco)toxicity profiles in the case of nanosize substances.

The question arises, then, naturally: how sustainable is nanotechnology and the derivate products? Can there be sustainable development and commercialisation of nano-chemicals, in line with the high level of human health and environmental protection pursued by REACH, when scientific information on toxicity impacts can be obtained only through tests involving the use of animals or animal cells? A preliminary answer could be that invasive and yet unreliable methods required for nanosubstances' testing might act in favour of the calls for limitations on the production of nanosubstances, coming from NGOs such as Friends of the Earth and ETC Group. Such limitations might represent a plausible alternative to the current indiscriminate diffusion of nanomaterials into the environment, to which the imperfect REACH framework seems to contribute significantly.

The forthcoming amendments to Annex XI now stipulate that the use of (Q)SAR, grouping and read-across, and the WoE approaches, shall be addressed separately for nanoforms covered by registration.[48] This is an important clarification that removes any doubt that structural similarity cannot be used as a criterion for grouping or reading across different forms of the same substance (e.g. bulk silver and nano silver). However, whether such approaches can be used to demonstrate the safety of different nanoforms of the same substance (e.g. 10 nm silver and 50 nm silver), remains unclear.

In addition to these amendments, ECHA has adopted a new nano-specific Appendix to its 'Guidance on QSARs and Grouping of Chemicals'.[49] This guidance was used by the OECD to develop, in collaboration with the JRC, a case study on the genotoxicity of two nanoforms of titanium dioxide (TiO$_2$). The study applied a slightly adapted version of the stepwise read-across Assessment Framework (RAAF) elaborated by ECHA and concluded in favour of the general practical application of the ECHA specific guidance, despite the fact that some 'nano-specific issues were identified for further specification of the RAAF for NMS, in particular the *concept of similarity* which cannot be based only on structural similarity for NMs'.[50] Furthermore, the GD by the ECHA has also been used in a study conducted by scientists at the EC's JRC to assess the genotoxicity of 19 different types of MWCNTs. The study[51] employed the principles of the ECHA's GDs on read-across methods for nanomaterials while supplementing them with chemioinformatics techniques, i.e. computer science models used to solve problems in the field of chemical research. In addition, the new RAAF was used to evaluate the uncertainties. The study was not performed for the purpose of conducting a hazard assessment but nonetheless the data yielded show that the MWCNTs analogues were not genotoxic, successfully demonstrating thus the applicability of the ECHA guidance in question for this specific purpose.[52]

It can be concluded hence that the new ECHA nano-specific Appendix in question represents another valuable effort in elucidating how such (Q)SARs and grouping might be applied in the case of nanomaterials. At the same time though, said Appendix is premised on the assumption that enough data (usually obtained through registration) will be available on main categories of nano-chemicals so as to allow the non-testing methods in question to be performed and used also for this class of chemicals. As the rest of this book will further demonstrate, this is not currently the case.

Procedures for the evaluation of testing proposals

The ECHA evaluates testing proposals on vertebrate animals in registration dossiers, according to the provisions set forth in Title VI of REACH. Publicity and transparency are important elements of the evaluation procedure since an open and transparent process allows involved subjects, including third parties, to share data or submit valid information or studies that might have already addressed the substance in question and/or the endpoints investigated by the proposed testing.[53] Hence, a period of 45 days' public consultation precedes the ECHA's decision on vertebrate animal testing.[54] During this period, the ECHA shall publish the name of the substance, the hazard endpoint for which animal testing is proposed, and the date by which any information from third parties is required.[55]

On the basis of the input received, the ECHA shall prepare a draft decision which might require the registrants/downstream users to carry out the test:

- as it is proposed;
- modifying the conditions under which the test is to be carried out;
- requiring one or more additional tests to be carried out in case of non-compliance of testing proposal with Annexes IX, X, XI.[56]

The ECHA can also reject a testing proposal.[57] When several registrants/downstream users have been submitting proposals for the same test, the ECHA shall grant a 90-day period for them to decide who will perform the test.[58]

Once a draft decision has been adopted, the ECHA shall notify the registrants/downstream users concerned, which have 30 days to comment on the draft. Following this period, the ECHA must send the draft decision in question, together with eventual comments received by registrants/downstream users, to the competent authorities of the Member States (MS CAs),[59] which have 30 days to comment on the draft and propose eventual amendments.[60] If amendments are proposed by MSs, the ECHA refers the draft, together with any amendments proposed, to the Member State Committee within 15 days of the end of the 30-day period referred to above.[61] The Agency shall forthwith communicate any proposal for amendment to the concerned registrants or downstream users and allow them to comment within 30 days. Any comment received must be taken into account by the Member State Committee.[62] The Member State Committee has 60 days to amend or adopt the decision unanimously;[63] otherwise the case is sent to the

Commission, which prepares a draft decision to be taken in accordance with the procedure referred to in Article 133(3).[64]

It is relevant to point out that the decision must be adopted unanimously; hence, the agreement of all Member States is necessary in order to avoid referring the matter to the Commission. A preliminary observation here concerns the probability of MSs to agree on decisions concerning testing of nano-chemicals. Given the diversity of approaches to nanosubstances on a national level,[65] it seems logical to assume that unanimous consensus can hardly be reached on this subject. In a best-case scenario, the Commission will be called in to rule on testing strategies affecting chemicals in nanoscale.

Generally speaking, the ECHA can adopt a decision on a testing proposal on vertebrate animals in two cases:

- pursuant to Article 51(3), if no proposals for amendments are made to the original draft decision at end of the 30 days period; and
- pursuant to Article 51(6), in case the MS Committee unanimously approves eventual amendments.

Considering the above-mentioned problem on the difficulties in generating registration data through non-testing methods, a first observation can be made on the 'narrowness' of the periods foreseen for the adoption of decisions on testing proposals under dossier evaluation procedures. Such terms can hardly be considered compatible with the complexity characterising different scientific aspects of nano-chemicals, including testing methodologies, and could eventually be questioned in front of the CJEU under the proportionality profile.

Another observation concerns the degree of discretion the ECHA has in assessing testing proposals submitted in accordance with Article 40(1) of REACH. Based on the outcome of the previous section on non-testing methods for nanosize chemicals, it seems logical to assume that because of current shortcomings and limitations of *in vitro* and *in silico* methodologies for this class of chemicals, the ECHA might be able to require testing on vertebrate animals 'more easily' for nanosubstances meeting the conditions set out in Annex XI.

In general, EU institutions' discretionary powers have already been recognised by the European Union Courts. In accordance with settled case law

> where EU authorities have a broad discretion, in particular as to the assessment of highly complex scientific and technical fasts in order to determine the nature and scope of the measure which they adopt, review by the European Union judicature is limited to verifying whether there has been a manifest error of assessment or a misuse of powers, or whether those authorities have manifestly exceeded the limits of their discretion.[66]

In particular regarding the ECHA's discretionary powers, the CJEU has ruled that

> ECHA has a broad discretion in a sphere which entails political, economic and social choices on its part, and in which it is called upon to undertake complex assessments. The legality of a measure adopted in that sphere can be affected only if the measure is manifestly inappropriate having regard to the objective which the legislature is seeking to pursue.[67]

There is little doubt that nanosubstances and the complexity of their assessment will entail political, social, and economic considerations from the ECHA's side. The ECHA acknowledges that it needs to be fully aware of the latest scientific developments when adopting judgments on the adequacy of information submitted by industry, when issuing regulatory opinions, or when providing guidance on the fulfilment of REACH's requirements. Being acquainted with the latest scientific progress concerning risks posed by nanomaterials is considered among the ECHA's top priorities.[68] Against this backdrop, it can be argued that tests involving animals will constitute a 'routine' choice when testing nanosubstances, as opposed to the general indication under REACH that such tests shall be required only as a 'last resort' rule. The implications on the legal plan would be that such decisions can hardly be challenged before the EU Courts for being manifestly inappropriate, when taking into account the scope of REACH which is to ensure a high level of protection of human and environmental health.

In general, while a very few current *in vivo* testing methods might be able to detect effects of nanosubstances on target organs such as the liver, spleen, and lungs, more sophisticated methods are needed in order to test effects on the nervous system and the blood-brain barrier – essential endpoints in human toxicology.[69] To date, the determination of dose-response relationships for target organs and cells can only be determined *in vivo*. However, the lack of standardisation on the concept of dose, with respect to specific characterisers of nanomaterials such as size, surface area and charge, number-size distribution, etc.,[70] certainly vitiates the very validity of existing *in vivo* methodologies for chemicals in nanoscale. Hence, the impression is that even the *in vivo* methodologies might hardly be successfully employed to satisfy REACH's testing requirements on several endpoints.

Another scenario that can be envisaged for nanoscale chemicals in connection to the testing proposal checking by the ECHA under the Evaluation procedure is one that involves Article 50(3) of REACH. Article 50(3) of REACH holds that upon receiving a draft decision from the ECHA, the producer/importer/downstream-user might decide to cease the production/import/use of the chemical in question. Notice shall be given to the Agency with the consequence that no further information needs to be provided. The flip side of this 'emergency exit' would be that the registration dossier becomes invalid. Hence, the ECHA, in requiring testing on specific end-points for nano-chemicals, might place a high burden on registrants. In line with the precautionary principle in REACH, it is for producers to demonstrate the safety of chemicals placed on the market, and nano-chemicals are no exception. Nevertheless, the above-stated reasons might make the performance of nano-testing difficult, if not impossible, arguably leaving no other choice to the producer than that of opting out by ceasing the production of that chemical. The invalidity of the registration dossier that follows such withdrawal is, however, reversible: a new dossier can be submitted and with that the entire process will re-start. The procedure in question can act as a de facto ban for nano-substances in REACH. However, the ECHA's checking mechanism implies that the information on the nanoscale nature of the chemical must, in the first place, be known to the ECHA, while the current REACH set of provisions does not require such information to be submitted. Hence, until the status of nanosubstances as *new for regulatory purposes* and the consequent need for specific separate registration and testing are established, this mechanism will rarely be invoked. The consequence would be that nanomaterials currently go undetected and untested under REACH.

Compliance check

Article 41(1) of REACH foresees the possibility for the ECHA to examine registration dossiers or different parts of them. Particular focus is placed on dossiers waiving/adapting standard registration requirements[71] and 'opt outs' from joint registration procedures, both in case of substances and intermediates.[72] Within 12 months from the starting of such a compliance check, the ECHA may draft a decision requiring registrant(s) to submit further information in order to bring the dossier in line with the relevant information requirements foreseen by REACH.[73] In the event that it is impossible to conduct an investigation on a dossier presented, REACH establishes that the ECHA shall perform such a check on a selected sample of dossiers, representing not less than 5 per cent of the total number of dossiers submitted for each tonnage band.[74] The Commission, after having consulted the ECHA, may vary the 5 per cent minimum by deciding through regulatory procedure with scrutiny (RPS).[75] However, given the pace at which the ECHA is fulfilling the 5 per cent obligation,[76] it is unlikely that the percentage is going to be increased in the near future. Arguably, a decision to subject all or part of potential dossiers for the registration of nanoscale chemicals to compliance check shall be taken through the regulatory procedure with scrutiny. Still, considering the evaluation is based on the data submitted with the registered dossiers, the lack of a legal obligation in REACH to specifically register the nanoform of a chemical suggests that the 5 per cent rule can hardly be enforced for chemicals of this nature. The compliance check of this category of substances becomes hence almost impossible. What the ECHA could perhaps do in the current text of REACH is to employ the prerogatives it has regarding the request of further testing pursuant to Article 41(3) of REACH. It can thus be imagined that the Agency might prepare a draft decision requiring registrant(s) to submit specific information, in case

- Of dossier(s) referring to both the nano and the bulk form of a chemical substance and when the registrant falls short of the indication to provide specific data on the nanoform, in line with the nano-specific indications contained in the Guidance Documents issued by the ECHA;[77]
- There is sufficient indication that the registered substance might be a nanomaterial, in spite of the absence of a clear statement in the registered dossier.

Even if the REACH legal text does not contain any reference to nano-chemicals, it is currently possible for registrants to inform the Agency of the fact that a certain nano-chemical is in nanoscale. This can be done by clicking the 'nano' box in the IUCLID. IUCLID 6 is a software tool used to store data on the hazardous properties of chemicals and to prepare and submit registration dossiers, in line with REACH legal obligations.[78] It must be stressed here that the current developments in REACH indicate that the ticking of the nano-box is done mostly voluntarily. According to the current practice, a nanosubstance can be registered either as a substance on its own or as form and/or multiple forms/compositions of a bulk substance.[79] A search of the IUCLID data entered for nanomaterials yields a remarkable shortage of data and dossiers (five in total) submitted for this category of substances.

According to the ECHA's 2013 report on Evaluation:

> ECHA has performed a number of compliance checks on dossiers covering, or suspected to be covering nanomaterials. These compliance checks have targeted the information requirements on substance identity and granulometry. Three final decisions had been sent in 2013 on dossiers covering nanomaterials, and the registrants have complied with these decisions. This demonstrates that *REACH applies to nanomaterials and can enable the generation of new data on these substances.* ... The outcome of these decisions will be published on ECHA's website as best practice examples.[80]

To this end, there have been three published reports of the Group Assessing Already Registered Nanomaterials (GAARN). Of note is the fact that such reports do not disclose the identity of the nano-chemicals subject to the evaluation in question.[81] The purpose of the GAARN is

> to build a consensus in an informal setting on best practices for assessing and managing the safety of nanomaterials under the REACH Regulation and thereby increase confidence and mutual understanding among stakeholders so that nanomaterials can be sustainably developed.[82]

The GAARN documents provide suggestions on how to conduct risk assessment of nano-chemicals in REACH. They conclude with 'the reminder of the legal obligation that registration dossiers need to be updated with new nano-specific studies as scientific developments are progressing'.[83] However, these documents take on the traits of friendly advice instead of a legally binding set of rules. Indeed, authoritative commentators have asked when the ECHA is going to enforce the obligations so clearly summarised in the GAARN reports.[84] Before elaborating on the concrete powers of ECHA to 'do more' about nano-chemicals within the range of powers and options the Agency is endowed with under REACH, it is important to turn our attention first to the existing criteria for compliance check in order to investigate their suitability for nano-chemicals.

Compliance-checking criteria

ECHA can make use of the following criteria in order to perform compliance checking:

1 *Legal criteria* for prioritisation of evaluating dossiers are laid down in Article 41(5). In accordance with this provision, the ECHA can evaluate the status of the substances (phase-in), the correct tonnage of production, the subsistence of CMR, PBT, vPvB, and other hazardous properties. In addition to this, dossiers concerning substances listed on the CoRAP [Community Action Rolling Plan] shall be prioritised.[85] In case of pre-registered substances,[86] Article 41(6) foresees the possibility for third parties to submit information; the dossier in question will as a consequence be prioritised in case:

    • The information submitted by third parties is contradictory to information in the dossier but may influence the outcome of the chemical safety assessment;
    • Or – the third party information addresses issues not yet considered in the dossiers(s) but may influence the outcome of the chemical safety assessment.[87]

The submitted information has to be reliable and relevant and 'can be any information pertaining to inherent properties, uses, worker, consumer and/or environmental exposure (incl. monitoring data) or fate'.[88] Arguably, NGOs or other scientific bodies could approach the ECHA with information on the nanoscale properties of a phase-in substance which might have been registered with no safety data on the nanoscale. In this case however, third parties bear the burden of demonstrating:

    • That the information on the nanoscale is of such relevance as to determine the outcome of the chemical safety assessment. Third parties shall in other words demonstrate the toxicity of the nanoform as compared to the registered bulk substance;

- Other causes for concern, provided they can prove a direct correlation between the reduction in nanoform and the emergence of such concerns.

Clearly, in a situation of great scientific uncertainty and insufficient testing methodologies for understanding toxicological profiles of nano-chemicals, it is unlikely that someone will contact the ECHA in order to submit additional information of this sort. Demonstrating how nano-related properties and data – not provided in the registration dossier which does not mention the nanoscale – are able to change the outcome of a CSA, is not a reasonable option in times of nanotoxicology and regulatory instruments shrouded in uncertainty.

2   *Random and concern driven criteria.* In the ECHA's view: 'random selection is considered the best means to render the selection of a registration dossier for compliance check unpredictable for a registrant and thus will help to ensure that the quality of the submitted dossiers increases over time'.[89]

Therefore, the random selection of dossiers allows the Agency to gather experience on typical reasons for non-compliance, which can then be employed for setting target criteria for the evaluation of problematic dossiers.[90] It must be noted that the Agency, in the first year after the enactment of REACH, could only use the random checking criteria, besides the legal ones laid down in Article 41(5)(a)–(c). The rationale behind this choice was that it would ensure the unpredictability of the ECHA's action, which in turn, was thought to encourage the submission of high quality dossiers. In addition, Article 41(7) substantiates that the Commission, acting through the regulatory procedure with scrutiny, may take a decision to 'amend or include further criteria in paragraph 5 [of Article 41] in accordance with the procedure referred to in Article 133(4)'. Hence, the Commission could in principle decide to

- increase/eliminate the 5 per cent threshold for dossiers referring to the nanoscale;
- establish that the existence of the nanoform alone (either on its own or as part of a dossier on the bulk substance) is sufficient to trigger prioritisation for evaluation under the compliance check.

Currently the ECHA can decide to evaluate dossiers where there is cause for concern. This includes substances with known or expected CMR, PBT, vPvB properties, sensitisers, substances which are hazardous for the environment, and substances with a high potential for exposure. In addition, administrative inconsistencies and anomalies within the dossier, or a combination of several concerns can trigger evaluation.[91] In this case though, the obligation to justify the compliance check on concern-related issues is on the ECHA and REACH does not offer any indication on how and to what extent the discretion can be exercised by the Agency.

Arguably, the ECHA might base the evaluation of dossiers referring to or suspected to refer to nanoscale hazardous chemicals, on the same criteria. However, in this case too the ECHA will have to justify in the light of REACH provisions, why such dossiers ought to undergo evaluation. The following section explains why this is the case.

ECHA's power in requesting additional information for nanosubstances

In order to better illustrate the powers of the ECHA to request nano-specific information under the existing text of REACH, the TiO_2 case and its recent settling by the ECHA's BoA is significant. The case concerns a 2014 decision by the ECHA to request for additional information on a TiO_2 registration dossier, adopting a decision pursuant to the procedure set out in Articles 50 and 51 of REACH. The dossier in question was submitted by Tioxide Europe Limited. The ECHA found that the registrants did not comply with the requirements of Article 10(a)(ii) of REACH as well as with Annex VI, section 2 and, as a result, requested the registrant to provide information concerning the *name and other identifiers of the substance, composition of the substance, and description of analytic methods used.*

The Appellants contested the decision on the basis that it

> is unlawful in so far as it requires the update of the Substance registration dossier with specific information related to phases of the Substance, *nano-forms*, and *surface treatment of nanoforms*, as part of the Substance identification information.[92]

The Appellants appealed directly to the current loopholes of REACH, namely the lack of any reference to the nanoform in both the legal text and the Annexes. The ECHA had, in the view of the Appellants, requested 'significantly more detailed information than is requested in Annex VI, Section 2'.[93] Hence, the Agency had, again in the Appellant's view, breached the principle of proportionality and infringed REACH in that such request had resulted in a manifest error of assessment. In addition, the appellants pointed out that their dossier on TiO_2 complied with the REACH requirements also with regard to the available GD on the identification and naming of the substances. It is true then that the GD on the *identification and naming of substances* does not offer guidance on nano-chemicals. What is more, it clearly stated that 'the current state of development is not mature enough to include guidance on the identification of substances in the nanoform in this GD'.[94]

As a consequence, there might be a real difficulty for the industry due to the lack of clear and standard parameters guiding the identification process in the case of nano-chemicals. With that being said, it must be recalled that industry has not been a great supporter of nano-amendments in REACH, holding that the current framework is generally capable of dealing with such chemicals as it currently is. Therefore, it seems more plausible to assume that the industry is trying to use the deadlock REACH has created in terms of enforceable legal duties to register and test nanomaterials, so as to get nano-forms of widely used substances commercialised without specifically testing the safety of the nanoform. This might allow circumventing REACH's obligations without in practice infringing the legal dictate of the Regulation.

In such a situation the ECHA's decision to request addition information on nanoforms would seem like the only way to know whether the substance in question is in nanoform. Yet, the ECHA decision was not upheld by its BoA. The reasoning of the BoA in annulling the ECHA decision on TiO_2 is significant: The ECHA, the BoA held, did not have the competence to ask nanomaterial-specific information on substance identification requirements under Section 2 of Annex VI, which is silent on nanosubstances. This is because neither the ECHA nor the BoA are in a position to interpret REACH in such a way as to amend or extend it. It is the legislature, the BoA concluded, that would need to amend the REACH Annexes accordingly, in case it sees a need for further information on the nanoforms.[95] As this specu-lation remains such, the possibility that a widely produced nano-chemical like TiO_2 might be actually used in nanoform without complying with safety requirements and (eco)toxicity data requirements in REACH, is alarming from an environmental protection standpoint.

The second example concerns another decision by the ECHA requesting information on the nanoform of registered surface-treated *silicon dioxide* (SAS), this time under substance evaluation in the CoRAP procedure, which was also annulled by the BoA (see the following).

Substance evaluation

One of the main reasons for adopting REACH was the slow and burden-some procedure governing the risk assessment of chemicals under the prec-edent chemical laws. The pre-REACH system placed this burden almost entirely on regulators, with the consequence that very few chemicals were fully assessed. The lack of data on chemical properties constitutes the major reason for the failure to assess and manage the risks to humans and the environment. It should be recalled that the previous chemical policy was essentially articulated in four phases: data collection, priority setting, risk assessment, and measures for risk reduction. From 1994 to 2001, the Com-mission passed four priority lists containing 140 existing substances to be assessed. By 2001, when the REACH proposal was being discussed, Member States had submitted a draft proposal for 88 of the 140 substances, and a complete risk assessment was concluded for only 56 substances.[96] Hence, making industry responsible for data generation and risk assessment is at the core of the paradigm shift operated by REACH. Nevertheless, MSs are still to some extent responsible for carrying out risk assessments, with the difference this time that RA will be based on the data provided by industry during the registration process.

Another feature inherited from the past system is that of prioritising. Article 44(1) foresees the possibility for the ECHA, in collaboration with MSs, to elaborate criteria for prioritisation of substances to be evaluated. Such criteria are generally risk-based, having particular regard for exposure information and the (overall) tonnage of production.[97] However, a certain margin for also taking into account intrinsic properties of chemicals, i.e. hazardousness, is offered by Article 41(1)(a).[98] It can be argued that nano-chemicals, especially those of low tonnage of production, might be prioritised using the criteria set out in Article 41(1)(a), while for HPV nanosubstances the legal basis for prioritisation would be Article 41(1)(b)(c).

The ECHA shall adopt a draft on substances to be prioritised, covering a period of three years and establishing substances to be evaluated each year. Information on risk to humans and the environment shall guide the ECHA's decision on this point. This first step is therefore hazard-based. Dossier evaluation results, information provided by registrants, or other appropriate sources might be used to determine such a risk. Such a list constitutes the draft of the CoRAP. Nevertheless, the burden of obtaining the relevant information indicating human and environmental risks is placed on the ECHA. Yet it remains unclear whether it is only the demonstration of actual risk that can determine the inclusion of a substance in the CoRAP or if, as is suggested in Article 44(1)(a), hazard-based considerations can also be employed. The need for clarity on this point directly affects the possibility for the ECHA to prioritise substances in nanoscale, because whereas for obtaining information on the hazardousness of certain nano-chemicals the ECHA could rely on scientific articles and studies performed outside REACH, in order to determine 'risk', the Agency must rely on data submitted with the registration dossier in order to determine volumes of productions and exposure. In both cases, however, the lack of a legal duty to separately register nano-chemicals negatively affects the ECHA's powers in prioritising chemicals in nanoscale: unlike authorisation and restriction, registration is a prerequisite of substance evaluation.

The draft adopted by the ECHA officially turns into a CoRAP only when the Member State Committee (MSC) issues a positive opinion in merit.[99] Substances listed in the CoRAP will be evaluated by MS CAs or pertinent institutions appointed for the occasion, in line with specific procedural rules outlined by REACH.[100] Among the situations that the rules in question deal with is the case where no MS is willing to evaluate a certain chemical on the CoRAP. In that eventuality, the ECHA shall ensure[101] that the substance is nevertheless evaluated. A hypothesis could be raised here with regard to potential nanosubstances included in a CoRAP. Given that MSs have 12 months (either from the start of the evaluation or, in case additional information was required from the registrant, after the submission of said information)[102] to evaluate an assigned substance, and given the complexity of assessing risks of nanosubstances in general, meeting this deadline might be highly problematic. The consequence would be that at the current state of the art, potential evaluations of chemicals in nanoscale will most likely fail due to 'exceeded term' for evaluation with the need to re-start the procedure all over again.

This assumption seems to find support in the overview on the presence of nano-chemicals in the CoRAP so far adopted. The CoRAP covering the period 2012–2014 listed *nano silicon dioxide* and *nano silver* to be evaluated by the Netherlands within 2012 and 2013, respectively.[103] In the following updated CoRAP for the period 2013–2015, only *nano silver* appeared on the list, with an extended deadline.[104] It can be speculated that due to the procedural rule of the 12-month period, the appointed MS had either requested further information, or simply failed to perform an evaluation within the deadline. Both nano silver and nano silicon dioxide had been added to the list due to the suspected toxicity of their different forms and their widespread use in consumer products. Interestingly, the CoRAP draft for the 2015–2017 period made no mention of *nano silver*. *Zinc oxide* and *Multi-Wall Carbon Nanotubes (MWCNTs)* represented the new entries to be evaluated by Germany, respectively within 2016 and 2017. Germany was also supposed to evaluate *nano cerium oxide* by 2017, while France did not manage to evaluate *titanium dioxide* by the established deadline of 2015.[105] The latest CoRAP draft contains two nanosubstances: the MWCNTs, synthetic graphite in tubular shape, already in CoRAP; and nano cerium dioxide. Both are expected to be evaluated by Germany within 2019 and 2020, respectively.[106]

Substance evaluation is of significant regulatory importance since the outcome of a substance evaluation procedure can be used by MS CAs for Authorisation, Restriction, and classification and labelling purposes.[107] Therefore, for nanosubstances subject to substance evaluation, the difficulty of assessing information in relation to risk to humans and the environment combined with a tight 12-month timeframe to do so, might seriously impede the possibility to utilise the outcome in other programmes of REACH such as the Authorisation and Restriction of chemicals. While it is true that each single phase under REACH (Registration, Evaluation, Authorisation, and Restriction) can well be considered as a stand-alone programme, REACH remains a stepwise regulation, meaning that it is upheld by logical and practical connections between the four phases so that data obtained under one phase feed into and facilitate the fulfilment of the legal obligations stemming from the consecutive phases. For nanosubstances, this stepwise approach is difficult to envisage and the above-mentioned hindrances in the evaluation process suggest that the REACH requirements are likely to operate intermittently, rather than as a continuum. This is much owed to the upstream shortcomings and the loopholes which have the potential to produce a domino effect in the enforcement of the subsequent provisions.

Overall, the prioritisation of substances to be evaluated is predominately a risk-based procedure, although a hazard-based approach is not completely ruled out.[108] MSs have considerable discretion in the evaluation process, including the right to require additional information from the registrant(s). It is reasonable to assume that the required information will respect general EU principles with the proportionality principle as a minimum. Therefore the question is: can MS CAs request information on nano-specific properties if a chemical on the CoRAP is suspected to be in nanoscale? A closer look at the procedure can help answer this question.

When an MS wants to include a certain chemical in the CoRAP for evaluation on the premise that it poses a risk to human health and the environment and hence necessitates prioritisation, the MS shall notify the Agency. REACH suggests that in doing so, the MS shall provide the information in its possession suggesting why such substance demands inclusion in the CoRAP. The ECHA, based on an opinion from MS Committee, shall decide whether to include the substance in the list. Either the MS who decided to include the substance in the CoRAP, or another MS who agrees, must evaluate the substance.[109] The evaluation shall be based on all the available information submitted on the substance in question and both of the other evaluations under title VI (dossier evaluation, compliance check). However, in order to ensure coherence in the evaluation process, Article 74 of REACH foresees that in case an evaluation decision has been previously taken, the request for additional information under Article 46 'may be justified only by a change of circumstances or acquired knowledge'. The registrant has nevertheless the right to appeal the decision for additional information to the ECHA's BoA, in case it finds that the request breaches REACH.[110] It is unclear whether the requirement of additional information on the nanoscale of a substance that has been previously evaluated (and especially when such substance has not been deemed an SVHC), is at the complete discretion of the MS or whether, in accordance with Article 47(1), the MS shall justify its request by providing information in its possession. In the second case, the burden placed on the MS is considerable, and such path is unlikely to yield significant results in terms of evaluation for nanoscale chemicals or nanoforms of existing/evaluated bulk chemicals.

Whenever reaching a decision to include a substance on the CoRAP, the MS shall document its conclusion and inform the ECHA on how it intends to use the information in regard to:

- the preparation of an authorisation dossier (pursuant to Article 59(3));
- the preparation of a restriction proposal (pursuant to Article 69(4));
- CLP purposes.

At this point the ECHA shall serve as intermediary between the interested registrant/downstream user and the MS who took the decision in question, facilitating the flow of information between these subjects. As in the case of dossier evaluation, registrants who cannot provide the required information have an 'emergency exit': they can inform the Agency of a decision to cease production. Hence, a producer/registrant reached by a request for additional information in case of a nano-scale chemical, could choose to opt out of the REACH system by ending the production of such a chemical.

However, the responses to the ECHA's requests for additional information on the nanoform have been rather different. A case in point here is that of synthetic amorphous silica (SAS), mentioned in the previous section. The decision to include SAS, a form of silicon dioxide (SiO_2) in the CoRAP was taken by the ECHA on the request of the Netherlands CA, which was evaluating the substance. Of note here is the fact that the evaluation from the Netherlands REACH Competent Authority was 'targeted to the characterisation of the substance, human health hazard assessment in relation to the inhalation route and exposure assessment of the registered synthetic amorphous silica'.[111]

The decision required the registrant to provide a considerable set of data and was grounded on the fact that 'only the Registrant(s) of the substance know the details of each of its forms necessary for their characterisation'. In the statement of reasons accompanying the decision, the ECHA justifies its request for data on the fact that the safety of SAS is not assessed for the nanoform and rejects the registrants' claim that it can be derived by the safety assessment of the bulk material. ECHA rejects also the claims that given its long history of use, SAS is to be considered safe. Hence 'although SAS may have been produced and marketed for decades, this does *not* provide a guarantee that SAS is a safe substance during its whole life cycle'.[112]

The text of the ECHA decision clearly demonstrates the regulatory struggle over nanomaterials under the nano-silent framework of REACH. The Agency repetitively points at the need for (eco)toxicity data on the specific and different nanoforms of the SAS. In line with the emerging principles of nanotoxicology, which establish that the toxicity profiles of chemicals in nanoscale are determined by parameters other than mass – for example, the surface area, the number-size distribution, the exact size of the nanomaterial, the surface reactivity and coating, etc. – the ECHA demanded specific tests to be conducted on these very specific parameters.

However, as the first part of this chapter illustrated, performing specific tests on nanomaterials under the current set of REACH provisions and its implementing regulation on testing methodologies might be an arduous task for a registrant. In some cases, testing on specific endpoints simply might not be materially possible due to the lack of validated materials and methodologies. It is therefore no surprise that the immediate reaction from the producers/registrants of SAS was to oppose the ECHA decision. Two cases were filed in this regard.[113] Among others, the appellants' argument for opposing the decision included the fact that

> [t]he Agency has based its decision very largely on its own classification of SAS as a nanomaterial, a classification that the Agency is not empowered to make and that in any event is irrelevant to the toxicity of SAS.[114]

Like in the TiO_2 case, the industry seems to appeal to the loopholes of REACH with regard to nano-chemicals' absence in REACH in order to avoid the difficult, expensive, and sometimes simply unavailable testing studies on the specific toxicity related to the nanoscale. This decision as well was annulled by the

BoA,[115] on the reasoning that the Agency had not demonstrated how the information on the nanoform would clarify the potential concerns identified on SAS, and thus breaching the principle of proportionality.[116] In other words, the BoA deemed the mere fact of a substance being in nanoform insufficient to justify a concern that could trigger substance evaluation. By so deliberating, the BoA made it clear that the burden to demonstrate the risk posed by the sole fact of the substances being nanoform, still lies with the ECHA in a situation where nothing in REACH refers to nanosubstances.[117] Importantly for the argument of this section, the applicants had also claimed that the decision to include the substance in the CoRAP was consequently illegal. The BoA declared this last claim inadmissible and dismissed it as it found that it was incompetent to decide on appeals against decisions to include substances on the CoRAP.[118]

Such decision is of crucial importance, since the evaluation of substances on the CoRAP is particularly relevant for the subsequent phases of REACH, such as Authorisation and Restriction. Nevertheless, the vital role played by the evaluation of a chemical (including for nano-chemicals) on CoRAP is impaired by the legal quibbles of the Evaluation phase which is highly, if not completely, dependent on Authorities' (the ECHA, MS CAs) ability to prove risks. This view seems to be confirmed also by the fact that even after a notification of ceased production pursuant Article 50(2)(3) of REACH, the ECHA still detains the power to ask for additional information if

- a competent authority prepares an Annex XV dossier concluding that there is potential long-term risk to human health or the environment justifying the need for further information;
- the exposure to the substance contributes significantly to such risk.[119]

As the number of suggested SVHCs to be prioritised might be very high, the ECHA shall establish clear criteria for prioritising substances to be included in the Candidate List. According to Article 58(3) ECHA shall prioritise substances that display PBT or vPvB properties or those having a widespread use or being produced in high volumes. Clearly, the intrinsic hazardous properties of certain chemicals combined with relevant quantity of production are used here as a proxy for potential risk to human health and the environment. However, for the very nature of nano-chemicals, such criteria are unlikely to help their evaluation on the CoRAP.

As we shall see in the following chapter, this might negatively affect the ability of stricter REACH regimes, such as Authorisation and Restriction, to successfully target nanoscale chemicals.

Summing up

This chapter has shown that the ECHA plays a central role in the correct implementation of the REACH obligations and in ensuring that the quality of data submitted under the Registration phase is appropriate and in line with what is required by the REACH provisions. As will be shown in Chapters 5–6 the quality of submitted data is particularly relevant for triggering of the application of stricter measures under Authorisation and Restriction for chemicals of concern. However, as far as nanoscale chemicals are concerned, the ECHA has virtually no powers to request registrants to provide information specific to the nanoform, if the registrants fail do so in their registration dossier. The BoA made this clear in the TiO_2 and the SAS annulments, where it ruled that the powers the Agency has in regards to REACH are broad but not unlimited. The Agency is bound by the text of REACH and cannot interpret it so as to extend its meaning or request information that the text does not mandate it to, like on the nanoform of registered substances. What is more, the ECHA cannot base the request for more data on the sole premise of the substance being in nanoform. Rather, it needs to demonstrate why the nanoform poses a risk that justifies the request for additional information. In other words, the burden of proof lies with the Agency. This situation might change with the coming into force of the amendments to the REACH Annexes, which will lay out specific requirements for the nanoforms of registered substances. Starting from 2020, the ECHA will arguably see its prerogatives in requesting additional information on the nanoform of registered substances strengthened – something that will hopefully compel the producers of such substances to include said information in the registration dossiers now, as a failure to do so will most likely be challenged by the ECHA in the rightful exercise of its powers, once it will be enabled by the newly modified Annexes to do so, i.e. from 2020 on.

However, for nanosubstances not subject to Registration (i.e. produced in quantities lower than the minimum threshold of $1 \, t/y$), doubt and questions persist. It is therefore important to investigate the applicability to nanosubstances of the third phase of REACH, the Authorisation phase, which has at its core a primarily *hazard-based* and *tonnage-free* model of regulation, in theory ideal for the regulatory needs of nanoscale substances. This investigation will take place in the following chapter.

Notes

1 REACH, Articles 40–43.
2 REACH, Articles 44–48.
3 REACH, Article 49.
4 REACH Articles 40 and 41.
5 See Decision of the Board of Appeal of ECHA, Case A-005–2011 *Honeywell v ECHA* [2013] para 123.
6 REACH, Article 40(1); Note that from 1 June 2015, Directive 67/548/EEC was repealed and replaced by Council Regulation (EC) 1272/2008 of 16 December 2008 on classification, labelling and packaging of substances and mixtures, amending and repealing Directives 67/548/EEC and 1999/45/EC, and amending Regulation (EC) No. 1907/2006 [2008] OJ L353/1.
7 According to Article 40(1) of REACH, the examination of the testing proposals, as part of the DE procedure, is performed in accordance with both Annex IX – which deals with standard information for substances produced in quantities of

100 t/y or more – and Annex X, which deals with standard information foreseen for substances in quantities of 1,000 t/y or more.

8 REACH, Title III.
9 Royal Society for the Prevention of Cruelty to Animals (RSPCA UK) Information Paper 'Replacement of Animals in Safety Brighter Outlook?' (Date unknown) 3; REACH, Articles 13 (2), 138 (9).
10 Council Regulation (EC) 440/2008 of 30 May 2008 laying down test methods pursuant to Regulation (EC) No. 1907/2006 of the European Parliament and of the Council on the Registration, Evaluation, Authorisation and Restriction of Chemicals (REACH) [2008] OJ L142/1.
11 Ibid., recital (5).
12 Ibid., Article 2.
13 This results from the working of recital (5) of Regulation, (EC) No. 440/2008:

> The principles of replacement, reduction and refinement of the use of animals in procedures should be fully taken into account in the design of the test methods, in particular when appropriate validated methods become available to replace, reduce or refine animal testing.

14 Katinka van der Jagt, Sharon Munn, Jens Tørsløv, and Jack de Bruijn (eds) 'Alternative Approaches Can Reduce the Use of Test Animals under REACH: Addendum to the Report: Assessment of Additional Testing Needs under REACH Effects of (Q)SARS, Risk Based Testing and Voluntary Industry Initiatives' (European Commission JRC 2004) 17.
15 Ibid. 18.
16 Council Directive 2010/63/EU of 22 September 2010 on the protection of animals used for scientific purposes [2010] L 276/33.
17 REACH, Article 25(1) and Annex VI (STEP-4).
18 The information gap concerned, in the case in question, Section 8.6.4 of Annex X of REACH.
19 Case A-005–2011 (n 5), para 90.
20 Article 13(1) of REACH; see in general ECHA, 'The Use of Alternatives to Testing on Animals for the REACH Regulation, Third Report under Article 117(3) of the REACH Regulation' (ECHA-17-R-02-EN June 2017).
21 ECHA, 'Guidance on Information Requirements and Chemical Safety Assessment Chapter R.6: QSARs and Grouping of Chemicals' (May 2008) 9.
22 Ibid. 10.
23 Ibid.
24 Ibid. 9, emphasis added.
25 Ibid.
26 Ibid. 11.
27 OECD, 'Principles for the Validation, for Regulatory Purposes, of (Quantitative) Structure-Activity Relationships Models' (November 2004).
28 Ibid.
29 SCENIHR, 'The Appropriateness of the Risk Assessment Methodology in Accordance with the Technical Guidance Documents for New and Existing Substances for Assessing the Risks of Nanomaterials' (21–22 June 2007) 48.
30 Ibid. 61.
31 Ibid. 39.
32 See Ceyda Oksel and Xue Z. Wang, 'Quantitative Structure-Activity Relationships (QSAR) Models' www.qualitynano.eu/uploads/School2013/Training-Materials/7.QSARs-Lecture_CeydaOksel.pdf accessed 19.02.2019.
33 OECD, 'Guidance on Grouping of Chemicals, Second Edition, Series on Testing & Assessment No. 194' (ENV/JM/MONO(2014)4, 14 April 2014) 11–12.

34 Ibid. 18.
35 An important part of the debate surrounding the usage of read-across techniques as an alternative testing method under REACH is that on the acceptance of extrapolation and/or interpolation of data within the same category of chemicals. This debate is relevant in the light of producer's responsibility and burden of proof concepts, as the two concepts (extrapolation and interpolation) require different amounts of data to be generated upstream, before the possibility to perform a read-across and consequently avoid testing on animals. However, the ECHA is more prone to considering a step-wise approach, requiring that read-across methods in REACH supplement shortcomings of other non-testing methods. Two decisions from ECHA BoA, Case A-001–2012 *Dow v ECHA* [2012] and Case A-006–2012 *Momentive Specialty Chemicals v ECHA* [2012], upheld the ECHA's rejection of read-across procedures submitted by the applicants. Such decisions have been questioned under the consistency profile, since, especially in the *Dow* case the BoA decided not to investigate the appellant's choice for read-across under the scientific profile. Contrary to this, in the previous Case A-005–2011 *Honeywell v ECHA* [2011], the BoA carefully scrutinised the scientific aspects of the case and provided advice on implementation and application of testing suggestions. A discussion on consistency issues can be found at: http://chemicalwatch.com/16541/ngo-platform-minimising-animal-testing-under-reach accessed 22.02.2019.
36 ECHA 2008 (n 21) 66.
37 SCENIHR 2007 (n 29), EFSA, 'The Potential Risks Arising from Nanoscience and Nanotechnologies on Food and Feed Safety' (2009) 958 The EFSA Journal 1.
38 Commission, 'Regulatory Aspects of Nanomaterials' (Communication) COM(2008) 366 final; Commission, 'Second Regulatory Review on Nanomaterials' (Communication) COM(2012) 572 final; Commission, 'Types and Uses of Nanomaterials, Including Safety Aspects' (Staff Working Document) SWD (2012) 288 final.
39 OECD, ENV/JM/MONO(2014)4 (n 33) 104.
40 Case C-14/10 *Nickel Institute* [2011] ECLI:EU:C:2011:503, para 70.
41 ECHA, 'Guidance on Information Requirements and Chemical Safety Assessment, Appendix R8–15 Recommendations for Nanomaterials Applicable to Chapter R.8 Characterisation of Dose [Concentration] – Response for Human Health' (ECHA-12-G-09-EN, May 2012) 7.
42 Ibid.
43 ECHA, 'Guidance on Information Requirements and Chemical Safety Assessment, Appendix R10–2 Recommendations for Nanomaterials Applicable to Chapter R.10 Characterisation of Dose [Concentration] – Response for Environment' (ECHA-12-G-10-EN, May 2012) 4.
44 Lucas Bergkamp and Nicolas Herbatschek, 'Information and Data Sharing Requirements' in Lucas Bergkamp (ed.), *The European Union REACH Regulation for Chemicals Law and Practice* (OUP 2013) 215.
45 An early reference to the *Weight of Evidence* approach is found in SCENIHR 2007 (n 29) 58, which states that when there is a considerable body of knowledge on the low toxicity of the chemical in bulk form, the negative findings from *in vitro* studies on the toxicity of the same chemical in nanoform, shall be 'weighted' to eventually decide whether to use limited or no additional *in vivo* testing at all.
46 Progress is being made regarding the development of in *vitro* methods. See in general Hanna L. Karlsson et al. 'Mechanism-based Genotoxicity Screening of Metal Oxide Nanoparticles Using the *ToxTracker* Panel of Reporter Cell Lines', (2014) 11:41 Particle and Fibre Toxicology 1.

47 *In silico* is a term that refers to anything that can be done through a computer in toxicology, including (Q)SARs. In merit, see Hannu Raunio, 'In Silico Toxicology – Non-Testing Methods' (2011) 2 Article 33 Front Pharmacol 1.

48 Commission (Draft Regulation) (EU) .../... of XXX amending Regulation (EC) No. 1907/2006 of the European Parliament and of the Council on the Registration, Evaluation, Authorisation and Restriction of Chemicals (REACH) as regards Annexes I, III, VI, VII, VIII, IX, X, XI, and XII to address nanoforms of substances, XXX [...] (2017) XXX draft, Annex Ares(2017) 4925011–09/10/2017, Annex XI, point 8 (a)–(f), 22–24.

49 ECHA, 'Appendix R.6–1 for nanomaterials applicable to the Guidance on QSARs and Grouping of Chemicals' (ECHA-17-G-17-EN, May 2017).

50 OECD, 'Case Study on Grouping and Read-Across for Nanomaterials Genotoxicity of Nano-TiO$_2$', ENV/JM/MONO(2018)28 8.

51 Karin Aschberger et al., 'Grouping of Multi-Walled Carbon Nanotubes to Read-Across Genotoxicity: A Case Study to Evaluate the Applicability of Regulatory Guidance' (2019) 9 Computational Toxicology 22.

52 https://euon.echa.europa.eu/view-article/-/journal_content/title/new-case-study-on-using-echa-s-read-across-guidance-for-multi-walled-carbon-nanotubes accessed 19.02.2019.

53 REACH, Article 40(2).

54 In specific, ECHA, pursuant Article 40(2) shall publish on its website 'the name of the substance, the hazard end-point for which vertebrate testing is proposed, and the date by which any third party information is required'.

55 REACH, Article 40(2).

56 REACH, Article 40(2)(a)(b)(c).

57 REACH, Article 40(2)(d).

58 REACH, Article 40(2)(e).

59 Article 3(19) defines CAs as 'authorities or bodies established by the Member States to carry out the obligations arising from this Regulation'. There are 40 CAs operating in EU Member States and EFTA States, meaning that seven States have more than one CA. The Commission identified at least three different areas of responsibilities for each national institution nominated as CAs. Environmental responsibilities topped such a ranking. CAs take active part in the Commission Expert Group 'Competent Authorities for REACH and CLP (CARACAL)', the aim of which is to facilitate cooperation between CAs, the Commission, and ECHA on the implementation of REACH, in the respective areas of responsibility.

60 REACH, Article 51(2).

61 REACH, Article 51(4).

62 REACH, Article 51(5).

63 REACH, Article 51(6).

64 REACH, Article 51(7).

65 To date France, the Netherlands, Belgium, Sweden, Denmark, and Norway have adopted national schemes for reporting nanomaterials. However, the frameworks for such a report and the mandatory nature of the provisions therein vary significantly from state to state. See in general A.M. Ponce Del Castillo, 'The European and Member States' Approaches to Regulating Nanomaterials: Two Levels of Governance' (2013) 7 Nanoethics 189.

66 Case C-326/05 P *Industrias Químicas del Vallés v Commission* [2007] ECLI:EU:C:2006:751 and Case C-326/05 P – *Industrias Químicas del Vallés v Commission* [2007] ECLI:EU:C:2006:751 Opinion of AG Ruiz-Jarabo Colomer, paras 75–76; Case C-425/08 *Enviro Tech (Europe)* [2009] ECLI:EU:C:2009:635, para 47; Case C-15/10 *Etimine* [2011] ECLI:EU:C:2011:504, para 60 and Case T-96/10 *Rütgers Germany and Others v ECHA* [2013] ECLI:EU:T:2013:109, para 99.

67 Ibid., *Rütgers Germany and Others v ECHA*, para 134.
68 ECHA-17-R-02-EN (n 20) 50. Interestingly, other areas of priority where the ECHA underlines the need to be fully aware of the latest scientific developments before adopting adequate decisions under REACH are those of endocrine disrupters and the 'cocktail effect' of chemicals; both requiring considerations on toxicity that transcend dose-response relationships based on mass only.
69 SCENIHR 2007 (n 29) 30.
70 Ibid.
71 REACH, Article 41(1)(b).
72 REACH, Article 41(1)(d).
73 REACH, Article 41(3).
74 REACH, Article 41(5).
75 Article 41(7) of REACH clarifies that the procedure to be followed by the Commission for varying the 5 per cent minimum for compliance check, is that of Article 133(4) of REACH, which in turn refers to Article 5a(1)(4), 7 and 8 of Council Decision 1999/468/EC of 28 June 1999 laying down the procedures for the exercise of implementing powers conferred on the Commission [1999] OJ L184/23.
76 Biwer, citing the ECHA's Multi-Annual programme for 2013–2015, notes that the Agency foresees to reach the 5 per cent for dossiers submitted by 2010, by the end of 2013 and start evaluating dossiers submitted in 2013 only in 2014–2015. See Arno P. Biwer, 'Evaluation' in Dieter Drohmann and Matthew Townsend (eds) *REACH Best Practice Guide to Regulation (EC) No 1907/2006* (Beck/Hart 2013) 420.
77 Specifically, starting from 2012 the ECHA issued several Appendixes to the different chapters of the 'Guidance on Information Requirements and Chemical Safety Assessment', which can be found here: http://echa.europa.eu/guidance-documents/guidance-on-information-requirements-and-chemical-safety-assessment accessed 20.02.2019.
78 IUCLID is also fundamental to ECHA's and MS CA's activity because it serves among others, as: the central data repository for all dossiers submitted; the basis for evaluating the risks of substances and requiring new information and basis for restricting and authorising the use of chemicals to manage risk. The software is based on the OECD harmonised templates in order to ensure consistency and in addition complies with the requirements of HPV Chemicals programme, US HPV Challenge programme, Japan Challenge programme, and EU Biocides. See: http://iuclid.eu/index.php?fuseaction=home.faq#106 accessed 20.02.2019.
79 See in general ECHA, 'IUCLID Guidance and Support: Nanomaterials in IUCLID 5' (February 2013).
80 ECHA, 'Evaluation under REACH Progress Report 2014' (ECHA-15-R-03-EN, February 2015) 37–38. Note however that the ECHA, 'Evaluation under REACH Progress Report 2015' (ECHA-15-R-20-EN, February 2016) does not contain any reference to nanosubstances. The report from 2017 does instead refer both to nanomaterials and to the new documents adopted by ECHA in this regard: see 'Evaluation under REACH: Progress Report 2017. 10 Years of Experience' (ECHA-18-R-05-EN, February 2018).
81 'Nanomaterials' *(ECHA)* http://echa.europa.eu/regulations/nanomaterials accessed 20.02.2019; also see ECHA: 'Best Practices on Physicochemical and Substance Identity Information for Nanomaterials' (1st GAARN meeting 29 May 2012); 'Assessing Human Health and Environmental Hazards of Nanomaterials: Best Practice for REACH Registrants' (Second GAARN meeting Helsinki 21–22 January 2013); 'Human Health and Environmental Exposure Assessment and Risk Characterisation of Nanomaterials: Best Practice for REACH Registrants' (Third GAARN meeting Helsinki 30 September 2013).

82 ECHA (Second GAARN meeting Helsinki 21–22 January 2013) 4.
83 ECHA (Third GAARN meeting Helsinki 30 September 2013) 10.
84 'ECHA Publishes "Best Practice" for REACH Nano Registrants' (*CW*) https://chemicalwatch.com/19019/echa-publishes-best-practice-for-reach-nano-registrants accessed 20.02.2019.
85 See Biwer (n 76) 421.
86 'Pre-registered substances' (*ECHA*) https://echa.europa.eu/information-on-chemicals/pre-registered-substances accessed 20.02.2019.
87 ECHA 'Guidance on Priority Setting for Evaluation' (August 2008) 29.
88 Ibid.
89 Ibid. 30.
90 Ibid. 30.
91 Biwer (n 76) 423.
92 Announcement of Appeal Case A-011–2014 *Tioxide Europe Limited v ECHA* [2014] 2.
93 Ibid.
94 ECHA, 'Guidance for Identification and Naming of Substances under REACH and CLP' (ECHA-16-B-37.1-EN, May 2017) 36.
95 ECHA-18-R-05-EN (n 80) 61.
96 Ralf Nordbeck and Michael Faust, 'European Chemicals Regulation and its Effect on Innovation: An Assessment of the EU's White Paper on the Strategy for a Future Chemicals Policy' (2003) 13 European Environment 79, 82.
97 REACH, Article 41(b)(c).
98 Article 41(1)(a) states that prioritisation can also be based on considerations on:

> hazard information, for instance structural similarity of the substance with known substances of concern or with substances which are persistent and liable to bio-accumulate, suggesting that the substance or one or more of its transformation products has properties of concern or is persistent and liable to bio-accumulate.

99 REACH, Article 44(2).
100 See Article 45(1)(2)(3) of REACH.
101 REACH, Article 45(2). It remains unclear, however, whether it is for the Agency itself to carry out the evaluation of a substance that MSs are not willing to perform, or if the ECHA can somehow bring the MS to comply with evaluation obligations in this case.
102 REACH, Article 46(3)(4).
103 ECHA, 'Community Rolling Action Plan (CoRAP)' (29 February 2012).
104 ECHA, 'Community Rolling Action Plan (CoRAP) Update Covering Years 2013, 2014 and 2015' (20 March 2013).
105 See for more details: ECHA, 'Draft Community Rolling Action Plan (CoRAP) Update for Years 2016–2018' (28 October 2015).
106 ECHA, 'Draft Community Rolling Action Plan (CoRAP) Update for Years 2019–2021' (22 October 2018).
107 REACH, Article 48.
108 REACH, Article 44(1).
109 REACH, Article 45(5).
110 REACH, Article 51(8).
111 ECHA, 'Decision on Substance Evaluation: For Silicon Dioxide, CAS No 7631–86–9 (EC No 23 1–545–4)' (March 2015).
112 Ibid. 9.
113 Case A-015–2015 *Evonik and Others v ECHA* [2015] and Case A-014–2015 *Grace GmbH & Co. KG, Germany v ECHA* [2015].
114 Case A-014–2015 *Grace GmbH & Co. KG, Germany v ECHA* [2015] 2.

115 ECHA, Decision of the BoA, Case A-*015–2015* [2017].
116 BoA, 'Summary of Decision Case number: A-015–2015 (Substance evaluation – Nanomaterials – Potential risk – 'Forms' of a nanomaterial – Proportionality – Error of assessment – Article 25 – Legal certainty)' [2017] 2.
117 Ibid.
118 ECHA-18-R-05-EN (n 80) 61.
119 REACH, Article 50(4)(a)(b).

5   Authorisation

Introduction

This chapter deals with the status of nano-chemicals under the Authorisation procedure in REACH. Authorisation represents one of the two 'command-and-control' mechanisms of REACH (the other being Restriction), which empowers the EU authorities to restrict and/or ban hazardous chemicals. Such chemicals are referred to in Article 57 as *substances of very high concern* (SVHCs). SVHCs cannot be placed or used in the EU market, unless an authorisation has been granted. This category of substances is set out in Article 57 and includes

> *(a)–(c)* Substances which are carcinogenic, mutagenic or toxic to reproduction of category 1 or 2 (CMR);
>
> *(d)–(e)* Substances which are persistent, bioaccumulative and toxic and very persistent and very bioaccumulative (PBT and vPvB);
>
> *(f)* Substances – such as those having *endocrine disrupting properties* or those having persistent, bioaccumulative and toxic properties or very persistent and very bioaccumulative properties, which do not fulfil the criteria of points (d) or (e) – for which there is scientific evidence of probable serious effects to human health or the environment which give rise to an equivalent level of concern to those of other substances listed in points (a) to (e) and which are identified on a case-by-case basis in accordance with the procedure set out in Article 59.

Once SVHCs are included in Annex XIV of REACH, they are, as a general rule, prohibited unless otherwise authorised. The onus of proof is in this case inverted: it is for the registrant, and in some cases, for the downstream users, to prove either of the following:

*   The risk is adequately controlled in line with the provisions of Annex I Section 6.4 and the substance is not a PBT, vPvB, non-threshold or other substance of equivalent concern; or
*   The socio-economic benefits outweigh the risks and no suitable alternatives or technologies are available.[1]

As noted in Chapter 2, because of their stringent nature and the consequent potential to affect the free circulation and commercialisation of chemicals and chemical-based goods within the EU/EEA, Authorisation provisions might be at the centre of a divergent interpretation of REACH.[2] The approach MSs will take with respect to the provisions set forth for authorisation purposes in REACH, may hence vary in degree, with consequent variation of the extent to which stricter national policies on chemicals regulation can still be maintained/adopted in the post-REACH era. Given the uncertain status of nanoscale chemicals in REACH, questions on the admissibility of stricter national measures for this class of chemicals are likely to be even more accentuated when considering regulatory options for chemicals in nanoscale under the Authorisation phase of REACH. In the following part, the options currently available for nano-chemicals' consideration under the authorisation set of rules are discussed, in an attempt to investigate whether Authorisation could constitute a possible regulatory tool for controlling environmental and human health risks associated with chemicals in nanoscale.

General aim and overview

Authorisation's aim is

> to ensure the good functioning of the internal market while assuring that the risks from substances of very high concern are properly controlled and that these substances are progressively replaced by suitable alternative substances or technologies where these are economically and technically viable.[3]

In a nutshell, Authorisation stipulates that SVHCs cannot be placed on the market/used unless they are authorised by the Commission. The de facto prohibition of substances identified as of VHC and placed on the Annex XIV list, can be lifted by following one of two routes: the adequately controlled risks route and the socio-economic one.[4] The essence of this phase is a direct expression of the *substitution principle*, which was promoted as one of the cornerstone elements of REACH. Indeed, one of the aims of REACH, according to the White Paper of 2001, is 'to encourage the substitution of dangerous by less dangerous substances where suitable alternatives are available'.[5] The number of dangerous substances that needed to be phased out, such as CMRs and POPs, was estimated to be 1,400 at the time the WP was adopted.[6] However, after the adoption of REACH the phasing-out process proved to be much slower than predicted given that only 138 substances were included in the Candidate List for authorisation by 2014.[7] Nevertheless, it is this Chapter's argument that the Authorisation phase could, in principle, still offer a regulatory option for nanosubstances as substances of particular concern. Reasons for this include the possibility to evaluate and rule on a group of substances with similar characteristics; the lack of a minimum threshold for triggering authorisation; and the open-ended provision of Article 57(1)(f), which might allow a greater margin of discretion in the process of identification and inclusion of hazardous substances in the Candidate List.

Although placing nanosubstances under Authorisation's rule might represent a daunting task for regulators, legislative guidance and support might come from other recent regulations adopted on the EU level, specifically in the food law area. Sectoral-specific regulations, such as those concerning FCMs, already consider nano-substances used in their realm of application, the same way as they consider other dangerous substances corresponding to some extent to what REACH defines as SVHCs.[8] One inseparable trait of Authorisation is its impetus for substitution. The submission of an application for authorisation based on one of the two routes requires manufacturers/importers/downstream users to evaluate the existence of less harmful alternatives. Applicants are hence responsible not only for generating the data in accordance with the route chosen, but REACH tries to engage such subjects on the substitution principle front too, making them responsible for the assessment of the existence of more sustainable or 'greener' alternatives. When safer alternatives are technically possible and economically feasible, an authorisation of a SVHC *can* be denied. However, the socio-economic considerations that together with the availability and suitability of alternatives should be taken into account when evaluating an authorisation request, might severely impair the ability of Authorisation to deliver significant results in terms of substitution. If it is considered that the substances in question are already deemed 'of particular concern', the choice of tying their phasing-out and replacement to economic feasibility considerations is questionable from a precautionary standpoint. But as this section aims to elucidate, the environmental benefits stemming from Authorisation are due not so much to the finalisation of the procedure, but rather to the preliminary sub-phases that precede authorisation decisions, namely:

- the identification of SVHCs; and, particularly,
- the inclusion of SVHCs in the Candidate List for Authorisation.

Each preliminary sub-phase will be analysed in order to try to understand how the legal requirements they stipulate for different stakeholders, can contribute to the goal of high levels of protection for humans and the environment in relation to SVHCs risks. Before that, though, a closer look at the central concept of substitution is necessary in order to be able to appreciate its applicability to nanoscale substances.

The substitution principle: a tricky concept for nano-chemicals

Broadly speaking, the substitution principle (SP) is a principle of common sense; it requires that dangerous chemicals be replaced with less dangerous alternatives whenever this is economically feasible and technically possible. Drawing upon hazard rather than risk, it implements the precautionary principle in the sense there is no need to wait for the materialisation of harm to occur in order to replace a dangerous chemical.[9] The SP made its first appearance in the Swedish law on workers' health and safety in 1949 and was consolidated in the law on chemical products in 1990.[10] Sweden has been promoting the principle ever since, and starting from 1989 the SP has been incorporated in a number of European directives such as Directive EEC 89/391[11] on health and safety of works in general and Directive 98/24/EC[12] on risks related to chemical agents at work, in particular.[13]

In addition, starting from 1999, the SP has been formally adopted as a basis for regulating hazardous substances in Norway.[14] Enshrined in Article 3a of the Product Control Act,[15] the *substitusjonsplikt* (substitution duty) requires that any activity using a product that contains a chemical which may be hazardous to health or the environment, shall assess whether there exist less risky alternatives. The less risky alternatives shall be used if the costs or the inconvenience are not unreasonable.[16]

On the EU level, the adoption of the Sixth Environmental Action Program which was based on Article 192(3) TFEU, acquiring thus the status of source of law,[17] requested that 'chemicals that are dangerous should be substituted by safer chemicals or safer alternative technologies not entailing the use of chemicals, with the aim of reducing risks to man and the environment'.[18] As Ludwig Krämer points out, this 'clearly constitutes the recognition of the substitution principle in EU environmental law' with the consequence that this principle might influence the interpretation of Articles 34, 36, 114, 192 or 193 TFEU – the principal provisions used as legal bases for EU legislation.[19] For instance, the CJEU recalled the substitution principle when reviewing the Swedish national ban on trichloroethylene in the *Toolex* case.[20] The Court held that although the ban adopted by Sweden amounted to a measure having an effect equivalent to a quantitative restriction,[21] it was nevertheless proportionate in the sense of Article 36 TFEU. In reaching such a conclusion the Court referred, *inter alia*, to the substitution principle, 'which consists in the elimination or reduction of risks by means of replacing one dangerous substance with another, less dangerous substance'.[22] The Swedish measure did provide indeed for individual exemptions to the general ban in case no safe replacement for the trichloroethylene existed, and provided that the applicant continued to seek alternatives that are less harmful for the public health and the environment.[23] And yet, even in the eventuality of authorised exceptions, the exposure to the substance in question should be kept at acceptable levels, the Court held.[24]

Later, the White Paper on chemical policy made substitution one of the principal goals to be implemented in REACH.[25] However, it is relevant from an environmental protection standpoint to mention here the fact that the conceptualisation of the substitution principle incorporated in the final text of REACH is a watered-down version of the original idea. Instead of the mandatory obligation to phase out an SVHC in presence of safer alternatives envisaged in the original REACH proposal, now the availability of safer alternatives may only determine a refusal to authorise an SVHC.[26] Substitution this way conceptualised is today the very essence of Authorisation in REACH and remains one of the main aims of the regulation, as emerges in Title VII. Yet, operational difficulties remain. For instance, like in the case of the PP, an agreed definition on the SP is currently lacking.

A reference to the concept of substitution can found in the UN Agenda 21, which urges the Governments to

> Adopt policies and regulatory and non-regulatory measures to identify, and minimize exposure to, toxic chemicals by *replacing them with less toxic substitutes* and ultimately phasing out the chemicals that pose unreasonable and otherwise unmanageable risk to human health and the environment and those that are toxic, persistent and bioaccumulative and whose use cannot be adequately controlled.[27]

A more concise definition is given by the CEFIC:

> Substitution is the replacement of one substance by another with the aim of achieving a lower level of risk.[28]

A more detailed definition is offered by Hansson, Molander, and Rudden:

> If risks to the environment and human health and safety can be reduced by replacing a chemical substance, mixture or product either by another substance, mixture or product or by some non-chemical technology, then this replacement should be made. All decisions on such substitutions should be based on the best available evidence. This evidence can be sufficient to warrant a substitution even if it only consists of hazard information and quantitative risk estimates cannot be made.[29]

In addition to definitional issues, the concept of 'less dangerous alternative' is a disputed one. On the one side, the industry sector, through CEFIC's positions, maintains that an alternative shall consist of another *substance*, while Hansson, Molander, and Rudden take a more comprehensive view contending that 'non-chemical technology' could also represent a less dangerous alternative. REACH endorses the second approach, ruling that the safer alternative can consist of 'substances or technologies'.[30] Considerations on this point become interesting from a legal as well as a technical point of view, if the chemicals subject to Authorisation are in nanoscale. While some of their risks to human health and the environment are recognised by several scientific opinions,[31] their contextual potential for remedying environmental problems,[32] and improving human health,[33] is also claimed. As a way of example, the Commission, while recognising that some of the risks associated with manufactured nanosubstances are not well understood, comes nonetheless to the conclusion that

> the benefits of nanomaterials range from saving lives, breakthroughs enabling new applications or reducing the environmental impacts to improving the function of everyday commodity products.[34]

Also, the US Environmental Protection Agency (EPA) recognises that 'the rapid development of nanotechnology and the increasing production of nano-materials and nano-products present both opportunities and challenges'.[35] With regard to the benefits of nanotechnology, EPA holds that

> nanotechnology can create materials and products that will not only directly advance our ability to detect, monitor, and clean-up environmental contaminants, but also help us avoid creating pollution in the first place.[36]

Some examples include:

- Remediation/Treatment of contaminated sites: Nano zero valent iron has been tested, the EPA holds, to treat aqueous dissolved chlorinated solvents in situ, while Silica-titania nanocomposites can be used for elemental mercury removal from vapours such as those generated from combustion sources.
- Development of sensors which can be used to detect harmful agents in the environment even in very low concentrations.
- Applications that address long-term sustainability: green manufacturing using nanotechnology, the EPA states, may deliver more sustainable products since it may, for example, reduce the need to use solvents, hence suggesting a possible function in line with the substitution principle.
- Substitute the use of dangerous metals on the premise that

> with nanomaterials' increased material functionality, it may be possible in some cases to replace toxic materials and still achieve the desired functionality (in terms of electrical conductivity, material strength, heat transfer, etc.), often with other life-cycle benefits in terms of material and energy use.[37]

In the same document, however, a broad investigation of the risk for humans and the environment follows the EPA's illustration of nano-benefits. Of particular concern is also the fact that the environmental fate of nanomaterials is not well understood.[38] Interestingly, on biodegradation of nanosubstances, EPA holds that 'many of the nanomaterials in current use are composed of inherently nonbiodegradable inorganic chemicals, such as ceramics, metals and metal oxides, and are not expected to biodegrade'.[39] Problems arise also about bioaccumulation: 'Environmental fate processes may be too slow for effective removal of persistent nanomaterials before they can be taken up by an organism.'[40] It seems therefore that nanosubstances might take on the traits of both an environmental problem and of its very solution, depending on the case. Veerle Heyvaert suggests, after the *Toolex* decision, the CJEU has shown 'a willingness to lower the hurdles for compatibility with the requirements of necessity and proportionality if the national restriction under scrutiny is an application of a new environmental principle; the substitution principle'.[41] However, Heyvaert also warns of the difficulty of applying the substitution principle successfully since in some cases a hasty resort to substitution may result in lower rather than higher levels of protection.[42] This might be one of the dangers of substituting dangerous chemicals with nano-alternatives, without fully understanding the risks that have already been pointed out in Chapter 1.

Overall, nanotechnology and the products of its application, are indicated as new and emerging greener alternatives, capable of solving some of the most pressing environmental issues (i.e. energy, climate change, heavy metal contamination, etc.). Such promising green attributes are however inextricably linked to those very same intrinsic properties – scale, grater surface area, greater reactivity, etc. – which have been held responsible for environmental damages and human health risks. Therefore, the Janus-faced nature of nanotechnology must be taken into account when its substitutive potential is advocated.

An increasing number of scientific studies on the hazardous nature of nano-chemicals are showing that the toxicity profiles of some substances in nanoscale correspond largely to the CMR and PBT categories of SVHCs contemplated by Article 57 of REACH. However, Article 57 does not mention nano-chemicals. Two questions arise here:

1   What parameters can be used for identifying nano-chemicals in the light of Authorisation rules?
2   Is there a risk that nanosubstances or nano-based technologies, albeit shrouded in uncertainties, might be embraced too early and perhaps too enthusiastically as safe alternatives to traditional (e.g. bulk scale) SVHCs under the REACH Authorisation programme?

With regard to the identification issue, nothing in REACH is nano-specific. Most problematic is perhaps the unsuitability of substance definition in REACH for nanoscale chemicals. Hence, the way nanosubstances are regulated in some sectoral-specific Regulations outside REACH – most notably the EU Regulations on certain food contact materials (FCMs) – might offer an insight on what status to assign them under REACH in general, and the Authorisation phase in particular. Regulations on intelligent and active FCMs[43] and on plastic FCMs[44] treat nanomaterials the same way as other dangerous substances, stipulating stricter norms for their use. For instance, CMR substances should not be covered by the concept of the *functional barrier* (FB) endorsed by both Regulations at issue. The FB barrier is a layer used for separating the FCM from the food, in order to prevent the migration of substances from behind that barrier and into the food.[45] This is so because behind the FB, non-authorised substances may be used, provided that they fulfil certain criteria and that their migration into food remains below a given detection limit, established at a maximum of 0.01 mg/kg. However, both Regulations exclude substances classified as CMR from the concept of FB. Specific authorisation is needed if any CMR substance is to be used behind a FB.[46]

In addition, both Regulations state that

> New technologies that engineer substances in particle size that exhibit chemical and physical properties that significantly differ from those at a larger scale, for example, nanoparticles, should be assessed on a case-by-case basis as regards their risk until more information is known about such new technology.[47]

Hence, the intention to treat nanomaterials at the same level of substances of particular concern emerges clearly from this provision.[48] Given the legal coverage of nanomaterials under these two Regulations, the questions that arise with regard to the status of nanosubstances under REACH are:

- Will the classification or at least the indication of a particular concern, in line with the PP – which is clearly endorsed in the General Food Law[49] – influence nanosubstances' status in REACH, in line with the precautionary approach therein?
- Is this implied equation of nanosubstances to those of particular concern (such as CMRs in the FCMs area) alone able to create a pressure for substitution[50] under the REACH framework without the need to initiate an authorisation process for nanosubstances?

Although the EU legislator has tried to avoid overlapping between REACH and other sectoral legislation, points of contact exist and for certain articles, i.e. FCMs, producers shall comply both with REACH and sectoral-specific regulations. What is relevant here is the ability of Authorisation, as it currently stands, to capture nano-chemicals displaying SVHCs criteria. In the following, the role of different stakeholders in different sub-phases of Authorisation is analysed. As de Sadeleer points out, licensing or restricting chemicals on the national and EU level might directly influence the internal market functioning.[51] Therefore, Authorisation (and Restriction) phase(s) are likely to be hit by interpretative divergences and the case of nano-chemicals might offer a first example in this direction. Are MSs free to restrict nano-chemicals? What would be MSs' prerogatives in order to include nanosubstances in the Authorisation list? The attempt to answer these questions necessarily requires an analysis of the roles and powers of MSs, the ECHA, and the Commission in the long and twisted procedures that lead to Authorisation of chemicals under REACH.

General preliminary considerations on nano–chemicals under Article 57(f)

Ensuring a good functioning of the internal market while encouraging the phasing out of dangerous chemicals through substitution with less dangerous alternatives represents the primary aim of the Authorisation phase.[52] This book takes the view that, certainly not until the Annexes' amendments come into force in early 2020, nano–chemicals' regulation is not harmonised by REACH rule of law because, according to the criteria delineated in Article 128:

- nano–chemicals can hardly be said to fall within *the scope* of REACH;
- they do not *comply* with REACH requirements; and,
- nano–chemicals do not comply with other EU legislation adopted to *implement* REACH, one above all: the testing methodologies Regulation.[53]

Indeed, several MSs have adopted national schemes that require, as a minimum, the disclosure of data on the presence of nano–chemicals on the market and their use. Pioneering in this regard, France has passed a national law for making its national report scheme mandatory for all companies trading nanosubstances in the country.[54] Article 128(2) of REACH allows for MSs to introduce/maintain national measures on nano–chemicals, stipulating that

> Nothing in this Regulation shall prevent Member States from main-taining or laying down national rules to protect workers, human health and the environment applying in cases where this Regulation does not harmonise the requirements on manufacture, placing on the market or use.

Contrary to what some scholars contend,[55] as has been shown, REACH does not appear to harmonise nano–chemicals; not only because its technological-neutral provisions seem rather obsolete for regulating the products of an advanced technology, but also because nothing in REACH was drafted with nano–needs in mind. In addition, the aforementioned TiO_2 case and the reasoning of the CJEU in the *Toolex* case[56] make it difficult to consider REACH as fully harmonising chemicals law for the case of nano–chemicals.

Notwithstanding the existing loopholes, Authorisation might still be the best equipped REACH phase for curtailing nano–risks, given that during the negotiation of REACH there were suggestions advanced by the EU Parliament on the need to include nano–chemicals in the category of substances warranting authorisation. The EU Parliament's Committee on the Environmental, Public Health and Food Safety held that

According to 'Science', the very small size of nanomaterials can modify the physico-chemical properties and create the opportunity for increased uptake and interaction with biological tissues. This combination can generate adverse biological effects in living cells that would not otherwise be possible with the same material in larger form. According to SCENIHR, information about the biological fate of nanoparticles (e.g. distribution, accumulation, metabolism and organ specific toxicity) is still minimal.[57]

On these premises, the amendment brought forward was that of including nanoparticles among the substances triggering Authorisation, as defined in Article 57(f) of today's version of REACH. Importantly, Article 57(f) deals with the identification of SVHCs such as non-threshold PBT and vPvB chemicals, endocrine disrupters, and other substances *of equivalent concern*. The rejected amendment aimed at the explicit introduction of nanoparticles under the category of *substances of equivalent concern*.[58] The open-ended provision of section (f) can be particularly relevant for capturing nanoscale chemicals under the Authorisation grid. However, due to the lack of a clear mentioning of nanoscale chemicals in the Article, the onus of proving that nano-chemicals do pose an equivalent concern to that of other SVHCs listed in Article 57, is placed entirely on the regulator. Therefore, in a moment of great scientific uncertainty, data paucity, and discordant debate on the risks posed by nano-chemicals, it seems difficult to envisage a common use of Article 57(f) for the identification of SVHCs.

Difficulties are exacerbated by the fact that in order to identify nano-chemicals as substances of equivalent concern, scientific evidence of 'probable *serious* effects' to human health or the environment, is required in accordance with Article 57(f). A shift towards more risk-based criteria seems to take place in the (f) section of Article 57 of REACH. Unlike sections (a)–(e), which enable identification of SVHCs on hazard-basis only, for potential chemicals of equivalent concerns, the threshold to meet is higher: the probable harmful effects must be considered as 'serious', although no further indication is given on how to measure the seriousness of effects. Moreover, the assessment of *equivalent concern* substances should be based on a case-by-case approach, making it difficult for nano-chemicals to fall under this provision as a specific class of chemicals, or as a sub-group of the same bulk substance (e.g. carbon nanoparticle or silver nanoparticles).

The ECHA Guidance on the identification of SVHCs offers hardly any useful insight on the intrinsic properties a chemical shall display in order to be eligible for posing an equivalent concern. It is the argument of this book, though, that other areas of EU law might offer a solution to the definition issue of SVHCs in relation to nanoscale chemicals. As already mentioned, under some food law sectoral regulations, nanosubstances are deemed to be equivalent to CRM chemicals, and as such are subjected to more stringent regimes such as a case-by-case authorisation granted only if applicants are able to demonstrate, through an RA, the safety for human health and the environment. One of the main hypotheses upholding this thesis is that REACH should mirror the criteria laid down in FCMs regulation for the identification of SVHCs also when it comes to nanosubstances. In this case, in light of the classification operated in the sectoral FCMs regulation, nanosubstances would hold the status of SVHC under Article 57(f) of REACH.

Legal coherence and consistency in the EU regulation of dangerous chemicals in terms of environmental protection is not the only reason to support a cross-fertilisation between REACH's identification of SVHCs and nanosubstances' classification in the FCMs area of EU law. In fact, the two sectors are, perhaps unsurprisingly, linked also on the plan of implementation and obligations they impose on chemicals producers/users in the EU. Generally speaking, REACH was designed to avoid or minimise overlapping with sectoral-specific law. This way, Article 56(5)(b) exempts SVHCs that are CMR or of other equivalent concern because of human health hazards only, from authorisation requirements if these substances are to be used in FCMs. The rationale behind this regulatory choice is that human health risks are dealt with under the specific FCM regulations. On the other hand, the implications of Article 56(5) are that:

> if a PBT or vPvB substance for reasons other than human health hazards is included in Annex XIV, its use in cosmetic products or in food contact material still needs to be authorised as the risks to the environment are not regulated in the specific legislation. If a substance of equivalent concern is included in Annex XIV, this use still needs to be authorised if environmental considerations motivate the inclusion. If on the other hand only human health motivates the inclusion, then this use is exempted.[59]

With the REACH legal text currently silent on nanotechnology while at the same time some FCMs expressly require data on the safety of the nanoform of chemicals used in their realm of application, controversies and legal inconsistency might arise for the following reasons. When applying to the EFSA for the clearance of a PBT/vPvB chemical used in a given FCM, the applicant will have to demonstrate that the nano-chemical in question does not endanger human health. However, if the same chemical is identified and included in the Candidate List due to environmental concerns, then, even if it is already authorised by the EFSA and already in use in FCM, it still needs to be authorised under the REACH framework. This is because while the FCM regulations manage human health risk in accordance with their specific set of rules, the environmental risks are not managed under the same rules. It is thus for REACH to control and manage such risks. Nevertheless, given that REACH is not nano-specific there is virtually no provision that can oblige the producer that performed the safety assessment of the nano-chemical based on the hazards emerging from the nanoscale in the realm of the FCM (which specifically requires it) to conduct the environmental risk assessment in REACH with data specific for the nanoscale. Hence, the human health risks will be based on toxicity data for the nanoscale, while the environmental ones, which are left to REACH rules, will, in all probability, be not. Therefore, there might be a situation where a producer obtains EU clearance for a nano-chemical used in an FCM by conducting tests on the nanoscale while providing data on the bulk form in order to obtain authorisation in REACH. The considerable costs of ecotoxicity testing and the strong limitations in this area of testing methods might make this scenario more than just a hypothesis.

This way, the crucial provision of Article 57(f) and the identification of substances of equivalent concern, useful to a potential inclusion of nano-chemicals under the Authorisation rule, are difficult to apply in practice. A solution might be offered by drawing a legislative parallel with the FCM regulations. Although the specific rules are intertwined and not straightforward, the consideration of nanosubstances as a class of chemicals at the same level of CMR SVHCs in the food law area, should not be ignored. Lastly, bringing nano-chemicals under the Authorisation rule, drawing the definitions of SVHCs endorsed in FCMs, might also help circumvent the problem of substance definition in REACH. This might offer temporary legal coverage to those nanosubstances of VHC, until REACH undergoes the necessary nano-review. The approved amendments to the REACH Annexes are expected to improve this kind of legal cross-fertilisation.

Procedural rules for the identification of SVHCs for Candidate List purposes

Pursuant to Article 59 of REACH, either the ECHA upon request from the Commission[60] or MSs[61] may prepare a dossier in accordance with Annex XV. Of note is the fact that the ECHA has no autonomous powers in identifying/ proposing SVHCs. Bergkamp et al. notice that as a general trend, proposals submitted by MSs in this regard considerably outweigh those submitted by the ECHA.[62] Hence, the identification of SVHCs appears to be a policy-driven process which not only mirrors national priorities in terms of danger-ous chemicals but is, precisely for this reason, highly dependent on MSs' willingness to act.

Given that the identification of such chemicals is the cornerstone of the Authorisation process, the EU legislature considered the empowerment of the ECHA with an independent right of initiative as a threat to the *Meroni* anti-delegation doctrine, albeit the Agency was conceived as a regulatory one, endowed with decision-making powers. The ECHA can, though, screen the registration dossiers for data indicating potential VHC, on the basis of the intrinsic properties, and eventually include substances in the so-called Community Rolling Action Plan (CoRAP) which specifies the substances that are to be evaluated over a period of three years. Thus, such substances can be assigned to individual MSs for evaluation in light of their inclusion in the Candidate List. However, so far, no nanosubstances have been successfully evaluated by MSs. Considering that one of this book's claims consists in arguing that Authorisation in REACH would, ideally, offer regulatory coverage for substances in nanoscale, it is relevant here to analyse the arguments in favour of this assumption.

A preliminary remark is warranted: in the current REACH framework, no chemicals in nanoscale have moved from the CoRAP into the Candidate List. As Chapter 4 and the example of the SAS showed regarding substance evaluation, inclusion on the CoRAP list was the farthest into the regulatory process that leads to Authorisation that a nanosubstance could get.[63]

Nano silver's case is an outstanding example of complex factors that determine the successful inclusion of a chemical in Annex XIV. At the outset, it can be observed that beside MSs' political will and national priorities on chemicals and environmental law, which inevitably influence Authorisation as such,[64] in the case of chemicals in nanoscale, technical difficulties shall not be underestimated. The ECHA provides the following explanation on the factors that might influence the preparation from MSs of a CoRAP evaluation dossier for chemicals in general:

> It should be noted that as the production of the information requested may, in some cases, take several years (e.g. in the case of long term studies and annual environmental monitoring) finishing a final evaluation report may also take several years from the adoption of the CoRAP.[65]

It is logical to presume here that given the fact that nano-chemicals' (eco)toxicity testing is shrouded in uncertainty, and methodological and material difficulties, which make the generation of data a very difficult task, more time would be needed for a report on nano-chemical evaluation in the CoRAP. This might be the reason why nano silver, which was to be evaluated by the Netherlands in 2014, is no longer on the CoRAP and is still not evaluated yet. Economic considerations might also have an impact on the choice of the appointed MS on whether to initiate nano-chemicals towards legally relevant Authorisation steps – namely the inclusion in the Candidate List and subsequently the listing in Annex XIV. However, there is no direct and automatic link between CoRAP evaluation and the initiation of an Authorisation/ Restriction procedure. This means that such stricter procedures may take place only as a follow-up to the evaluation in question and only if MSs or the Commission decide to initiate such processes.

Once the SVHC has been properly identified, it may be included in the Candidate List. This requires the preparation – either by the MSs or the ECHA acting upon a Commission request – of risk management options (RMO) before an Annex XV dossier is prepared. An important element in this procedure is the Registry of Intentions (RoI), which is public on the ECHA website. The function of the RoI is to inform the interested parties of the intentions of the regulators with regard to Annex XV dossiers, allowing the interested parties to prepare their contribution in this regard.[66] The RoI has three sections: the active intentions, the submitted but pending Annex XV dossiers, and the withdrawn intentions after evaluation by MSs or the ECHA.[67] What is relevant, and at the same time problematic for chemicals in nanoscale, is the fact that if an Annex XV dossier is prepared, it must include scientific evidence supporting why a substance has been identified as an SVHC and why it should be included in the Annex XIV Candidate List for authorisation.[68] Once such a dossier has been prepared, the Agency shall publish it on its website, inviting interested parties to submit comments within a specified deadline.[69] If the ECHA does not receive or make comments within 60 days, it will include the substance in the Candidate List, which is a pre-requirement for the eventual inclusion of SVHCs in the List of Substances Subject to Authorisation, i.e. Annex XIV of REACH.[70]

In case the ECHA receives or makes comments on the identification of the SVHC, it shall refer the dossier to the Member State Committee (MSC) within 15 days from the end of the 60-day period mentioned above. If, within 30 days from the referral, the MSC does not reach a unanimous agreement on the identification, the question is sent to the Commission which shall prepare a draft for the identification within three months of receipt of the opinion of the MSC.[71]

It can be concluded here that the different national policies and approaches to risks posed by nano-chemicals might create difficulties within the MSC for reaching a unanimous opinion. Hence, should the identification of a nano SVHC come all the way up to the Commission's final decision, it appears difficult to envisage a propensity of the Commission to grant the SVHC status to nano-chemicals, given its known general reluctance to enact specific legal rules for nanoscale chemicals. The scientific evidence provided in the Annex XV dossier must be so convincing as to leave little discretion to the Commission.

However, as this book seeks to demonstrate, such scientific certainty is simply not possible at the current state of the art of nano-chemicals. Therefore, the burden of proof is again shifted in Article 59 from industry to authorities that wish to subject nano-chemicals to Authorisation's stringent norms.

Prioritising criteria for substances on the Candidate List and their inclusion in Annex XIV: changing the rules in the middle of the game and the consequences for nanosubstances

Once an SVHC is identified in accordance with Articles 57–59 of REACH, the chemical is included in the Candidate List of substances (of very high concern) for Authorisation. Up to this moment, no legal obligations on the status of the substance are triggered. Substances on the Candidate List, may, following a decision from the Commission, be included in Annex XIV of

REACH, representing the List of Substances Subject to Authorisation. The Prioritisation of Candidate List substances is thus a fundamental step towards a successful inclusion in the final Authorisation List, i.e. Annex XIV. Considering the continuous postponement of various nanoscale substances' CoRAP evaluation, including, remarkably, that of nano silver,[72] the following analysis of the legal duties and tasks for the inclusion of a substance on the Candidate List is particularly relevant.

The Commission is empowered to include the substance in Annex XIV, after a recommendation by the ECHA. However, the criteria elaborated by the ECHA with regard to the prioritisation process leave room for discretion, agreements and, in the ECHA's own words, to arbitrary considerations. More precisely, the ECHA stated that

> These conventions can be science based with regard to the selection and combination of relevant criteria but the *scoring* of the criteria remains *to some extent arbitrary* and based on agreement as it *is hardly possible to provide 'scientific' justifications for assignment of particular weighting factors*, scores or the chosen way to integrate complex bits of different kinds of information in order to draw the overall conclusions. As *there is no (at least no absolute) 'scientific truth'* on how to reasonably combine and weight different kinds of complex information, opinions on the optimal approach may therefore be divergent and the end result does at its best reflect a procedure considered acceptable by a broad majority.[73]

This passage has been removed from the new[74] ECHA GD on prioritisation. However, the scoring system has been maintained. Following the general prioritisation criteria set out in Article 58(3) of REACH, the ECHA specifies that the assessment of priority needs to be performed on a substance-specific basis, as inclusion in Annex XIV is done per substance, not per use.[75] The Agency has thus elaborated a scoring/categorising system for each of the three criteria for prioritisation laid down in Article 58(3), in the following fashion:

1 Inherent properties

Here the different categories of SVHCs included in Article 57 are scored and categorised. For instance, substances belonging to the categories of 57(a) or/and 57(b) or/and 57(c) or/and 57(f) are considered of *low* priority and assigned a score of 1; whereas substances falling under the categories at 57(f), e.g. EDCs, are considered of *medium* priority and assigned a score of 7; and so on, until the categories of substances at Article 57(e) and (d) *and* that present also (at least) one other SVHC property, are considered of *high* priority and assigned a score of 15.[76]

2 Volume

Here the annual volumes of productions are assigned a score in proportion to the amount of production. For instance, a tonnage of 'no volume' is assigned a *zero* category of priority and a 0 score; a tonnage of < 10 t/y a *very low* category of priority and a score of 3; and so on, up to the ≥ 10,000 t/y tonnage which is assigned a *very high* category and a 15 score.[77]

3 Wide-dispersive uses (WDU)

Here the wide dispersiveness of uses is assessed primarily on the basis of the actors involved, i.e. Industrial use (IND), Professional use (PROF), Consumer use (CONS). The underlying assumption here is that 'the control of releases and the wide-spreadness of a use are inversely proportional in relation to the use type, i.e. moving from consumer to professional to industrial uses, the expected control of releases increases and the expected wide-spreadness decreases'.[78] The scoring thus is the following: (IND) *low* and 5; (PROF) *medium* and 10; (CONS) *high* and 15.[79]

The assessment should always include a *verbal description* which illustrates why a particular score has been allocated, because the verbal descriptions are 'of particular importance to transparently and comprehensibly describe the reasoning for a given score'.[80] The total final score used for prioritisation purposes is represented by the total sum of the scoring under each of the three criteria above.

It can be concluded thus, that, in line with what has been observed on substance evaluation in the CoRAP, in the prioritisation process, certain declared approaches are weakened by sub-procedures and operational rules that change the rules of 'the regulatory game' significantly. An example is the return of the volumes of production criterion as crucial to successfully subjecting SVHCs to Authorisation rules. As explained so far, this is particularly burdensome for nanoscale chemicals, which act through a toxicity mode that is not measured as a function of mass/volumes of exposure.

The impression is that in order to win the strong opposition to Authorisation's new approach, the EU legislature had to compromise on procedural rules, which in turn, watered down the overall aim of the Authorisation. While the facade of Authorisation is that of a phase with a strong precautionary imprint, centred on the complete reversion of the onus of proof, the reality of its procedural operation is rather different. Member States and the ECHA are central actors for initiating the Authorisation process and requiring the necessary information for the finalisation of the process. However, once the process is initiated, the responsibility for accelerating it and making sure that substances are included in the Annex XIV list gradually shifts towards the Commission and MSs' political agendas. This might be particularly problematic for regulating nano-chemicals given that there is no common EU understanding of their uncertain risks for humans and the environment. Thus, a 'regulatory limbo' is created as a result of the shift from the general *hazard-based* approach announced in the Authorisation Title in REACH, to the actual *risk-based* one of the procedural (prioritisation) sub-phase. The risk is that such internal shifting might halt the inclusion of substances in Annex XIV. Hence, certain chemicals might remain indefinitely on the Candidate List due to poor data or lack of agreement for prioritising them, creating a regulatory deadlock.

As Scott notes for the decision-making process in REACH in general, 'an initial burden of proof, in a form or another, always rests on the regulator' as it cannot act without at least some evidence of risk.[81] When it comes to nanosubstances, assuming that some of them can make it through the CoRAP evaluation or be otherwise identified as SVHCs and enter the Candidate List, it remains doubtful whether prioritisation would apply to many low-volume nano-chemicals to begin with. Problematic can also be the case of nano-chemicals for which hazardousness is not linked to PBT/vPvB intrinsic properties, as the prioritisation requires.

As a result, it can be concluded that a major overhaul of the prioritisation criteria, so as to encompass a greater spectrum of hazard-linked criteria and/or to eliminate the reference to the mass-related exposure, is needed. The intermittency currently characterising Authorisation's operation ought to be corrected. Consistency within the phase and between its sub-phases is fundamental, and a rethinking of the coordination between risk and hazard criteria is necessary, if products of advanced technologies – and nano-chemicals are a clear example of this – and non-threshold chemicals in general, are to be brought under the REACH regulatory umbrella.

Inclusion in the List of Substances Subject to Authorisation

Although nano-chemicals have not yet made it further than CoRAP listing, it is now important to examine what is the implication of inclusion in Annex XIV. It must be recalled that once a substance is listed in Annex XIV, its use is de facto banned, unless authorisation for use has been granted. When the Commission decides to include an SVHC in Annex XIV, a *sunset date* is established, and if no authorisation has been requested/obtained within such a date, the substance is deemed to be prohibited. Scott notes that the EU legislator must always adduce some evidence of risk when it comes to restrictions and authorisation. Such evidence threshold, says Scott, differs according to what is being evaluated: for the identification of SVHCs the legislator needs only to provide data on the 'harm-causing' potential of the substance (i.e. intrinsic hazardous properties), whereas if the regulatory standard is based on risk (i.e. the probability that hazards materialise), then exposure data will be also required. However, the distinction between risk and hazard-based criteria becomes quite blurred with the unfolding of the sub-phases which lead to the final inclusion in Annex XIV list (see above). Be this as it may, it is for the Commission, following the ECHA's recommendation, to include a substance from the Candidate List to Annex XIV. The decision in question shall specify the following information:

- Identity of the substance;
- Intrinsic properties as an SVHC;
- Transitional arrangements concerning:
  - the date(s) from which the placing on the market and the use of the substance shall be prohibited unless an authorisation is granted (hereinafter referred to as 'the sunset date') which should take into account, where appropriate, the production cycle specified for that use;
  - a date or dates at least 18 months before the sunset date(s) by which applications must be received if the applicant wishes to continue to use the substance or place it on the market for certain uses after the sunset date(s); these continued uses shall be allowed after the sunset date until a decision on the application for authorisation is taken;
  - if appropriate, review periods for certain uses;
  - exemptions, if any, and the conditions for such exemptions.[82]

Once a chemical has been included through a Commission decision on the list of Annex XIV, it can continue to be used until the sunset date. After that, if no successful authorisation request has been presented, the substance is considered to be banned from the EU market.

In order to obtain authorisation, a producer/importer and also downstream user, acting as applicants, should submit a dossier to the ECHA, including, among other things, the following elements:

- An analysis of alternatives considering their risks and the technical and economic feasibility of substitution and including, if appropriate, information about any relevant research and development activities by the applicant;
- Where the analysis in question shows that suitable alternatives are available, a substitution plan including a timetable for proposed actions by the applicant.[83]

It may also include:

- A socio-economic analysis;
- A justification for not considering risks to human health and the environment arising from emission of substances from an installation which was granted a permit in accordance with the IPP Directive, and the discharges of a substance from a point source regulated by the Water Framework Directive.[84]

It emerges clearly that the data flow, both from the other phases of REACH and from other EU legislation, is vital to a successful assessment of chemicals hazards, and, eventually, to a successful authorisation request. This flow of data is currently not materialising for nanomaterials in REACH. Additionally, few other EU regulations are nano-specific; the two mentioned here, i.e. the IPPD (now IED) and the WFD, are not.

Another demanding provision in terms of authorisation request is that on the socio-economic analysis. The procedure is similar to that followed for restriction purposes, for which we refer to Chapter 6.

The producer may apply for an authorisation based on one of the two routes provided for by REACH:

i The adequately controlled risks route

Here the applicant must demonstrate that the risk to human health or the environment from the use of a substance arising from the intrinsic properties specified in Annex XIV is adequately controlled (see Chapter 7 for a detailed analysis on how the adequately controlled risks concept is defined in REACH) in accordance with Section 6.4 of Annex I.

In addition, the applicant should demonstrate that there are no safer alternatives or, in case such alternatives exist, that she is submitting a substitution plan.[85]

ii The socio-economic route

Here the applicant must show that the socio-economic benefits from the use of the substance outweigh the risks connected with its use and there are no suitable alternative substances or technologies that are economically and technically viable. This route must be followed for PBT, vPvB, non-threshold CMRs, and non-threshold chemicals of equivalent concern, which cannot be authorised in accordance with the first route.

In both cases, it is for the applicant to provide data in support of the route it is advocating. Hence, in case a nano-chemical makes it into the Candidate List, depending on the hazardous profiles that were determinant to its entry, it will be for the applicant to demonstrate one of the two routes, generating the necessary data to this end.

The authorisation dossier will then be assessed by the ECHA's Committee for Risk Assessment (RAC) and the Committee for Socio-economic Analysis (SEAC) which will perform a conformity check of the dossier to authorisation requirements in REACH. Within ten months from the submission of the dossier, the RAC and SEAC should present their draft opinions to the ECHA. The opinions shall respectively contain an RA assessment on human health and environmental risks, as well as the assessment of RMM contained in the dossier, and if there are relevant risks associated with the identified alternatives, an assessment of such risk for the RAC; and an assessment of socio-economic factors and the availability, feasibility, and suitability of alternatives, and third-party contributions for the SEAC.[86] The draft opinions from the RAC and SEAC are then sent to the applicants for comments, and depending whether there have been comments, the final opinion is sent to the Commission, the MSs, and the applicant, and the non-confidential parts are published on the ECHA's website for consultation.[87] The final decision is taken by the Commission, taking into account the opinions from the RAC and SEAC and their conclusions. One provision of particular relevance for nanoscale chemicals here is that the Commission decision must refrain from granting authorisation, if the authorisation constitutes a relaxation of an existing substance under REACH.[88] The Commission's decisions on Authorisation cannot be appealed to the ECHA BoA. Hence, an action ought to be brought before the CJEU in accordance with Article 263 TFEU, which, contrary to an appeal filed with the ECHA's BoA, has no suspensive effects.

The black-listing effect of the Candidate List

As stated earlier in this chapter, the positive implications of a procedure like Authorisation for the protection of human health and the environment derive from the transparency and information function of some of its sub-phases.

For instance, although the obligation to seek authorisation – and the consequent de facto prohibition to use and place the concerned substance on the EU market before an authorisation is granted – is only triggered at the moment of inclusion on the final list of Annex XIV, positive effects in terms of environmental and human health protection may well arise as the result of the mere inclusion of a substance in the Candidate List, pursuant Annex XIII criteria.

Notoriously, the inclusion in the Candidate List gives way to a *black-listing effect*[89] which might accelerate, or even anticipate, substitution with safer alternatives, before decisions to do so are enacted by regulators. The black-listing effect can also arise by the parallel activity of NGOs working to identify and 'catalogue' dangerous intrinsic properties, uses, and even existing alternatives of substances that meet the SVHC criteria of Article 57 of REACH, but that the Commission has not yet included in the Candidate List.

Outstanding in this regard is the International Chemical Secretariat, ChemSec. This is a non-profit organisation formed in 2002 by four Swedish environmental organisations: the Swedish Society for Nature Conservation, the WWF Sweden, Nature and Youth Sweden, and Friends of the Earth Sweden – which now form the board of ChemSec. In a multiparty dialogue among industry, regulators, and other stockholders involved in the chemical sector, ChemSec seeks to facilitate and speed up the transition to a world free of hazardous chemicals.[90]

The main instrument serving this aim is the *Substitute It Now! (SIN) List* which contains an extensive number of substances identified as SVHCs in accordance with the REACH Article 57 criteria.[91] Like Authorisation in REACH, the aim of the SIN List is to spark innovation through substitution of SIN chemicals with less hazardous alternatives. Even the SIN database[92] mirrors the ECHA one of SVHCs to some extent, but its content is more detailed, more user-friendly than the ECHA one and can be searched through several filters,[93] making it easier for consumers to check the presence of concerning chemicals in specific products, e.g. textiles or electronics. Although SIN information draws heavily upon the ECHA's work and data when it comes to substances already on the Authorisation track (which might be already on the CoRAP, the Candidate List, or even in Annex XIV), the way information is presented is clearer and more straightforward on the SIN database. In addition, in the case of the ECHA, the displayed information decreases when the substance passes from the Candidate to the Authorisation List, for instance. In terms of consumers' information this means that a thorough investigation of various lists must be performed in order to acquire relevant data on the products where the substance is used, the identity of the producers, and, eventually, the safer alternatives that may exist. Differences on the practical access to information are all but negligible when it comes to the environmental benefits deriving from informed consumers' choice. The average consumer might find it difficult to navigate the ECHA's multiple lists, assuming he has the required knowledge to distinguish between different elements of Authorisation (CoRAP, Candidate List, and Annex XIV List) and their legal implications.

These practical pitfalls might become a serious hindrance to the right to know if it is considered that for SVHCs present in articles, there is no direct obligation to inform consumers. Article 33 of REACH stipulates that, while suppliers have a duty to inform recipients of articles containing SVHCs in a concentration above 0.1 per cent weight by weight (w/w), consumers must make a formal request in order to obtain information on the safe use of the substance. While the rationale behind this legislative choice remains obscure the following question arises: where shall the consumer look for information on the presence of SVHCs in order to file a formal request to the supplier, and have information on the safe handling of the object, with the name of the substance as a minimum? One place to look for such information might be the ECHA's website. This is why, offering a clear, user-friendly access to the various Lists of Authorisation is important and can compensate for other deficiencies and loopholes elsewhere in REACH.

But the real contribution of the SIN List is with regard to those substances which are not subject to any of the Authorisation steps, and yet are fully compatible with the definition of SVCHs in accordance with the criteria laid down in Article 57 of REACH. Identification and listing of such chemicals on these bases includes the advantage of anticipating regulatory decision-making, offering industry some predictability, and enabling substitution in due time. The SIN List is a clear example on how voluntary initiatives can contribute to the acceleration of the regulatory process in complex subject matters, highly dependent on broad and comprehensive scientific expertise. Particularly valuable is the work of ChemSec when it comes to substances like endocrine disrupting chemicals (EDCs), for which there is little political consensus on how to regulate, nor are there valid criteria for their evaluation and inclusion in the authorisation list(s). The transparency of the ChemSec website on the use of EDCs in products and the available safer alternatives, is important at a time when the attempt to regulate EDCs at the EU level is proving to be a difficult war of science and policy.[94]

The latest update on Authorisation

Notwithstanding the aforementioned pitfalls of the Authorisation procedure and disregarding the concerns voiced by NGOs and consumers associations on such pitfalls, the Commission has decided to take a completely different position, almost antithetical to what has been advocated for improving Authorisation. Right now, on the Commission's agenda is the idea of introducing 'simplifications of the authorisation process'.[95] The Commission makes it very clear that improvement of authorisation means to make 'it simpler, less costly and more predictable'.[96] For industry.

The paper[97] adopted specifically with regard to Authorisation simplification, is puzzling. It presents a set of solutions for 'special cases' in light of a general simplification of the burden borne by the industry in terms of both data to be provided and economic costs to be sustained as a consequence. There are three areas and/or parameters to be streamlined through simplification:

1 The use of low-volume SVHCs included in Annex XIV, which according to the Commission, would be

> the clearest specific case for seeking simplified solutions, mainly due to the disproportionality of the cost of preparing a full-scale authorisation application in those cases compared with the potential benefits for human health and the environment in terms of reduced risks related to its substitution by another substance or technology.[98]

2 The legacy spare parts concerning the application for authorisation of SVHCs intended for articles that were placed on the market and whose production stopped or will stop before the sunset date ('legacy spare parts'). There are two driving concerns for such simplification:

> On the one hand, the cost of preparing an application for authorisation is disproportionately high, in view of the limited (and decreasing) volumes of spare parts intended for articles that are no longer produced. On the other hand, the economic and technical difficulties of searching for substitutes for such uses.[99]

3 Special cases of simplification procedure for certain uses of SVHCs within the supply chain when

the end-product is subject to a type approval/an authorisation requirement under another piece of EU legislation and where the use of an alternative will require re-approval or re-authorisation.[100]

A comparison between these options and the shortcoming of the Authorisation procedure analysed in this section, yields such a contradiction that one has to question whether the Commission is really aware of the demands of the civil society on REACH. One point is striking: the suggestion to further exempt lower volumes of production from authorisation rules, either partially or totally. It is important to recall here that Authorisation is a tonnage-free phase of REACH, i.e. it applies regardless of the quantity of production, meaning it applies also to substances not subject to Registration because they are produced in quantities below 1 t/y. This is at the very core of the Authorisation regime. However, as shown, while the tonnage considerations do not affect the identification and the inclusion of SVHCs in the Candidate List, they make a return in the prioritisation of Candidate List substances to be included in the Annex XIV. For such inclusion, which triggers the legal duty to apply for an authorisation, exposure considerations based on volumes of production are reintroduced. The result might be that very dangerous chemicals, e.g. EDCs, might not be prioritised because the volumes of production might be relatively low. However, the irreversible harms of EDCs are not related to their quantity of exposure. Therefore, the hitch created by the re-introduction in the last sub-phase of the Authorisation procedure (i.e. prioritisation of Candidate List chemicals) is all but negligible in terms of high levels of environmental and health protection.

Notwithstanding this significant flaw, Authorisation, as currently designed, contributes to the attainment of the high protection aim not only through the conclusion of the procedure and the inclusion of the hazardous chemical in Annex XIV. What is proven to be one of its main novelties, rather, is the inclusion of the SVHCs in the Candidate List, triggering important information duties, including the consumer right to know (albeit upon request) which SVHC is used in a given product. Information and transparency have shown also to be important drivers for phasing out SVHCs and substituting them with safer alternatives. The fact that such duties are triggered regardless of any consideration whatsoever on the quantity of production, is one of the most powerful available tools for addressing the risks of complex and novel chemicals like EDCs or nanoscale ones which, precisely because of their low volumes of production, can escape the Registration and Evaluation phases of REACH, while still presenting high risks at any quantity of exposure.

What the Commission's suggestion on the low volumes would bring, in case it is approved, is an elimination of even this possibility to know about the use of such harmful chemicals. This would deprive Authorisation of its very essence, turning it into a nugatory concept. Moreover, in order to reduce the burden for industry, the burden for the authorities will necessarily increase, given that it would be for the ECHA and/or MSs to prove why an exempted low-volume chemical deserves a thorough consideration for authorisation purposes. This further weakens the precautionary principle, which had in the volume-free and the reversion of the onus of proof characteristics of Authorisation, one of its major expressions in REACH. The fact that the Commission is even suggesting such an option, in a moment when regulatory debate on nano-chemicals and EDCs is highly critical to the current concept of dose and the volume-based triggers in REACH, is inexplicable – except in the view of profit logics and neoliberal deregulatory tendencies. Likewise, the other two suggestions are likely to have a detrimental impact on the health and environment protection aim, as they aim to weaken the requirements applicable to SVHCs in articles. Also here, in clear contrast with what the CJEU has recently ruled on the SVHCs in articles, the Commission seeks to exempt or lighten the obligation triggered by the use of very dangerous chemicals in articles. What is more, it tries to do so by appealing to justifications or necessities that are to be found nowhere in the REACH text.

This initiative was still ongoing at the time this book was being finalised.

Summing up

Authorisation is considered the biggest contribution that the REACH set of rules and provisions can offer to the aim of high levels of human health and environmental protection. When nanosubstances' case is used to analyse the procedures that make up this third phase of the Regulation, features that make Authorisation an outstanding and quite independent programme under the REACH framework emerge clearly.

To start with, no minimum threshold is required for triggering authorisation, thus making it possible to apply its provisions to chemicals, like nanoscale ones, for which toxicity for humans and the environment is not represented by the volumes of production. No-threshold substances entailing stochastic damages include, among other things, endocrine disrupters. While this last category is taken into account by Article 57(f) of REACH, nanosubstances are not. However, the open end of the norm suggests that nanochemicals might well fall within the 'equivalent concern' rule and thus be considered for authorisation. The possibility to adapt the definition represents the second feature that makes Authorisation potentially applicable to nanochemicals. This is particularly so because no need for previous registration is required in order to initiate the procedures of Title VII. Finally, the initiation of the process is hazard-based (also given the lack of a minimum threshold and exposure scenarios).

However, a closer look at the meticulous and burdensome processes that lead to inclusion in Annex XIV unravelled a series of loopholes which might undermine the potential of this phase for the protection of human health and the environment. As a general note, the process is far more policy-based, political, and consensus-driven than it appears from the

REACH text. The role of MSs is still relevant for the identification of SVHCs and their inclusion in the Candidate List, as the prerogatives within the CoRAP and Member State Committee showed, leading to the reflection of national approaches to risk in the Authorisation process. Moreover, when it comes to the inclusion of substances in Annex XIV (i.e. List of Substance Subject to Authorisation) ECHA's powers in the processes are limited due to the non-delegation of powers (*Meroni*) doctrine. This is also seen by the fact that the Commission, which has the last say on such inclusion, does not limit its decision on rubber-stamping ECHA's recommendations but, more often than not, alters technicalities pertinent to individual substances.[101]

Therefore, although at the time of its establishment it was a novelty, the Authorisation procedure, as it currently stands, is not having the revolutionary impact it was expected to. Despite the attempts from the EU Parliament to bring nano-chemicals under the Authorisation rule, the 2006 proposed provisions did not make it into the final text of REACH. This is because Authorisation in particular, and the legal text of REACH as a whole, are the product of severe and unprecedented lobbying (both inter- and intra-EU) which led to the watering down of many original provisions. For instance, the mandatory obligation to substitute hazardous chemicals when safer alternatives exist was reduced to the simple possibility to refuse granting an authorisation in such an eventuality. Concessions on key and strategic elements of the original REACH regime were also made, like the increase of the minimum threshold for registration from 10 kg/y to 1 t/y and the obligation to carry out a CSA and prepare a CSR only at 10 t/y of production. Perhaps the main drawback of Authorisation is that of assigning a certain relevance to the volumes of production within its stepwise structure, which limits the possibility to capture under Authorisation's rule all those very dangerous chemicals produced in low volumes. In addition, the requirement to perform a socio–economic analysis before including an SVHC in the Authorisation List, is questionable and needlessly burdensome: the substances in question are proven to have deleterious effects on human health and ecosystems; therefore, insisting on the socio–economic considerations would, at best, be unethical. It can also be considered as a general lack of care[102] from the regulator's side with regard to the duty to holistically protect ecosystems and human life as part of them.

Finally, if the ongoing reform to streamline authorisation is going to pass, the regulatory status of deleterious chemicals in REACH, e.g. EDCs and nanosubstances, would become even more uncertain. The proposal to exempt low-volume chemicals and certain articles from the REACH obligations would create a free zone where, paradoxically, the most concerning and harmful chemicals would be allowed to be used without any obligation to comply with health and safety data requirements.

Notes

1 REACH, Article 60.
2 Nicolas de Sadeleer, 'The Impact of Registration, Evaluation and Authorisation of Chemicals (REACH) Regulation on the Regulatory Powers of the Nordic Countries' in N. de Sadeleer (ed.) *Implementing the Precautionary Principle, Approaches from the Nordic Countries, EU and USA* (EarthScan 2007) 330, 332.
3 REACH, Article 55(1). Note the reversion of the words' order as compared to the aim of REACH under Title I, Article 1(1), which reads:

> The purpose of this Regulation is to ensure a high level of protection of human health and the environment, including the promotion of alternative methods for assessment of hazards of substances, as well as the free circulation of substances on the internal market while enhancing competitiveness and innovation.

4 REACH, Article 60(2)(4).
5 Commission, 'Strategy for a future Chemicals Policy' (White Paper) COM (2001) 88 final 5.
6 Ibid. 16–17.
7 Ragnar Lofstedt, 'The Substitution Principle in Chemical Regulation: A Constructive Critique' (2014) 17 Journal of Risk Research 543, 548; as of January 2019, the number of substances on the ECHA Candidate List is 197, available at: http://echa.europa.eu/candidate-list-table accessed 23.01.2019.
8 See Commission Regulation (EU) 10/2011 of 14 January 2011 on plastic materials and articles intended to come into contact with food [2011] OJ L12/1 and Commission Regulation (EC) 450/2009 of 29 May 2009 on active and intelligent materials and articles intended to come into contact with food [2009] OJ L135/3.
9 See Greenpeace, 'Safer Chemicals within Reach: Using the Substitution Principle to Drive Green Chemistry' (February 2005) 6.
10 Lofstedt (n 7) 544.
11 Council Directive 89/391/EEC of 12 June 1989 on the introduction of measures to encourage improvements in the safety and health of workers at work [1989] OJ L183/1. Though no explicit reference is made here to the SP, the Directive rules at Article 6(2)(f) that 'replacing the dangerous by the non-dangerous or the less dangerous' is part of the duty of prevention that employers must implement.
12 Council Directive 98/24/EC of 7 April 1998 on the protection of the health and safety of workers from the risks related to chemical agents at work (14th individual Directive within the meaning of Article 16(1) of Directive 89/391/EEC) OJ L13111, states at Article 6(2) that

> substitution shall by preference be undertaken, whereby the employer shall avoid the use of a hazardous chemical agent by replacing it with a chemical agent or process which, under its condition of use, is not hazardous or less hazardous to workers' safety and health, as the case may be.

13 Lofstedt (n 7) 545.
14 See Hans Christian Bugge, *Environmental Law in Norway* (Kluwer Law International 2011) 40.
15 Lov om kontroll med produkter og forbrukertjenester (produktkontrolloven), LOV 1976–06–11 nr 79 (1977).
16 Bugge (n 14) 40.
17 Ludwig Krämer, *EU Environmental Law* (7th edn, Sweet & Maxwell 2011) 7–8.

18 Article 17(1) and Recital (25) of Council Decision1600/2002/EC of 22 July 2002 laying down the Sixth Community Environment Action Programme [2002] OJ L242/1.

19 Krämer (n 17) 8.

20 Case C-473/98 *Toolex* [2000] ECLI:EU:C:2000:379.

21 Ibid. para 35.

22 Ibid. para 47.

23 Ibid. paras 46–47.

24 Ibid. para 48.

25 Commission, 'Strategy for a future Chemicals Policy' (White Paper) COM (2001) 88 final 8.

26 Gunnar Lind, 'The Only Planet Guide to the Secrets of Chemicals Policy in the EU: REACH – What Happened and Why?' (Inger Schörling 2004) 83.

27 Agenda 21: Programme of Action for Sustainable Development, 1992–06–14, U.N. GAOR, 46th Sess., Agenda Item 21, UN Doc A/Conf.151/26 (1992), §19.49 (c), emphasis added.

28 CEFIC, 'Paper on substitution and authorisation under REACH' (2005) 1, emphasis added.

29 Sven O. Hansson, Linda Molander, and Christina Rudén, 'The Substitution Principle' (2011) 59 Regulatory Toxicology and Pharmacology 454, 456, emphasis added.

30 REACH, Article 55(1).

31 See among others SCENIHR, 'The Existing and Proposed Definitions Relating to Products of Nanotechnologies' (29 November 2007); SCENIHR 'Risk Assessment of Products of Nanotechnologies' (19 January 2009); SCENIHR, 'Scientific Basis for the Definition of the Term "Nanomaterial"' (6 July 2010); SCENIHR 'Nanosilver: Safety, Health and Environmental Effects and Role in Antimicrobial Resistance' (10–11 June 2014); EFSA, 'The Potential Risks Arising from Nanoscience and Nanotechnologies on Food and Feed Safety' (2009) 958 The EFSA Journal 1; EFSA, 'Guidance on the Risk Assessment of the Application of Nanoscience and Nanotechnologies in the Food and Feed Chain' (2011) 9 EFSA Journal 2140; The Royal Society and The Royal Academy of Engineering, *Nanoscience and Nanotechnologies: Opportunities and Uncertainties* (The Royal Society 2004).

32 OECD, 'Nanotechnology for Green Innovation' (2013) No. 5 OECD Science, Technology and Industry Policy Papers.

33 See the European Medicines Agency 'Reflection Paper on Nanotechnology-Based Medicinal Products for Human Use' (EMEA/CHMP/79769/2006, 29 June 2006).

34 COM (2012) 572 final, section 3.

35 EPA, 'Nanotechnology White Paper' (100/B-07/001, February 2007) 21.

36 Ibid. 22.

37 Ibid. 27.

38 Ibid. 33.

39 Ibid. 36.

40 Ibid. 37.

41 Veerle Heyvaert, 'Balancing Trade and Environment in the European Union: Proportionality Substituted?' (2001) 13 J Environmental Law 392, 392.

42 Ibid. 405.

43 Regulation (EC) 450/2009.

44 Regulation (EU) 10/2011.

45 Ibid., recital (27).

46 See Regulation (EC) 450/2009 Article 5 (c)(i) and Regulation (EU) 10/2011, Recital (27).

47 Interestingly, Regulation (EU) 10/2011, Recital (27) and Regulation (EC) 450/2009, Recital (14) contain the same exact provision regarding substances to be excluded by the FB concept.

48 This intention emerges even more clearly at Article 5(c)(ii), stating that 'substances deliberately engineered to particle size which exhibit functional physical and chemical properties that significantly differ from those at a larger scale' cannot be used behind an FB, unless authorised on a case by case basis.

49 The Precautionary Principle is clearly evoked in Article 6 and 7 of Council Regulation (EC) 178/2002 of 28 January 2002 laying down the general principles and requirements of food law, establishing the European Food Safety Authority and laying down procedures in matters of food safety [2002] OJ L31/1.

50 Lucas Bergkamp and Nicolas Herbatschek, 'Regulating Chemical Substances under REACH: The Choice between Authorization and Restriction and the Case of Dipolar Aprotic Solvents' (2014) 23 RECIEL 221 241.

51 de Sadeleer (n 2) 331–351.

52 REACH, Article 55.

53 Council Regulation (EC) 440/2008 of 30 May 2008 laying down test methods pursuant to Regulation (EC) No. 1907/2006 of the European Parliament and of the Council on the Registration, Evaluation, Authorisation and Restriction of Chemicals (REACH) [2008] OJ L142/1, which is completely silent on nanotechnology.

54 See in general Jean-Philippe Montfort, 'The French Nano Decree: A Model for Europe?' (NIA Symposium, 19 December 2012) www.mayerbrown.com/files/uploads/Documents/French_Nano_Decrees.pdf accessed 20.02.2019.

55 Jean-Philippe Montfort et al., 'Nanomaterials under REACH: Legal Aspects' (2010) 1 EJRR 5158.

56 *Toolex* (n 20).

57 ***II RECOMMENDATION FOR SECOND READING on the Council common position for adopting a regulation of the European Parliament and of the Council concerning the Registration, Evaluation, Authorisation and Restriction of Chemicals (REACH), establishing a European Chemicals Agency, amending Directive 1999/45/EC of the European Parliament and of the Council and repealing Council Regulation (EEC) No. 793/93 and Commission Regulation (EC) No. 1488/94 as well as Council Directive 76/769/EEC and Commission Directives 91/155/EEC, 93/67/EEC, 93/105/EC and 2000/21/EC (7524/8/2006–C6 –0267/2006–2003/0256(COD)), FINAL A6–0352, Amendment 79, 51.

58 Ibid.

59 ECHA, 'Guidance on Inclusion of Substances in Annex XIV (List of Substances Subject to Authorisation)' (August 2008) 21. The updated Guidance reiterates the exempted categories in question, see ECHA, 'Preparation of Draft Annex XIV Entries for Substances Recommended to Be Included in Annex XIV General Approach' (21 August 2014), Annex I, 9.

60 REACH, Article 59(1).

61 REACH, Article 59(2).

62 Nicolas Herbatschek, Lucas Bergkamp, and Meglena Mihova, 'The REACH Programmes and Procedures' in Lucas Bergkamp (ed.), *The European Union REACH Regulation for Chemicals Law and Practice* (OUP 2013) 153.

63 'Substance Evaluation – CoRAP' (*ECHA*) http://echa.europa.eu/information-on-chemicals/evaluation/community-rolling-action-plan/corap-table accessed 20.02.2019.

64 See in this regard de Sadeleer (n 2) 331–351.

65 'Q&As' (*ECHA*) http://echa.europa.eu/qa-display/-/qadisplay/5s1R/view/reach/corapandsubstanceevaluation accessed 20. 02.2019.

66 Gauthier van Thuyne and Fee Goossens, 'Authorisation and Restrictions' in Dieter Drohmann and Matthew Townsend (eds) *REACH Best Practice Guide to Regulation (EC) No 1907/2006* (Beck/Hart 2013) 450.

67 Ibid.
68 Ibid.
69 REACH, Article 59(4).
70 Van Thyne and Goossens (n 66) 451.
71 REACH, Article 59.
72 It must be recalled here that the deadline for evaluation was 2016. The Netherlands did not manage to evaluate the substance which was not included in the next CoRAP.
73 ECHA, 'General Approach for Prioritisation of Substances of Very High Concern (SVHCs) for Inclusion in the List of Substances Subject to Authorisation' (28 May 2010) 3, emphasis added.
74 ECHA, 'General Approach for Prioritisation of Substances of Very High Concern (SVHCs) for Inclusion in the List of Substances Subject to Authorisation' (10 February 2014).
75 Ibid. 4.
76 Ibid. 7.
77 Ibid. 8.
78 Ibid. 8–9.
79 Ibid. 9.
80 Ibid. 10.
81 Joanne Scott, 'REACH and the Evolution of EU Administrative Law', Comparative Administrative Law conference 7–9 May, Yale Law School, 12. Available at www.law.yale.edu/academics/papers.htm accessed 27.06.2016.
82 REACH, Article 58(1).
83 REACH, Article 62(4).
84 REACH, Article 62(5).
85 Van Thyne and Goossens (n 66) 456.
86 See ECHA, 'Guidance on the Preparation of an Application for Authorisation' (ECHA-11-G-01-EN January 2011) 16.
87 REACH, Article 64.
88 Van Thyne and Goossens (n 66) 459.
89 See in this regard Kerstin Heitmann and Antonia Reihlen, 'Case Study on "Announcement Effect" in the Market Related to the Candidate List of Substances Subject to Authorisation' (Ökopol GmbH Institute for Environmental Strategies 2007) 13.
90 www.chemsec.org/about-us/who-we-are accessed 20.10.2016.
91 www.chemsec.org/what-we-do/sin-list accessed 20.02.2019.
92 http://sinlist.chemsec.org/options/3-114 accessed 20.02.2019.
93 The current filters include: Health & Environmental concerns; Uses; REACH Status; Appearance date on SIN List; Production volume; SIN Groups; Producers.
94 See in general Nertila Kuraj, 'Complexities and Conflict in Controlling Dangerous Chemicals: The Case of Regulating Endocrine Disruptors in EU Law', in Eléonore Maitre-Ekern, Carl Dalhammar, and Hans Christian Bugge (eds), *Preventing Environmental Damage from Products: An Analysis of the Policy and Regulatory Framework in Europe* (CPU 2018).
95 European Commission, 17th Meeting of Competent Authorities for REACH and CLP (CARACAL) 26–27 March 2015, 'Streamlining and Simplifications of the Authorisation Process' (13 March 2015 Doc. CA/16/2015).
96 Commission, 'Regulatory Fitness and Performance Programme (REFIT): State of Play and Outlook Accompanying the Document Better Regulation for Better Results – An EU Agenda' (Staff Working Document) SWD (2015) 110 final, 8.
97 See Commission, 'Streamlining and Simplification of Authorisation' (Commission's paper) (Doc. CA/16/2015, 13 March 2015).

98 Ibid. 2.
99 Ibid. 3.
100 Ibid. 4.
101 See in general: Christoph Klika, 'The Implementation of the REACH Authori-sation Procedure on Chemical Substances of Concern: What Kind of Legiti-macy?' (2015) 3 Politics and Governance 128.
102 Care is particularly relevant to decision-making pertaining to highly uncertain and potentially catastrophic technologies and materials. Nanotechnology and the products of its application are considered to pose a threat to the very existence of the planet and all forms of life on it. Therefore, the lack of a willingness to address risk early enough and with an appropriate degree of concern (care) can be considered as a general failure in precaution as care. See in general Chapter 8.

6 Restriction

Introduction

Often referred to as the 'safety net' of REACH, *Restriction* represents the fourth and final phase of the regulatory programme put forth by REACH. Restriction seeks to provide a last option for addressing those chemicals risks which managed to slip through the regulatory grids of the other phases of REACH – most notably of Authorisation.

At the outset, it is useful to state that the measures envisaged in the Restriction phase are not revolutionary compared to the previous EU law on the banning of dangerous substances. As the following will undertake to demonstrate, Restriction in REACH reiterates one main controversial feature of the past regime, that of the burden of evidentiary proof resting entirely with the authority proposing the restriction. Nonetheless, a few novelties can be observed. As we now know, before the enactment of REACH the restriction of the marketing and use of dangerous substances in the EU was governed by Directive 76/769/EEC.[1] The REACH restriction list replaces the Directive's list, which means that existing restrictions (e.g. asbestos) are carried over in REACH. Further, REACH extends the possibility to restrict not only the use and placing on the market of dangerous chemicals, but also their production. In addition, REACH provides for the restriction of dangerous chemicals in articles, which was not contemplated in the previous regime. But perhaps the most innovative feature of the REACH Restriction regime, as compared to the previous system of chemicals regulation, is owed to the fact that Restriction is placed at the far end of the REACH regulatory continuum. This means that as a result of the data generated for Registration, Evaluating, and eventually Authorisation purposes, greater information would be arguably available to authorities to use for Restriction purposes.

Contact points with Authorisation

There exist different contact points and procedural similarities between Authorisation and Restriction. For instance, Restriction, too, is a 'command and control'[2] form of regulatory model. Additionally, just like Authorisation,

Restriction sets out norms for dealing with the risk management of highly hazardous chemicals under the double precondition that they pose an 'unacceptable risk to human health or the environment' and that 'there is a need to address such risk on Community-wide basis'.[3]

Yet, before restricting such dangerous chemicals, REACH stipulates that socio-economic considerations and the availability of alternatives should be taken into account. This legislative choice appears – as previously observed for the Authorisation phase – doubtful, given that restrictions represent a sort of last resort management option for risks which are already deemed to be *unacceptable*. The unacceptability of risk is not defined anywhere in the *legal text* of the Regulation (except for in the regulatory toxicology formulas used in the Annexes and GDs; see Chapter 7 for a detailed analysis of such formulas). As it can be deducted from the wording of Article 68 and as some authors[4] have already observed, risks that are *not adequately controlled*, in accordance with what is stipulated by Annex I of REACH,[5] can well be deemed to be unacceptable. However, the concept of unacceptability is not necessarily limited to this category of risks. Be that as it may, the burden of demonstrating unacceptable risks remains with the authority.

In relation to nano-chemicals, Restriction might offer a valid risk management tool, in case other options in REACH are not applicable. However, a first difficulty in this regard concerns the status of such chemicals in REACH and other EU law. Currently there is no differentiation between the *nano* and *bulk* forms of a chemical. As Chapter 3 illustrated, the current definition of substance in REACH does not take into account the nano-form of a chemical. Consequently, such hindrance is taken up by the subsequent phases of REACH which are all built on the concept of *substance*. The same is valid for Restriction. In a hypothetical scenario, the authority would first need to know/establish that the hazardous chemical it plans to restrict is indeed in nanoform and that such nanoform is posing an unacceptable risk to humans or the environment. As a consequence, the onus of proof – which in Restriction lies always with the authorities – becomes particularly burdensome when the substance to be restricted is in nanoscale. Such difficulties have prompted the research of alternative pathways for bringing nanoscale chemicals under the more stringent norms of Authorisation and/or Restriction.

A recent attempt to bring the nanoforms of titanium dioxide under the CLP category of carcinogenic substances can be used as an example of such difficulties. France submitted a proposal to introduce all forms of TiO_2, including the nanoscale one, to Annex VI of the CLP Regulation as Category 1B carcinogen (*Carc. Cat 1BH350i*) for *humans* when inhaled, based on the motivation that 'TiO2 can enter into nucleus and directly interact with DNA'.[6] This assessment was based primarily on animal testing evidence. Such classification was sought for both *fine particles* and *nanomaterials* of TiO_2 without any distinction in terms of morphology, crystal phase, and surface treatment.[7]

The Report that the ECHA prepared and submitted for public consultation on this proposal stated:

> TiO_2 is considered poorly soluble particles and the main proposed mechanism of carcinogenicity by inhalation is thus based on the low solubility and biopersistency of the particles leading to pulmonary inflammation then oxidative stress. Secondary genotoxicity and cell proliferation result in carcinogenicity. Nevertheless, possible *direct genotoxicity cannot be excluded.*

Based on available evidence and information in the registration dossier (e.g. mechanism of carcinogenicity, characterisation of the particles), the proposed scope for the Annex VI entry is: '*Titanium dioxide in all phases and phase combinations; particles in all sizes/morphologies*'.[8]

The proposal comes at a time when there is considerable discussion on the regulatory status of TiO_2 in REACH. As previously explained, the ECHA's request to the registrants of titanium dioxide to update the registration dossier with specific information, related, among other things, 'to phases of the Substance, *nanoforms*, and *surface treatment of nanoforms*, as part of the Substance identification information',[9] was annulled by the BoA. It is clear that this was an attempt (now failed) by the Agency to try to initiate a regulatory pathway for the nanoform of TiO_2, a substance that according to an increasing number of scientific studies, displays concerning toxicological profiles.[10]

Similarly, France, which has been in charge of the evaluation of TiO_2 on the CoRAP since 2014 and has not managed to meet the deadlines, tried to go another way. By proposing mandatory classification of TiO_2 as a Category 1B carcinogen the aim was to eventually bypass the CoRAP procedure altogether given that the classification of a chemical under the CLP Regulation[11] has direct consequences for its regulatory status in REACH. In particular the SVHCs, which include CMR chemicals among others (e.g. a 1A/1B carcinogens) can be subjected to authorisation or restriction rules in REACH. Another consequence would be that the use of SVHCs (particulate and nano TiO_2 in this case) in consumers' products and articles would be restricted. However, in this case, too, the opposition from industry was immediate. That same industry that was fighting the ECHA's request for information on the nanoform of TiO_2 in registration dossiers attacked the proposed French classification on grounds of test methodologies' limitations and lack of sufficient data to uphold such classification. More specifically, the Titanium Dioxide Manufacturers Association (TDMA) objected that the tests on rats on carcinogenicity by inhalation used for classification purposes are not a suitable model for human studies.[12]

In the wake of such developments, the ECHA's Committee for Risk Assessment (RAC) concluded that based on the data provided by France, TiO_2 warrants a Category 2B (*Animal*) carcinogen classification.[13] The distinction between what was asked and what was granted is all but marginal.

Whereas the French proposal sought to classify TiO_2 as a substance which is *presumed* to cause cancer to humans directly, what the RAC granted, is, in fact, a less severe classification, which designates TiO_2 only as a substance *suspected* of causing cancer to animals. These subtle linguistic nuances and small numeric differences do in fact translate to enormous differences in terms of consequences for human health and environmental protection: France's suggestion, had it been granted by the RAC, would have had the ability to bring TiO_2 under the SVHC category, with an eventual restriction or inclusion in the Candidate List and, most importantly, would have bypassed the lengthy CoRAP procedure altogether. What the RAC accorded has no such consequence for the substance's status in REACH.

It must be noted that the annulment of the ECHA decision to request information on the nanoform of registered TiO_2 dossiers, coupled with the RAC decision to assign TiO_2 a classification category that is not sufficient alone to bring the substance under the Restriction (or Authorisation) rule, is problematic, especially if the widespread use of the substance is considered. Given that the tonnage band registered in EU for TiO_2 is 1,000,000–10,000,000 tons per annum,[14] knowing whether the substance is being produced in nanoform and whether it is as such in need of a separate registration in REACH, might have significant consequences in terms of environmental and health protection data generation. The tonnage band in question is indeed the largest foreseen by REACH and, as such, requires the generation of a wide and comprehensive data set on toxicity to humans and the environment. It remains thus difficult in the present state of the art to see how data specifically referring to the nanoform of TiO_2 and its risks can be obtained under REACH. The modification of the Annexes will arguably make it easier for the ECHA to justify an eventual decision requesting data on the nanoform (although doubts persist on this) but this will not happen before 2020.

What is more, even the less-severe classification of TiO_2 is being met with further opposition. The Commission, which after the RAC opinion is in charge of deciding on the regulatory measures on TiO_2, instead of adopting such measures, asked the MSs whether the RAC opinion is to be translated as such in the CLP Regulation, or rather, if it should be modified so as to include footnotes that differentiate between various forms of the substance – derogating therefore the obligation to classify and label as carcinogenic forms of TiO_2 other than the powder ones. Various NGOs were said to be highly critical of this dangerous departure from the science-and-evidence-based approach of the RAC classification opinion.[15] This book takes the view that this proposal by the Commission is not only deplorable from a human health and environmental protection standpoint, but it represents a great interference with scientific evidence, which the Commission seeks to replace with policy considerations. Such a move is not only dangerous but may well be illegal. The lobbying[16] from industry in the case of TiO_2 has been unprecedented (comparable only perhaps with that on EDCs), with the intent being to further weaken the implications in terms of higher levels of protection aims of a classification, which is already less severe than the one originally sought by France. To derogate to the current awarded classification with the consequence, among others, of exempting certain forms of TiO$_2$ from being labelled as carcinogenic – albeit only as Category 2B – strongly limits the right to know of consumers and the transparency of information on which such right is premised. The sum of these coordinated actions and decision is that nano TiO$_2$ remains currently out of REACH.

Finally, whatever the final conclusions will be on the fate of TiO$_2$ in the CLP, it can be predicted that they might be influenced by or read in the light of the recent CJEU decision on the coal tar pitch, high temperature (CTPHT) classification, which will not be further examined in this book.[17]

Given the current situation, the following offers a closer look at Restriction procedures in REACH, in order to investigate whether they can be applicable to nanoscale chemicals.

Restriction: the ordinary procedure

Restriction procedures are loaded with procedural, administrative, and legal requirements. The right of initiative in this case belongs to the Commission, the ECHA, and individual MSs. This section elaborates on the ordinary restriction procedure.

When the Commission deems it necessary to issue a restrictive measure for a given chemical, it can initiate such a proposal through the ECHA. Article 68(1) allows for the Commission to require the Agency to prepare a dossier in accordance with the requirements of Annex XV, when risks posed by a chemical are not adequately controlled and need *to be addressed on a Community-wide basis*.[18] The ECHA might also prepare a restriction dossier on its own initiative, but in this case Article 68(2) sets as a precondition that the substance in question is an SVHC listed in Annex XIV, for which the *sunset date* therein has been reached without any authorisation granted. At this point, the ECHA can prepare a dossier in accordance with Annex XV requirements. Lastly, MSs can initiate a restriction procedure if they have grounds to believe that the substance to be restricted poses a risk that is not adequately controlled and there is a need to address such risk on a Community-wide basis. Hence when nano-chemicals are concerned, the ECHA initiative for restriction is bound to the presence of nanosubstances on Annex XIV and the expiring of the sunset therein. However, as explained in the previous section on Authorisation, there are currently zero nano-scale chemicals on Annex XIV. Potential candidates include nano silver and some other metallic oxides. For the time being though, the ECHA initiative for restricting hazardous nano-chemicals is rather unlikely in the near future.

However, regardless of whether the ECHA is acting on its own, on the behalf of the Commission, or whether an MS has put forward a proposal for restriction, the dossier shall comply with the requirements laid down in Annex XV and contain, among others:

- The identity of the substance, the uses to be restricted and a summary justification;
- Information on hazards and risks which shall be described based on an assessment of the hazards and risks according to the relevant parts of Annex I and shall be documented in the format set out in Part B of that Annex for the Chemical Safety Report. Of note here is that neither Annex I nor the CSR are nano-tailored;
- Evidence that implemented RM measures, including those foreseen in article 10 and 14 of REACH, are not sufficient;
- Analysis of the alternatives, including health for humans and the environment related to the use of alternatives, their economic and technical feasibility, etc.;
- Information submitted by interested parties;
- Justification not only of the fact that action is needed on a Community-wide basis but also the fact that restriction is the most appropriate Community-wide measure in this respect, based on the following criteria:

    i *effectiveness*: the restriction must be targeted to the effects or exposures that cause the risks identified, capable of reducing these risks to an acceptable level within a reasonable period of time and proportional to the risk;
    ii *practicality*: the restriction must be implementable, enforceable and manageable;
    iii *monitorability*: it must be possible to monitor the result of the implementation of the proposed restriction.[19]

- *Socio-economic* analysis (SEA) in accordance with Annex XVI. A comparison should be performed on the 'net benefits to human health and the environment of the proposed restriction may be compared to its net costs to manufacturers, importers, downstream users, distributors, consumers and society as a whole'.[20] Such an analysis is also imposed by Article 69(2)(b) and should be performed in accordance with the procedures indicated in Annex XVI. The list of the impacts that the authority performing an SEA *may* take into account includes:

    - Impact on all other actors in the supply chain, downstream users and associated businesses in terms of commercial consequences such as impact on investment, research and development, innovation, one-off and operating costs (e.g. compliance, transitional arrangements, changes to existing processes, reporting and monitoring systems, installation of new technology, etc.) taking into account general trends in the market and technology;
    - Impacts on consumers. For example, product prices, changes in composition or quality or performance of products, availability of

products, consumer choice, as well as effects on human health and the environment to the extent that these affect consumers;

- Social implications, for example job security and employment;
- Availability, suitability, and technical feasibility of alternative substances and/or technologies, and economic consequences thereof, and information on the rates of, and potential for, technological change in the sector(s) concerned. In the case of an application for authorisation, the social and/or economic impacts of using any available alternatives.
- Wider implications on trade, competition and economic development (in particular for SMEs and in relation to third countries) of a granted or refused authorisation, or a proposed restriction. This may include consideration of local, regional, national or international aspects;
- In the case of a proposed restriction, proposals for other regulatory or non-regulatory measures that could meet the aim of the proposed restriction (this shall take account of existing legislation). This should include an assessment of the effectiveness and the costs linked to alternative risk management measures;
- In the case of a proposed restriction or refused authorisation, the benefits for human health and the environment as well as the social and economic benefits of the proposed restriction. For example, worker health, environmental performance and the distribution of these benefits, for example, geographically, population groups;
- An SEA may also address any other issue that is considered to be relevant by the applicant(s) or interested party.[21]

An observation that can already be made here in the case of a hypothetical SEA for chemicals in nanoscale is connected to the difficulty to justify a restriction of a chemical in the light of Annex XVI-based criteria. Nanotechnology and the products of its application are endorsed as key solutions to current and future EU economical and societal challenges. The so-called *Key Enabling Technologies* (KETs) consist mainly in nano-scale materials and substances and such is their assumed importance for the growth and prosperity of the EU.[22] Such documents endorse the vision of nanotechnology and nanomaterials as factors of paramount importance for the transition to a knowledge-based and low carbon resource-efficient economy and their function as innovation-drivers and jobs and growth promoters, which: 'play an important role in the R&D, innovation and cluster strategies of many industries and are regarded as crucial for ensuring the competitiveness of European industries in the knowledge economy'.[23] It is hence logical to assume that attempts to restrict the use of nano-chemicals would lead to difficulties to justify such restrictions under SEA considerations. The socio-economic impacts of a proposed restriction considered during the performance of an SEA – such as those on jobs security and innovation, for instance – would need to be weighed against identical goals that the target substance aims to achieve. Considering the problematics surrounding toxicity, risk and health impacts of nano-chemicals, the attempt to restrict nano-chemicals with a successful SEA test seems rather unrealistic for the time being.

The next step in the route to restriction requires the authorities to submit the dossier in question to the Committee for Risk Assessment (RAC) and the Committee for Socio-economic Analysis (SEAC) which shall check the conformity with Annex XV requirements.[24] The Committees shall deliver a conformity opinion within 30 days of receipt of the dossier. In case the dossier does not conform, the Committees shall inform the ECHA/MS of the reason for non-conformity in written form within 45 days of receipt. At this point the ECHA/MS have 60 days to bring the dossier in conformity with Annex XV requirements or the restriction proposal drops.[25] Of note here is that despite the option of the RAC and SEAC, the Commission has the final say on the appropriateness of the proposed restriction as a measure for controlling unacceptable risks to humans and/or to the environment. The process is a transparent one, and the ECHA is required to publish all relevant steps of the procedure. In addition, the ECHA must maintain a *registry of restriction purposes* – a list[26] of substances for which a dossier conforming to the requirements of Annex XV is being considered, either by the Agency or a Member State, for restriction purposes.[27] In addition, Article 69(6) requires the ECHA to publish the restriction dossiers on its website in order to allow for six months' public consultation and comments.

The RAC has nine months for delivering an opinion on the appropriateness of the suggested restriction measures in reducing human and/or environmental risks posed by the substance in question. Article 70(1) foresees that the opinion of RAC shall be based on 'relevant parts of the dossier' presented by the ECHA/MS and that it shall take into account the comments submitted by interested parties during the public consultation period of six months. In turn, the SEAC has 12 months to deliver its opinion on the conforming proposal dossier. Again the opinion shall draw upon relevant parts of the presented dossier and the comments submitted during public consultation. Interestingly, the draft of the SEAC option shall be published on the ECHA's website in order to allow for 60 days of public consultation. The final opinion of the SEAC shall take into account the comments received.[28] The deadline for the SEAC to deliver its opinion can be extended to another 90 days in case its opinion diverges significantly from the RAC one. REACH does not further specify what happens in case of irreconcilable opinions. Within three months from the expiry of such period, regardless of whether the SEAC has reached an opinion or not, the Commission, in accordance with Article 73, shall prepare a draft for amending Annex XVII.

In both the RAC and SEAC opinion-drafting process it is the Commission which has the final say. What is more, the Commission draft may differ significantly from the initial proposal or disregard the RAC and/or SEAC opinion(s). In this case the Commission shall justify its choice by annexing a detailed explanation of the reasons that influenced its choice. Settled case law on the EU level has specified that EU institutions might depart from scientific opinions but in doing so they are obliged to provide a statement of reasons that should be 'of a scientific level at least commensurate with that of the opinion in question'.[29] As Scott notes, the *Pfizer* case confined this 'right to disagree' with scientific opinions adopted by risk assessment committees.[30] REACH extends this duty also to other committees such as the SEAC, engaged mainly in the RM phase.

The decision of the Commission to add a new restriction in Annex XVII or amend an existing one therein, shall be taken in accordance with Article 133(4) of REACH. It is useful to recall here that Article 133(4) refers the decision-making procedures laid down in Council Decision 1999/468/EC, and specifically that of Articles 5a(1)–(4) and Article 7.[31] Article 5a was added in 2006,[32] putting the Parliament on equal footing with the Council in the regulatory procedure with scrutiny (RPS) but still leaving both Parliament and the Council 'under' the Commission's rule, which can still override negative opinions from these supervision bodies.[33] The merit of Article 5a is that of attributing to the Parliament the 'ex post' veto on implementing measures adopted through co-decision.[34]

Today the adoption of delegated acts is subject to the dictate of Article 290 TFEU and the novelties are significant. However, there has been 'no automatic alignment from RPS to Delegated acts'.[35] Therefore, the RPS continues to exist as a procedure in committees including those dealing with restriction (and authorisation)[36] decisions under the REACH dictation. With the Parliament as a legislator equal to the Council, the chances are that the nanotechnology issue under REACH restriction (and also authorisation) procedure will find greater support. The position of the Parliament on nano-regulation is known[37] and it is logical to assume that while uncertainty and ignorance on toxicity and health impacts of nano-chemicals linger, the Parliament will advocate stricter regimes for nano-chemicals of concern.

It is relevant to point out here that when drafting a restriction proposal, the ECHA (either on its own initiative or on behalf of the Commission) and MSs shall refer to any dossier, chemical safety report, or risk assessment submitted to the Agency or Member State under this Regulation.[38] Hence, the risk assessment is not performed 'from scratch' but relies heavily, if not completely, on data submitted under other REACH phases. The formulation of the legal text does not clearly prevent the ECHA from performing an RA with its own means and resources but it remains unclear how such an option could be operated in practice.

What seems to hold true also for Restriction is that REACH is a stepwise regulation where different programmes and procedures – albeit differentiated and autonomous to some extent – depend on data submitted upstream by means of registration and dossier preparation. Such data feed the regulatory process and the environmental protection scope that REACH's framework enables. Toxicity and exposure data provided in registration dossiers, SDS, and the preliminary RA and RM considerations therein are transmitted in a cascading effect mode in the subsequent phases of Evaluation, Restriction, and Authorisation. There is hence little doubt that the data submitted under the REACH command are of crucial importance for environmental and human health protection measures.

In the case of nanomaterials, however, the crucial importance of data flow in REACH becomes highly problematic. The lack of a status of nano-chemicals as 'new for regulatory purposes' makes it discretionary for industry to submit nano-specific data on toxicity and risk related to the intrinsic properties chemicals display when reduced in nanoscale. Therefore, the inability of REACH to impose *general, certain, and enforceable* legal duties in terms of nanoscale chemicals registration, testing, and risk appraisal, strongly hinders the ability of more stringent REACH programmes to deliver high levels of human health and environmental protection for this class of chemicals. This is particularly the case for certain steps of the Authorisation procedure and the Restriction one, where the risk-anchored decision-making implies a considerable burden of proof for the Commission, the ECHA, or the MSs wishing to subject nano-chemicals to authorisation or restriction measures. If a general and certain duty to register is not foreseeable for nano-chemicals, what kind of data on toxicity, exposure, and risk should the legislator use when considering RM on hazardous nano-chemicals?

The rhetoric of these arguments inevitably conducts this analysis in the realm of decisional models based on risk and hazard. As Chapter 2 pointed out on the legislative battle for nano-chemicals' inclusion in the REACH framework from its genesis,[39] the precautionary subjection of nanosubstances as a class of chemicals to Authorisation rules was rejected by the Council. The rejection of this amendment is significant also for Restriction considerations. As stated earlier in this section, the ECHA can act in its own right to initiate a restriction proposal. However, the choice of the hazardous substance in this case is confined to those on the Candidate List for authorisation and for which a sunset date has been reached without gaining authorisation. Hence, had the Parliament amendment on nano-chemicals made it through the legislative bargaining on the REACH adoption, the ECHA's powers to initiate a restriction procedure could have been extended also to nano-scale chemicals.

Although data submitted under REACH are the vital lymph that runs through the whole process of chemicals regulation and, as such, represent supporting information for enacting sound environmental and human health protection measures, this is not the exclusive source of scientific evidence legitimating RM measures under the restriction procedure.

Article 69(4) of REACH reads:

> The Agency or Member States shall also refer to *any relevant risk assessment submitted for the purposes of other Community Regulations or Directives.* To this end other bodies, such as agencies, established under Community

law and carrying out a similar *task shall provide information* to the Agency or Member State concerned on request.[40]

Arguably, the ECHA might benefit greatly by such an option in the case of nanoscale substances. Given the paucity of data regarding (eco)toxicological profiles of chemicals in nanoscale, the previous endeavour of other EU agencies operating in different areas of EU legislation might assist the ECHA in the RA to be performed in light of a potential restriction. Interestingly, no limitations are made with regard to the areas of EU legislation the ECHA can turn to for risk assessment results which can then be used for restriction purposes in REACH. Thereby, in the case of nano-chemicals, the ECHA may make use of RA performed in the realm of whatever EU legislation is already nano-specific. Food and food contact materials but also cosmetics and biocides may provide valuable input in this regard. In the following we analyse specific cases that illustrate such a possibility.

i Nano TiN in FCMs

The first example concerns the EFSA's authorisation of titanium nitride (TiN) in nanoscale for use in PET bottles. In 2008 the Panel on Food Contact Materials, Enzymes, Flavourings and Processing Aids (CEF), based on data dossier on the safety assessment submitted by the industry, concluded that the use of this nanosubstance in quantities of 20 mg/kg would not give rise to exposure and hence no toxicological concern existed. The legal basis for the EFSA action was constituted by Regulation (EC) No. 1935/2004 which, as a framework regulation in the area of FCM, establishes the duty for industry to conduct and provide the EFSA with a prior safety assessment of substances intended to be used in FCM. The legal and technical details for such a procedure are laid down in Regulation (EU) No. 10/2011[41] on plastic FCM, which is nano-specific. As a consequence industry has the duty to carry out an RA based on the intrinsic properties displayed in nano-scale, as demonstrated in the nano TiN used in PET bottles.

Similar considerations were made by the same EFSA panel in 2012 for the use of nano TiN in thermoformed PET sheets/films for alimentary uses. In this case the applicant did not provide new data, but only new information specific to the new uses. The EFSA concluded that no migration was observed in this case either and granted clearance for the new uses of the substance.[42]

ii Colloidal nano silver

Another example is again provided by the EFSA's ruling on colloidal silver in nanoscale to be used as a dietary supplement. Here the Panel on Food Additives and Nutrient Sources added to Food (ANS) concluded that 'due to the lack of an appropriate dossier supporting the use of silver hydrosol, the safety of silver hydrosol and the bioavailability of silver from silver hydrosol cannot be assessed'.[43]

The ECHA could draw important lessons from these two cases and consult the dossiers prepared by industry in relation to such materials, should TiN and nano silver come to attention for restriction purposes. As this book was being finalised, a new assessment of an application on the safety of colloidal nanosilver was concluded by the EU's Scientific Committee on Consumer Safety (SCCS). The request came from the Commission, which had received 63 notifications on the use of colloidal silver in nanoform in cosmetic products pursuant to Article 2(1)(k) of Regulation (EC) No. 1223/2009. The Opinion concluded that

> Although other information is available in open literature relating to the toxicity of nano silver, their relevance with respect to the materials in this submission has not been considered by the Applicants. Due to a number of major data gaps, the SCCS is not in the position to draw a conclusion on the safety of colloidal silver in nano form when used in oral and dermal cosmetic products.[44]

Once again, an independent EU scientific body underlines the fact that scientific data are available regarding certain risk profiles of commonly used nanomaterials and that somehow such data keep being overlooked. The fact that such data might still be inconclusive or incomplete, shall not constitute an argument for claiming an absence of risk. Such approach is a clear expression of the PP, which represents a powerful tool for dealing with the worrisome risks of nano silver, which is suspected, among other qualities, of having the ability to mediate antibiotic resistance in cells (see point *iv* below).

iii Nanosubstances in cosmetics

Additional RA dossiers and data which might supplement the ECHA's own assessment during restriction procedures are also those performed in the context of the new EU cosmetics regulation.[45] Article 6 of the Regulation stipulates the possibility for the Commission to request a scientific opinion from the SCCS[46] on the risk and safety of nanoscale substances used in cosmetic products.[47] From 2009 on the SCCS has delivered scientific opinions on the safety evaluation of, among others, nano titanium dioxide (nano TiO_2),[48] nano zinc oxide (nano ZnO),[49] nano carbon black,[50] and nano amorphous silica (nano SAS).[51] Such documents expressed a positive outcome for the dermal-route usage of the nanomaterials in question, thus allowing their incorporation in cosmetic products. However, the same opinions generally contained a sort of disclaimer of precautionary imprint, reminding the Commission and the EU legislator that the outcomes are 'based on the currently available scientific evidence' and that should new evidence emerge in the future, the SCCS might revise its opinions. Following this approach, the SCCS revised the opinions on nano carbon black, nano TiO$_2$, and nano zinc so as to clarify that the safety assessment performed for the dermal exposure of such chemicals through cosmetics products does not apply to the exposure to the same chemicals via 'sprayable applications/products'.[52] For nano ZnO the revised text clearly states that 'the use of ZnO nanoparticles in spray products that could lead to exposure of the consumer's lungs to nano ZnO by inhalation cannot be considered safe'.[53] The ECHA might benefit from such a document and the RA data therein in order to feed the REACH programmes' procedures and elaborate appropriate RM measures.

iv Nano silver opinion

Another EU non-food scientific committee that has been particularly active in the field of nano RA is SCENIHR. The most recent opinion from SCENIHR concerns the assessment of nano silver safety.[54] The conspicuous document investigates the potential risks posed by exposure to nanoscale silver in different environmental media (like soil and water) and through a range of consumers' products inholding nano silver. In its opinion, the SCENIHR analyses the hazards nano silver might pose to human health, the environment, and the alleged antibacterial resistance triggered by nano silver, in a life-cycle perspective.

Given the difficulties encountered in the process of trying to bring nano silver under the Authorisation programme in REACH, Article 69(4) might offer a possibility for the ECHA to bypass Authorisation and eventually adopt restrictions for determinate uses of the substance based on the outcomes of the SCENIHR opinion.

Following Article 69(4), the ECHA might consult also the European Medicine Agency (EMA), which may supply the ECHA with valuable data on toxicology profiles of nano-chemicals and risk assessment consideration, given its pioneering work in this regard. Also, the fact that the EMA is a regulatory agency — and so is the ECHA — might perhaps confer a greater legitimacy to its contribution to the ECHA's decision pursuant to Article 69(4).

However, regardless of whether the ECHA makes use of the procedures put forth at Article 69(4), the decision-making mechanism laid down at Articles 68–73 remains a fundamentally risk-based one. It is the responsible authority (the Commission/ECHA or MSs) which must demonstrate the risk deriving from an SVHC (in nano and/or bulk form) and the need for regulatory measures to manage risks which are not being adequately controlled by manufacturers, importers, and users.[55] For chemicals in nano-scale this might turn out to be a particularly burdensome task. To this end, the following section examines the other restriction procedure under REACH, the so-called 'fast-track' one, in order to investigate whether simplified RA performances are possible in

REACH and if yes, to what extent can said procedures serve the pursuit of a high level of protection of human and environmental health also in the case of nanosubstances.

Fast-track procedures for restriction: a return to hazard-based criteria?

Given the great uncertainty that still surrounds the risk assessment of nano-scale chemicals and the consequent concrete difficulty in performing such an assessment, it becomes relevant to explore other options for eventually subjecting hazardous nano-chemicals to restriction measures other than the one centred on risk-based criteria.

To this end, the Restriction phase provides for an alternative procedure which shifts the decisional balance towards a more hazard-based assessment. Article 68(2) of REACH states that for substances on their own, in preparation, or in article, which are CMR of category 1 and 2 *and* could be used by consumers, and for which restrictions to consumers' use are proposed by the Commission, a restriction decision is to be made in accordance with Article 133(4) of REACH, hence through the regulatory procedure with scrutiny. What could perhaps be particularly relevant for nano-chemicals which fulfil the conditions set out in Article 68(2) is the fact that in this case, Articles 69–73 and the articulated and burdensome procedures therein do not apply.

In practical terms this means an alleviation of the general burden of proof which Restriction generally places on the regulator. The reason justifying the by-passing of the ordinary terms and assessment seems to reside in the fact that for this category of substances 'sound scientific basis has already been provided either within the classification procedure or during the international agreement procedure'.[56]

Hence, for nanomaterials displaying CMR properties the Commission could follow this fast-track procedure and include them in Annex XVII. However, the exercise of this option is difficult for the case of nano-scale materials, given that to date there are no nanomaterials which hold the CMR status in EU legislation (not yet at least, see the TiO_2 evaluation case above). Nonetheless, it is worth recalling here that the EU FMCs legislation equates nanomaterials to CMR substances. Consideration on the potential CMR nature of certain nanomaterials invites reflection on how this point is currently addressed in the food law area, where, as we know, there exist a number of nano-specific regulations. In this regard, the German Federal Environment Agency commissioned a study to the authoritative *Fraunhofer Institute* on the carcinogenicity and mutagenicity profiles of a number of nanomaterials.[57] The examined nanomaterials represent a well-known cluster of substances which have been under the EU legislators' attention for a while now and include: nano carbon black, nano TiO_2, nano iron oxide, nano silver, and SWCNTs and MWCNTs. A general conclusion of the study was that

The amount and quality of cancer studies as well as studies on genotoxicity of nanomaterials are insufficient to assess the carcinogenicity of nanomaterials. On the other side cell proliferation in the lung as a consequence of inflammation may be an important precursor of cancer.[58]

Indeed, in 2008, the Commission amended[59] REACH so as to remove carbon and graphite in nanoscale from Annex IV of REACH. Such Annex lists substances that are exempted from the registration, evaluation, and downstream users' duties provisions of REACH because sufficient information is known about these substances and they are considered to cause minimum risk.[60] The German study also found that CNTs can 'migrate to the pleura like asbestos fibres'.[61] The association of CNTs with asbestos fibres is nothing new since a growing number of studies have pointed out structural similarities which suggest similar (eco)toxicological profiles. Already in 2009 the SCENIHR stated that

> [w]hen nanotubes were found to have similar characteristics to some types of hazardous asbestos, it was demonstrated that similar inflammatory reactions can be induced by these specific nanotubes as induced by asbestos.[62]

Another nano-chemical which is thought to pose particular threats to human health and the environment and, as such, is in need of tailored regulation, is nano silver. The German study concluded that '[nano] silver was identified as the most toxic nanomaterial within our selection of nanomaterials'.[63]

The question naturally becomes: why is the Commission hesitating to regulate specific nanomaterials when institutional, legislative, and even scientific conditions emphasise an urgent need to control environmental and human health exposure of potentially hazardous nano-chemicals? One plausible answer to this question is that despite a general reallocation of the evidentiary burden of proof on industry, Restriction rules in particular (but Authorisation rules as well), still burden authorities with some demonstration of risks before a stringent measure can be enacted. Restriction would in principle empower authorities to restrict hazardous chemicals, regardless of the quantity of production. And yet, the procedures REACH prescribes for restriction purposes impose a substantial work load for preparing restriction dossiers. As the ECHA has pointed out, challenging information demands from the RAC and SEAC make it particularly difficult for MSs to supply such information for restriction purposes.[64] For nano-chemicals, the informational burden is an important one. One way of addressing such hindrances, as some stakeholders have suggested, is to allow for restriction to be based on incomplete information.[65] Another suggestion is that the RAC and SEAC 'could not only consider the strength of proof of the risk and the socio-economic benefit of a restriction, but also the strength of the evidence for the absence of risks'.[66] Both suggestions would in principle make it easier for the fast-track procedure of Restriction to apply to and thus allow for the restriction of nanosubstances of unacceptable risks.

Summing up

That REACH was not designed with nano-specificities in mind, is particularly visible in the Restriction procedure, which is mainly inherited from the old pre-REACH regulatory system. Potentially, the fast-track restriction procedure could be used by the Commission to regulate those nanomaterials having CMR properties, without waiting for a full and complete scientific demonstration of such risks, which might never arrive. In general, although there might still be considerable uncertainty on the factors that influence CMR or other toxicity profiles of nanoscale,[67] the EU fully-flagged precautionary principle allows for decision-making without the necessity to wait for full proof of the causal link between the nano-scale and the toxicity profiles ensuing as a consequence of it. To do otherwise would mean to ignore the existence of the PP as a regulatory tool and its potential for ensuring high levels of human health and environmental protection. For a number of nano-chemicals such as TiO_2, CNTs, and nano silver, the decision to postpone regulatory measures is a failure to pursue the high levels of human health and environmental protection that REACH seeks to achieve. It should not be forgotten that REACH itself endorses the PP both as a general principle that underpins all of its provisions[68] and with regard to the general EU's need to protect public health and the environment,[69] and also in relation to SVHCs, as a guiding principle in subjecting such chemicals to careful monitoring.[70] Hence, the current *paralysis by analysis*[71] is not justifiable from a precautionary perspective. It is time for the EU chemicals law to depart from the 'too little too late'[72] policy and legislative line that has characterised nano-chemicals' status so far. If REACH truly was to be lifted up to that 'best possible framework'[73] for managing nano-chemicals' risk that the Commission refers to in its policy document, then a thorough and timely re-negotiation of its key provisions is urged. The sole amendments to the Annexes and the nano-specific provisions that will come into force in 2020 are insufficient in this regard.

Complicating matters further is the fact that REACH is a modern law, informed and held up by a long and highly technical scientific Regulation[74] on the test methods, which represent the legitimate basis for the measures adopted pursuant to REACH. The scientific background against which the REACH legal operation unfolds has its pivotal element in *regulatory toxicology*. The next chapter takes a closer look at the science-law interface in REACH and its functioning in the case of nanoscale chemicals. The aim is to investigate whether the current framework of regulatory toxicology, to which the REACH rule of law is vitally tied, is capable of detecting and controlling nano-risks.

Notes

1 Council Directive 76/769/EEC of 27 July 1976 on the approximation of the laws, regulations and administrative provisions of the Member States relating to restrictions on the marketing and use of certain dangerous substances and preparations [1976] OJ L262/201.
2 Lucas Bergkamp and Nicolas Herbatschek, 'Regulating Chemical Substances under REACH: The Choice between Authorization and Restriction and the Case of Dipolar Aprotic Solvents' (2014) 23 RECIEL 221, 221.
3 REACH, Article 68(1).
4 See Nicolas Herbatschek, Lucas Bergkamp, and Meglena Mihova, 'REACH Programmes and Procedures' in Lucas Bergkamp (ed.) *The European Union REACH Regulation for Chemicals Law and Practice* (OUP 2013) 147.
5 REACH Annex I clarifies that the risks for the environment are not adequately controlled when the ratio PEC/PNEC for each environmental (and exposure/DNEL) compartment is greater than one. For a detailed discussion on the significance of such ratio and its problematic, we refer to the next chapter, Chapter 7. See also the ECHA 'Guidance on Information Requirements and Chemical Safety Assessment Part E: Risk Characterisation' (ECHA-2016-G-04-EN, May 2016) 8–9.
6 ECHA, 'CLH Report Proposal for Harmonised Classification and Labelling Based on Regulation (EC) No 1272/2008 (CLP Regulation), Annex VI, Part 2 Substance Name: Titanium Dioxide' (May 2016) 138.
7 Ibid. 69.
8 Ibid. 4, emphasis in the original.
9 See Case A-011–2014 *Tioxide Europe Limited v ECHA* [2014] 2.
10 Cam Walker, 'Independent Testing Finds Illegal and Potentially Harmful Nanoparticles in Common Food Products' (*Friends of the Earth Australia*, 17 September 2015) www.foe.org.au/articles/2015-09-17/independent-testing-finds-illegal-and-potentially-harmful-nanoparticles-common accessed 01.13.2019.
11 Council Regulation (EC) 1272/2008 of 16 December 2008 on classification, labelling and packaging of substances and mixtures, amending and repealing Directives 67/548/EEC and 1999/45/EC, and amending Regulation (EC) No 1907/2006 [2008] OJ L353/1.
12 'TiO2 Producers Dispute Science behind Proposed Carcinogen Classification' (*CW*, 2016) https://chemicalwatch.com/51856/tio2-producers-dispute-science-behind-proposed-carcinogen-classification accessed 25.01.2019.
13 ECHA/RAC, 'RAC Opinion Proposing Harmonised Classification and Labelling at EU Level of Titanium Dioxide' (CLH-O-0000001412–86–163/F, 14 September 2017) 40.
14 ECHA, May 2016 (n 6) 15.
15 'Classify all Titanium Dioxide Forms as Suspected Carcinogens' (*CW*, 2018) https://chemicalwatch.com/68516/classify-all-titanium-dioxide-forms-as-suspected-carcinogens-ngos-urge accessed 15.01.2019.
16 'Beyond the Pale on Titanium Dioxide' (*CEO*, 2018) https://corporateeurope.org/power-lobbies/2018/07/beyond-pale-titanium-dioxide accessed 15.01.2019.
17 Case C-691/15 P – *Commission v Bilbaína de Alquitranes and Others* [2017], ECLI:EU:C:2017:882.
18 The reference to the need for such a risk to be addressed on a Community-wide bases is substituted here with the simple need to address the risk.
19 REACH, Annex XV.
20 REACH, Annex XV.
21 The list represents the content of Annex XVI of REACH and the indicated impacts shall be taken into account when performing an SEA both for Authorisation and Restriction purposes.

22 Commission, 'Preparing for our Future: Developing a Common Strategy for Key Enabling Technologies in the EU' (Communication) COM (2009) 512 final, emphasis added.
23 http://ec.europa.eu/enterprise/sectors/ict/key_technologies/index_en.htm accessed 04.03.2017.
24 REACH, Article 69(4).
25 REACH, Article 69(4).
26 At the time of writing, the list contained five entries: 'Submitted Restrictions under Consideration' (*ECHA*) http://echa.europa.eu/web/guest/restrictions-under-consideration accessed 25.01.2019.
27 REACH, Article 69(5).
28 REACH, Article 71(2).
29 Case T-13/99 *Pfizer* [2002] ECLI:EU:T:2002:209 para 8.
30 Joanne Scott, 'REACH and the Evolution of EU Administrative Law', Comparative Administrative Law conference 7–9 May, Yale Law School, 7. Available at www.law.yale.edu/academics/papers.htm accessed 27.06.2016.
31 Council Decision 1999/468/EC of 28 June 1999 laying down the procedures for the exercise of implementing powers conferred on the Commission [1999] OJ L 184/23.
32 Council Decision 2006/512/EC of 17 July 2006 amending Decision 1999/468/EC laying down the procedures for the exercise of implementing powers conferred on the Commission [2006] OJ L 200/11.
33 See Pamela Lintner and Beatrice Vaccari, 'The European Parliament's Right of Scrutiny over Commission Implementing Acts: A Real Parliamentary Control?' (2005) 1 EIPASCOPE 15, 23, available at http://aei.pitt.edu/5941/1/scop05_1_3.pdf accessed 22.02.2019.
34 The other two rights are the right of information (Article 7 of Decision 1999/468/EC) and the right to pass a non-binding resolution if the Parliament considers that the Commission has exceeded its delegation powers (Article 8 of Decision 1999/468/EC). See in this regard Alan Hardacre and Mario Damen, 'The European Parliament and Comitology: PRAC in Practice' (2009) 1 EIPA-SCOPE 13, available at: http://aei.pitt.edu/12375/1/20090709111448_Art2_Eipascoop2009_01.pdf accessed 19.02.2019.
35 For a good overview on the passage see Alan Hardacre and Michael Kaeding, 'Delegated & Implementing Acts: The New Comitology' (2013) 5 EIPA Essential Guide 1, 15, available at: www.eipa.eu/files/repository/product/20130904094203_Comitology_Brochure5EN_web.pdf accessed 10.02.2019; Thomas Christiansen and Mathias Dobbels, 'Comitology and Delegated Acts after Lisbon: How the European Parliament Lost the Implementation Game' (2012) 16 (13) European Integration online Papers (EIoP) 1.
36 Christoph Klika, 'The Implementation of the REACH Authorisation Procedure on Chemical Substances of Concern: What Kind of Legitimacy?' (2015) 3 Politics and Governance 130.
37 Parliament resolution of 24 April 2009 on regulatory aspects of nanomaterials (2008/2208(INI)), P6_TA(2009)0328 [2009] OJ C184E/82.
38 REACH, Article 68(4).
39 See in this regard the discussion on the legislative amendments to the REACH legal draft in Chapter 2. A general obligation to bring nano-chemicals as a group under a generalised obligation to seek and obtain authorisation before production and use was rejected and pulled out of the final approved text of REACH.
40 REACH, Article 69(4), emphasis added.
41 Commission Regulation (EU) 10/2011 of 14 January 2011 on plastic materials and articles intended to come into contact with food [2011] OJ L12/1.
42 For the detailed EFSA reasoning see: EFSA Panel on Food Contact Materials, Flavourings, Enzymes and Processing Aids, 'Scientific Opinion on the Safety

Evaluation of the Substance, Titanium Nitride, Nanoparticles, for Use in Food Contact Materials' (2012) 10(3):2641 EFSA Journal.

43 EFSA, 'Scientific Opinion: Inability to Assess the Safety of a Silver Hydrosol Added for Nutritional Purposes as a Source of Silver in Food Supplements and the Bioavailability of Silver from this Source Based on the Supporting Dossier' EFSA Journal (2008) 884, 887.

44 SCCS, 'Opinion Colloidal Silver (Nano)' (SCCS/1596/18 Final, 24–25 October 2018) 29.

45 Council regulation (EC) 1223/2009 of 30 November 2009 on cosmetic products [2009] OJ L 342/59.

46 Scientific Committee on Consumer Safety (*EC*) http://ec.europa.eu/health/scientific_committees/consumer_safety/index_en.htm accessed 01.03.2019.

47 For a brief overview see Frank Henkler et al., 'Risk Assessment of Nanomaterials in Cosmetics: A European Union Perspective' (2012) 86 Archives of Toxicology 1629, 1641–1646.

48 SCCS, 'Opinion on Titanium Dioxide (Nano Form) 24 COLIPA n° S75' (SCCS/1516/13, 22 July 2013).

49 SCCS, 'Opinion on Zinc Oxide (Nano Form) COLIPA S 76' (SCCS/1489/12, 18 September 2012).

50 SCCS, 'Opinion on Carbon Black (Nano-Form)' (SCCS/1515/13, 12 December 2013).

51 SCCS, 'Opinion on Silica, Hydrated Silica, and Silica Surface Modified with Alkyl Silylates (Nano Form)' (SCCS/1545/15, 20 March 2015).

52 SCCS 'Opinion for Clarification of the Meaning of the Term "Sprayable Applications/Products" for the Nano Forms of Carbon Black CI 77266, Titanium Oxide and Zinc Oxide' (SCCS/1539/14, 23 September 2014).

53 Ibid. 10.

54 SCENIHR, 'Opinion on Nanosilver: Safety, Health and Environmental Effects and Role in Antimicrobial Resistance' (2014).

55 Bjorn G. Hansen and Mark Blainey, 'REACH: A Step Change in the Management of Chemicals' (2006) 15 RECIEL 270, 279.

56 Article 65, Commission, 'Proposal for a Regulation of the European Parliament and of the Council Concerning the Registration, Evaluation, Authorisation and Restriction of Chemicals (Reach), Establishing a European Chemicals Agency and Amending Directive 1999/45/EC and Regulation (EC) {on Persistent Organic Pollutants} {SEC(2003 1171}' COM (2003) 644 final.

57 Katrin Schröder et al., 'Carcinogenicity and Mutagenicity of Nanoparticles – Assessment of Current Knowledge as Basis for Regulation' (Texte 50/2014, Report No. (UBA-FB) 001725/E 2014).

58 Ibid. 67.

59 Commission Regulation (EC) 987/2008 of 8 October 2008 amending Regulation (EC) 1907/2006 of the European Parliament and of the Council on the Registration, Evaluation, Authorisation and Restriction of Chemicals (REACH) as regards Annexes IV and V [2008] OJ L268/14.

60 'Commission Review of REACH Annexes' (*EC*) http://ec.europa.eu/environment/chemicals/reach/reviews_en.htm accessed 22.02.2019.

61 Schröder et al. 2014 (n 57) 34.

62 SCENIHR, 'Risk Assessment of Products of Nanotechnologies' (19 January 2009) 9.

63 Schröder et al. 2014 (n 57).

64 See ECHA, 'Workshop on REACH(ing) the WSSD 2020 Goals' (Workshop proceedings, 4 April 2016) 15, 12–13.

65 'REACH FORWARD Priorities for Effective Regulation. Discussion Paper Policy Conference – Final Version.' (June 2016) 16, 8.

66 Ibid.
67 Different studies point at different factors and intrinsic properties which determine the toxicity profiles of chemicals in nanoscale. For instance, size-driven toxicity is not linear in the sense that the 'smaller the more toxic' but rather, the exact size determines the toxicological profiles. In addition the coating of a nanoparticle might have a relevant role in toxicity. Last but not least, the type of nanomaterial (zinc, silver, iron, etc.) strongly influences toxicity in nanoscale.
68 REACH, Article 1(3).
69 REACH, recital (9).
70 REACH, recital (69).
71 Steffen F. Hansen and Anders Baun, 'When Enough Is Enough' (2012) 7 Nature Nanotechnology 409.
72 Steffen F. Hansen, 'Regulation and Risk Assessment of Nanomaterials – Too Little, Too Late?' (Department of Environmental Engineering Technical University of Denmark 2009).
73 Commission, 'Second Regulatory Review on Nanomaterials' (Communication) COM (2012) 572 final, 11.
74 Council Regulation (EC) No. 440/2008 of 30 May 2008 laying down test methods pursuant to Regulation (EC) No. 1907/2006 of the European Parliament and of the Council on the Registration, Evaluation, Authorisation and Restriction of Chemicals (REACH) [2008] OJ L 142/1.

7 Toxics of the law

Understanding the underlying scientific foundations of REACH and their suitability for nanoscale risk

Introduction

To be able to speak about environmental problems today one ought to master the language of risk, for the way this concept is understood, approached, and dealt with by regulators in different jurisdictions and across different legal cultures, is central to the normative discourse on environmental regulations. The regulation of nanotechnology risks is no exception. As Elizabeth Fisher puts it:

> The term 'risk' and its accompanying language are not only common inclusions in legislation, policy, case law and academic commentary, but are also increasingly framing the environmental law discourse. Indeed *it is now common for environmental problems to be characterized in terms of risk and the bulk of environmental regulatory law to be thought of as risk regulation.*[1]

Therefore, this is a chapter on the process of risk analysis and risk understanding as it specifically applies to the chemicals regulation area. The aim is to elucidate the very first steps of the regulatory process entrusted with the generation of 'raw' scientific data to be used as a legitimate basis for environmental measures. To this end, the discerning of the scientific paradigms governing the risk assessment procedures, placed at the heart of modern chemicals legislation, serves as a necessary gateway to the broader and multifaceted discourse on (environmental) risks and the uncertainty often plaguing such risks. It would be arduous to have any kind of analysis on the legal coverage of nanoscale chemicals in REACH without first understanding the science at the base of its legal framework and, in general, the interplay between science and law.

In REACH the science supporting the regulation is contained in the Annexes, the ECHA guidance documents (GDs), and, importantly, in legislative acts the Commission adopts in order to implement the provisions of REACH. Regulation (EC) No. 440/2008[2] dealing with test methods, represents a chief legal instrument for the implementation of the data requirements put forth by REACH. Its provisions are heavily influenced by the work of the

Organisation for Economic Co-operation and Development (OECD) on chemicals science harmonisation and standardisation, and by international law developments on the subject.

Most of the legalistic discourse that has formed around the regulation of chemicals' risks and harm, disregards, or at best only briefly mentions, the technical and scientific concepts that enable a modern law like REACH to function. As a result, the procedures and principles employed to establish the safety standards remain jealously guarded by those in disciplines other than law. Therefore, this book as a whole and this chapter in particular, seek to bridge the gap between these two constitutive areas of chemicals regulation, science and law, starting from the assumption that they are intertwined, over-lapping, and perhaps interdependent – and yet distinguishable each in their own purpose and role in chemicals risk regulation. It is one of this chapter's arguments that only by engaging properly with the science behind REACH can we trace an accurate mapping of the current shortcomings and loopholes for both bulk and nanoscale chemicals. From here, the leap to the conceptu-alisation of necessary legislative revisions to be undertaken in order to bring nano-chemicals under the REACH framework, is arguably shorter and more efficient.

The analysis here offered proceeds in three steps. First, it introduces the basic concepts and principles of *regulatory (environmental and human health) toxi-cology* which govern the risk assessment (RA) phase in most Western chem-icals legislations. Here an analysis of the concepts of *hazard* and *risk* within the RA model of REACH will be meticulously presented, together with some reflection on the nature and magnitude of nano-risks. Second, this chapter elaborates on the scientific and technical arguments on how uncertainty is viewed, measured, and accounted for within the scientific models of RA employed by modern chemicals law such as REACH. Finally, it will be observed that there seems to be a reluctance on the side of the EU legislator to take precautionary action and to do so early enough and with enough steadiness so as to concretely pursue the ambitious aim of high levels of human health and environmental protection that REACH declares to have at the centre of its massive regulatory machinery. This chapter will try to identify the main scientific, even before legal, constraints, that might be hin-dering precautionary rulings on nano-chemical risk regulation in REACH. It is important to stress once more that in a highly technical subject such as nanotechnology, understanding the law-science interface is 'a necessary evil'. As such, this chapter represents also the chief interdisciplinary element of this book.

Understanding how safe is safe enough

Toxicology is the science concerned with the study of poisons and toxic effects. When the risk analysis is conducted *by* or *on behalf of* governments or intergovernmental organisations (e.g. OECD) the toxicology contained in the

RA is referred to as *regulatory toxicology*.[3] Hence, regulatory toxicology is a subdiscipline which, through standard-setting and appropriate regulations, seeks to protect humans and the environment from the negative toxic effects of different agents, including chemical substances.[4]

In the regulatory jargon of REACH, the 'adequately controlled risk' concept is the yardstick for discerning 'safe' chemicals from 'harmful' ones. In REACH, risks are generally thought to be adequately controlled when exposure levels to the substance are kept below the *derived no-effect levels* (DNELs) for human health and the *predicted no-effect concentrations* (PNECs) for the environment.[5] As a consequence, such concepts are of primary regulatory relevance given that compliance with established DNELs and PNECs allows for a certain chemical to be produced and commercialised freely on the EU market.[6] Conversely, higher exposure levels than a given DNEL/PNEC determine either a ban, or a reversion of the onus of proof, in that the producer must justify why humans and the environment shall bear significant risks. It must be noted that the data used in toxicology in order to determine DNELs and PNECs values or exposure estimations always include uncertainties which inevitably might lead to an over- or under-estimation of risk.[7] In the case of nano-chemicals, though, the uncertainties come into play much earlier in the process of calculating DNELs or PNECs, i.e. already in the characterisation of hazards, which, as it will be shown, is a necessary precondition for a successful risk assessment. This nano-specific uncertainty builds on the general uncertainty that permeates toxicology as such, with the result that for the assessment of nano-risks, the inherent structural flaws of regulatory toxicology are further exacerbated. In order to make meaningful nano-specific RA consideration hence, a general analysis on how regulatory toxicology currently operates is necessary. The question thus arises: what are regulators talking about when they talk about hazard, dose, exposure, DNELs/PNECs, and other paradigmatic concepts of toxicology? The core rule of regulatory toxicology and the chemicals laws informed by it, such as the American Toxic Substances Control Act (TSCA) and REACH for instance, is the simple formulation from Paracelsus:

> Alle Dinge sind Gift und nichts ist ohne Gift, allein die Dosis macht es, dass ein Ding kein Gift ist.[8]

This rule, usually condensed in the adage *sola dosis facit venenum* (the dose makes the poison) indicates that all chemicals have the potential to be toxic, depending on the quantity of their intake. In regulatory toxicology this is expressed with the following formula:

Risk = f (Hazard × Exposure)

The hazard(s) represents the intrinsic property(ies) of a chemical, which cannot be altered. Therefore, in the case of very toxic chemicals, the only way to prevent risks and hence harm to humans and the environment, is to reduce exposure to the chemical in question. This awareness is at the core of *hazard-based* regulation models, which stipulate that for very dangerous chemicals, for which no exposure is deemed tolerable and/or no safe dose can be established, the only effective regulatory measure is the de facto ban of the substances in question. Such ban operationalises a strong version of precaution in that it is for those claiming that risks can be controlled or should be tolerated, to provide the scientific (and/or socio-economic) justification supporting such claims. A correlated (but not necessarily exclusive, as it may well apply also to risk-based models, see below) concept here is that of *qualitative assessment* where the hazards rather than the risks are assessed, and where methods other than numeric estimations are employed in characterising risks. The result is a more descriptive model of risk assessment where judgments about the chemical's toxicity profiles and threshold are only based on some initial empirical data, without however being limited to such data.

However, a zero exposure is not possible, unless a total ban on production is imposed. A stop in production of hazardous chemicals would require a radical change of the industrial sector and the modern lifestyles that today are heavily dependent on the production and use of a large number of chemicals. Hence, in order to protect human and environmental health, chemical laws around the globe operate within the contours of the above-mentioned formula, by seeking to control the other variable, that of exposure, so that the overall risks will be kept at acceptable levels. Clearly, the better the hazardous properties of a chemical are understood and the better exposure can be monitored, measured, and quantified, the higher the chances for regulators to appraise risks and respond to such risks with adequate regulatory actions. Put it differently, such *risk-based* regulatory models presume an ability to control risk through exposure control and the application of safety factors (the 'f' in the given formula). In practical terms, the legislator (or industry, depending on who, according to the law, has the legal duty to perform testing in order to provide data on safety/risk) ought to be able to clearly point at the intrinsic properties of a chemical which are responsible for its toxic profiles and qualify such profiles (i.e. ecotoxicity, reproductive toxicity, carcinogenicity, bioaccumulation, etc.). Finally, the regulating entity should be able to understand what route and degree of exposure to the hazards this way characterised can lead to the materialisation of harm for humans and for the environment.

A correlated feature of such model of regulation is the *quantitative* approach to risk assessment, according to which risks and uncertainties can be quantified in numerical terms. Simply put, the hazard-based regulatory models make use of mainly qualitative/descriptive RA approaches, whereas risk-based models make use of mainly quantitative/mathematical ones. In risk appraisal, chemicals regulations today generally operate through precise numeric values (hence through a *quantitative* approach), such as the *no-observed-(adverse)-effect level* (NO(A)EL) and *lowest-observed-adverse-effect level* (LOAEL), *predicted environmental concentration* (PEC), *predicted no-effect concentration* (PNEC) and *derived no-effect level* (DNEL), or even the *acceptable daily intake* (ADI). Importantly though, 'toxicology as a biological and experimental discipline does not provide such precise data [value numbers attributed to NOEAL/PNEC/ DNEL]'.[9] How can the legislator deduce such numbers? And through what conceptual models? The following elaborates on how the current models of regulatory toxicology – including their inherent deductions and assumptions – came about.

The National Research Council's Reports

The models for assessing chemicals risk are those put forward in two reports from the US National Research Council (NRC). The first report, known as the *Red Book* on risk assessment,[10] advocates for a clear separation of the Risk Assessment phase from that of Risk Management, suggesting that

> regulatory agencies take steps to establish and *maintain a clear conceptual distinction between assessment of risks and consideration of risk management alternatives*; that is, the scientific findings and policy judgments embodied in risk assessments should be *explicitly distinguished* from the political, economic, and technical considerations that influence the design and choice of regulatory strategies.[11]

In this report, the NRC points at the necessity of having a detailed written RA which explains how the assessment was performed, before embarking on legislative measures. Explaining the choices and strategies that inform experts' reasoning in the assessment process, would, in NRC's view, help to maintain a 'sharper distinction between science and policy in the assessment of risk'[12] advocated greatly (albeit not exclusively) throughout the document. This approach seems to be justified by the need to 'guard against the inappropriate intrusion of risk management considerations' in the assessment of facts.[13] In other words, the role of regulators in the RA process is seen with suspicion as it might negatively interfere with the scientific reasoning, which ought to take place on a separated plane from that where the policy choices are made by risk managers. Hence, the Red Book defines *risk assessment* as 'the use of the factual base to define the health effects of exposure of individuals or populations to hazardous materials and situations',[14] adding that 'For some observers, the term is synonymous with *quantitative risk assessment* and emphasizes reliance on numerical results. Our broader definition includes quantification, but also includes qualitative expressions of risk.'[15]

Risk management is instead defined as 'the process of weighing policy alternatives and selecting the most appropriate regulatory action, integrating the results of risk assessment with engineering data and with social, economic, and political concerns to reach a decision'.[16] In the Red Book, RA is articulated in four phases, and regulators worldwide currently employ the following definitions within their legal systems:

- *Hazard identification*: The determination of whether a particular chemical is or is not causally linked to particular health effects.
- *Dose-response assessment*: The determination of the relation between the magnitude of exposure and the probability of occurrence of the health effects in question.
- *Exposure assessment*: The determination of the extent of human exposure before or after application of regulatory controls.
- *Risk characterisation*: The description of the nature and often the magnitude of human risk, including attendant uncertainty.[17]

The 1983 NRC Red Book has been viewed by regulators worldwide, perhaps wrongly so,[18] as advocating a clear-cut distinction between science and democracy; between a scientific RA and a policy-driven RM. Or, as the NRC would observe in a subsequent document, this report remains today 'best known for popularizing the distinction between risk assessment and risk management and raising the issue of how best to *keep these functions separate, yet coordinated*'.[19]

The alleged dichotomy was reiterated by the authoritative British Royal Society[20] and recalled in different case law in the US during the 1990s, despite the fact that the actual approach in the Red Book was in fact something more nuanced than a clear-cut distinction and most importantly, despite the distance taken from this drastic division in a subsequent NRC report entitled *Understanding Risk*.[21] In this late version,[22] the NRC recognised that 'science is not necessarily neutral and objective in its ways of framing problems'[23] and as a consequence, it called for an *analytic-deliberative approach* to RA which devotes greater attention to the RA variables other than scientific data and models; rather, the way scientific uncertainty should be tackled, understood, and handled in the RA process and the public participation in such a process, were presented as crucial factors which ought to be taken into account when asserting a specific risk. In so doing, the regulatory process would be based in a more *creative approach*[24] which would allow for greater participation of different stakeholders and, as a consequence, enable a more inclusive and democratic decision-making strategy on risk.

More specifically, the *creative approach* seeks to dismiss the previous approach taken in the Red Book, where risk characterisation, the final and crucial step in the RA process, needed 'no additional scientific knowledge or concepts' and 'only a minimal amount of judgment'.[25] The 1996 NRC report concluded that this inaccurate view of RA in general and that on the risk characterisation step in particular, permeated the work of different agencies in regulating risks, including ecological ones. Therefore, the view of risk assessment as a summary of solely scientific considerations is found to be 'seriously deficient' by the 1996 NRC report and, hence, in need for a more robust conceptualisation. Under the new conceptualisation, RA and its final phase, risk characterisation, should among other things, 'reflect both *analysis* and *deliberation*, with appropriate input from the interested and affected parties', meaning that both the scientific and rigorous methods developed by science experts *and* discussion, reflection, and communicative persuasion should be valued. This way, 'deliberation frames analysis and analysis informs deliberation'.[26] Despite these new elements in the 1996 NRC report advocating a risk characterisation reflecting both analysis and deliberation, the distinction between science and democracy has not only remained but, through a number of case laws in the US, the WTO, and finally on the EU levels has been assumed to be immutable.[27]

This book adheres to the view that the *analytic-deliberative* (AD) approach, as suggested in the 1996 NRC report, would be preferred to the current vision of strict separation between science and policy. However, in order for it to be optimal, the AD approach would need to be applied to the RA process as a whole. That is, the AD approach should kick in much earlier in the RA process, starting with hazard identification. As far as nano-chemicals are concerned, an AD approach would be particularly relevant also in the subsequent phases of dose–response relationship and exposure assessments.[28] In addition, this chapter argues for the need for lawyers and representatives of humanities[29] in general to become involved in the risk assessment process, starting from the collection of data. Given the type and magnitude of nano-related risk, this need is even more acute for the risk appraisal process of such chemicals. In order to substantiate such claims a thorough analysis of the technical-scientific background against which a complex legal architecture of REACH is built, is warranted. Therefore the following investigates the science that stands behind those administrative and legal provisions that, based on the analysis of Chapters 3–6, are already considered to be problematic for the regulation of nanoscale chemicals under the REACH umbrella.

Whose toxicology after all?

Before navigating the depths of regulatory toxicology in order to have a grip on concepts that REACH employs in its legal reasoning such as dose, exposure, and hazard, it is important to first sketch the contours of regulatory toxicology as a discipline, and identify the international actors involved in the generation of such science.

If toxicology is the science that deals with poisons and toxic effects, *regulatory toxicology* (RT) is 'a subdiscipline concerned with the question of how man and the environment can be protected from toxic effects'.[30] Much of RT is hence devoted to making appropriate regulations and setting suitable standards.[31] However, while the data-gathering process and the criteria employed therein are necessarily scientific in nature, the regulatory aims to be served by the analysis, understanding, and assessment of such data, involve socio-political considerations. It can be said hence that RT's function is to offer a solid empirical basis to the legal-political goal of human health and environmental protection. The entire process of regulating chemical risks is shaped by a multidisciplinary, multilevel, and multi-actor context. Historically speaking, toxicity testing for regulatory purposes became mandatory only after the 1960 thalidomide (*Contergan*) tragedy in Germany.[32] Industrial chemicals testing other than drugs took hold only in the following decades: the 1969 EC Dangerous Substances directive and its 7th amendment of 1981, the 1976 US TSCA, or the 1974 Japan Chemical Substances Control Law are some of the major laws passed by the major chemicals-producing nations worldwide.

The first difficulties encountered by the establishment of national standards for chemicals safety related to the differences in approach, guidelines, methodologies, and the consequent repercussions these had on trade and competition. Therefore, harmonisation was seen as the key element in order to achieve a balance between two often competing aims: that of health and environmental protection standard-setting and that of trade and competition barrier-elimination.

The role and limitations of harmonised OECD testing guidelines

When it comes to testing for regulatory purposes, complete harmonisation of test guidelines has been achieved in all areas of toxicology under the OECD.[33] Starting with the adoption and the publication of the *OECD Test Guidelines for the Chemicals* (TGs), regulatory safety testing of all chemicals became mandatory for OECD members[34] on such harmonised basis. Importantly, the OECD TGs – which operate through the *mutual acceptance of data* (MAD) of testing data produced by OECD members following the TGs guidelines – are accepted not only for toxicity testing but also for physicochemical properties and environmental safety (including bioaccumulation and degradation) assessment.[35] As a result, chemicals testing for REACH purposes must be conducted in accordance with the harmonised OECD TGs and the *good laboratory practice* (GLP).[36] The GLP is a prerequisite for successful MAD.[37] From a purely legal prospective, OECD guidelines are considered to be 'soft law' instruments.[38] However, as is commonly the case on an international law level, soft law can 'harden' and this can happen, among other ways through 'cross-references from one institution to another, the recalling of guidelines adopted by other apparently concurrent international authorities, recurrent invocation of the same rules formulated in one way or another at the universal, regional and more restricted levels'.[39] With the adoption of REACH, only OECD-approved TGs are accepted in Europe[40] and the ECHA specifies on its website that 'requirements on ecotoxicity, toxicity and physical-chemical properties are generated using [the OECD harmonised] test guidelines'.[41]

Of note here is the fact that testing concerning the toxicity of drugs, pesticides, cosmetics, and food and feed additives are *not* harmonised under the OECD guidelines. The exclusion of these areas from the harmonisation process assumes significant relevance in the case of testing nano-scale chemicals, especially those used in cosmetics, food contact materials (FMCs), food additives, and biocides. For instance, chemicals used in the food law area do not need to comply with REACH's safety requirements for what concerns their human health risks. This is because they will be tested for human health effects under sector-specific legislation enacted in the EU. Nevertheless, environmental safety is not dealt with under said specific legislation, i.e. the plastic FCM regulation, the food additives regulation, etc., which means that chemicals used in FCMs or food additives still need to comply with the REACH provisions and testing requirements on environmental toxicity. In addition, in case a chemical is listed in the REACH List of Substances Subject to Authorisation (Annex XIV of REACH) because of *human health* hazards (e.g. carcinogenic, mutagenic, or toxic to reproduction (CMR) properties) its use in FCMs will be exempted from an authorisation requirement in REACH, due to the fact that human health risks are managed under the specific sectorial legislation. However, if the inclusion in Annex XIV of REACH is owed to the *environmental* hazards the substance poses (e.g. PBT/vPvB), then the authorisation in REACH shall be obtained before the substance is used in FCMs. Logically these intertwined rules are elaborated in such a manner as to avoid overlapping and duplicated obligations. This different allocation of testing responsibilities, though – human health to the sector-specific EU registration and environmental toxicity to the REACH – bears significant implications in terms of safety considerations. This for two main reasons:

1   First, in the absence of harmonisation, for chemicals used in drugs, cosmetics, FMCs, biocides, and food additives, OECD members are free to use their own criteria and testing standards in assessing risks, setting the 'safety bar' at a level they deem appropriate. Additionally, as the following shall demonstrate, the chosen safety standards depend to a great extent on the chosen testing models and their underlying assumption on how, for instance, to account for uncertainty and ignorance.

2   Second, and most importantly for this book's aim, the EU sectoral regulations on biocides, cosmetics, FCMs, and food additives, are all *nano-specific* which means that the testing of their human health risks is in principle performed specifically for their nano-related physicochemical properties. However, REACH, which still applies for the environmental risks of chemicals used in such areas of application, will contain nano-specific provisions only by 2020, and even then, only in the Annexes and not in the legal text (like the sector-specific regulations in question do).

This discrepancy might give rise to legal uncertainty, inconsistency, and fragmentation. As we shall see in the following, the different scientific principles applicable to nanotoxicity are likely to exacerbate the consequences of what seems to be a lack of legal coherence in regulating chemicals' risks in the EU.

ECHA's Guidance Documents

It is one of the ECHA's prerogatives to prepare, keep, and update a number of technical Guidance Documents (GDs) in order to clarify REACH requirements and facilitate compliance. The GDs are considered to be instruments of soft law. They often contain a legal notice[42] clearly reminding the user that the only text of reference with regard to legally binding obligation remains REACH. However, with the adoption of the Lisbon Treaty and the new Article 263 TFEU therein, acts of EU agencies have become amenable to judicial review.[43] Notwithstanding legal notices and disclaimers, as Scott observes, 'non-binding shall not be equated with an absence of legal effects'.[44] It has already been pointed out that to date, the number of case laws concerning the conspicuous ECHA GDs on REACH, has been rather limited.[45] It has also been speculated that this might be so either because the GDs are not problematic from a legislative standpoint or because the cases that ended up in Court were not the best suited to challenge the legal nature of the GDs (or a mix of the two reasons).[46] To date, the ECHA has attached seven nano-specific appendixes to some of its GDs with six of them containing recommendations to be followed by registrants of nanosubstances during information gathering, chemical safety assessment (CSA), and the preparation of the chemicals safety report (CSR).[47] No doubt that such information will be welcomed by diligent producers wishing to comply with the REACH requirements, even in the absence of legal norms imposing a legal duty to do so. In addition, they might serve the scope of fostering data generation on nano-risks. As examined in Chapter 4, four ECHA decisions to request information on the nanoform of certain registered chemicals were annulled by the BoA.[48] The industry's main argument, upheld by the BoA, was the lack of provisions in REACH that would allow the ECHA to advance such a request and the contextual lack in the ECHA's GDs of technical advice on how to identify nanomaterials. Indeed, the ECHA's *Guidance on Identification and Naming of Chemicals*, a necessary starting point for every registration dossier, states:

> The current developments in nano-technology and insights in related hazard effects may cause the need for additional information on size of the substances in the future. The current state of development *is not mature enough to include guidance on the identification of substances in the nano-form in this guidance document.*[49]

It is important to note that while this book was being finalised, the ECHA adopted a number of new nano-specific Appendixes to its GDs and updated some of the existing ones.[50] Nonetheless, the proposed Appendix 4 to *Guidance on Registration*, containing recommendations on how to define nanomaterials, has not been adopted yet.[51] Of note is the fact that the Draft Appendix in question, in line with the 2011 Recommendation on the definition of the term 'nanomaterial', which is itself currently under review, seeks to offer a definition of the term 'nanoform' for registration purposes. It identifies in *size, shape,* and *surface chemistry* three of the key elements common to all nanomaterials.[52]

In the present situation, the lack of specific information about nanoforms covered by REACH registration dossiers and persistent scientific gaps as to the suitability of test methods for nanoforms of substances, are pointed out as the major hindrances to an appropriate regulation of nanosubstances within REACH.[53] Furthermore, the lack of an explicit legal obligation to register nanoforms separately in REACH and the lack of a definition of nanomaterial/nanoform therein, cause a general shortage of data that impedes the registration of nanosubstances in REACH.[54] A closer look at REACH's scientific models helps understand why this is so.

REACH implementing legislation: Regulation EC No. 440/2008 on test methods

When it comes to test methods, REACH is complemented by Regulation EC No. 440/2008,[55] which contains a long and elaborate list of tests to be performed for different endpoints[56] for both human health and environmental toxicity. The test methods are based on the OECD TGs on the same endpoints. Hence, the soft law rule of the OECD documents is hardened through transposition in EU law by way of regulation, a secondary law instrument, directly binding on MSs. As mentioned earlier, this Regulation is not nano-specific. As a general indication in said Regulation, the EU legislature is supposed to update its testing methods in line with new developments that might take place on the OECD level. As far as the latest developments on nanosubstance testing are concerned, no nano-related updates have been made so far. On the contrary, an important amendment in this regard, containing 'four new and one updated method for the determination of ecotoxicity and environmental fate and behaviour; nine methods for the determination of toxicity and other health effects including four inhalation toxicity test methods', clearly excludes the application of such methods for chemicals in nanoscale by specifying that

> This test method is not specifically intended for the testing of nanomaterials/This Test Method is not intended for the testing of nanomaterials.[57]

Nevertheless, in a press release from 2015, the OECD reassured the member governments and the consumers on the fact that tests used on standard chemical compounds 'are *in the most part* suitable for use on nanomaterials'.[58] The statement claimed that the conclusion was based on a seven-year experimental testing programme during which 11 commercially available nanomaterials were tested using over 110 existing testing methods. In addition, the press release further stated, 780 studies were conducted on the physicochemical properties of nanomaterials in order to eventually fill the data gap in the understanding of nanomaterials. The OECD concluded:

> The tests showed that the standard test guidelines used for normal chemical substances are in the most part suitable for use on nanomaterials. Changes to the Test Guidelines to better understand the intrinsic properties of nanomaterials are now providing a clear framework for OECD countries to move forward in the examination of nanomaterials.[59]

However, a quick search of the dossiers prepared for 11 commonly used nanomaterials, including nano silver and CNTs, leaves some perplexity as to the actual use of such data in the performance of risk assessment under the existing regulatory frameworks, including REACH. What seems more concerning from a regulatory standpoint is the fact the OECD accompanies the publication of the dossiers on its website with the following disclaimer:

> The dossiers found on this website *are for information only and are not to be used as a reference, standard or validation regarding the safety of specific nanomaterials*. The dossiers contained within this site were chosen to show the efficacy and accuracy of standard test guidelines and was *not intended for use in the determination of risks associated with the use or application of nanomaterials*. The data contained within these dossiers is raw data and has not been evaluated by either the programme sponsors or the WPMN. Any conclusions found within the [*sic*] these dossiers are the responsibility of the researchers who made them.[60]

A quick search of the dossiers yields several inconsistencies, data gaps, missing information and deficiencies on how the testing was conducted and the results collected. A similar responsibility-avoiding disclaimer is found in each single dossier. For example, the few dossiers on *nano silver* state:

> The programme focused on answering scientific questions in the field of the OECD test guidelines but not to provide conclusions on the hazard or risk of the materials selected. *The absence of data for some endpoints* may be a gap for some endpoints but for other endpoints there may not if the data was not considered necessary. Although the programme ensured a broad participation of many stakeholders *it was not intended to arrive at any pre-defined regulatory datasets requirements or risk assessment decisions*.[61]

In fact, a recent study commissioned by the Centre for International Environmental Law (CIEL) concluded that the OECD dossiers on nanomaterials are of little to no value for risk assessment purposes. The study analysed 11,500 pages of OECD dossiers on 11 nanomaterials and all characterisation and toxicity data on three specific nanomaterials – fullerenes, single-walled carbon nanotubes, and zinc oxide. The conclusion is that the claims on the existence of sufficient data on nanomaterials were 'not only false, but dangerously so'.[62]

Furthermore, in some cases the tests required by the REACH standard programme were absent from REACH's implementing regulation on test methods (Regulation (EC) No. 440/2008), in spite of their inclusion in the OECD guidelines.[63] In the presence of such a fragmented and rather desolated technical and legal overview, the understanding of the use of science in law becomes even more important. The following elaborates thus on the models underpinning the existing toxicity test methods as they currently (are deemed to) apply to nano-chemicals, and their implications in terms of human health and environmental protection. The analysis seeks to cast some light on the numerous limitations and loopholes of said methods and models, in the belief that nanoscale chemicals are only uncovering and emphasising deep flaws that have always been present in regulatory toxicology. These flaws and limitations are in a way intrinsic to the very foundations and conceptualisation of regulatory toxicology and the use regulators make of the data this way derived for human health and environmental protection purposes.

It is hoped that the nano-related challenges will bring a radical paradigmatic shift in the well-established but ill-functioning foundations of regulatory toxicology.

Risk assessment deconstructed

When dealing with the structure of RA models currently in place, two aspects must be underlined from the outset. First, the RA model the EU currently adopts is that derived from the NRC Red Book, where RA is the product of a staged analysis. The starting point for such an analysis is the *identification of hazard*, where hazards are understood as the intrinsic properties of a chemical which cannot be altered. In order to be able to perform an RA and hence enable the legislator to regulate nano-related risks, a good understanding of nano-related hazardous properties is of crucial importance. Once such hazards are rightly understood and characterised, the study of the *dose-response relationship* follows. However, in order to assess such a relationship, exposure data should be available, at least to some extent. As to the *dose* concept, in the Red Book it was thought not to pose particular difficulties due to the general acceptance of dose expressed as a linear function of mass (usually expressed in gr or mg). Precisely at this stage, the regulatory powers first kick in: when regulatory standards are based on risk control, the law will be concerned with controlling such risks by keeping exposure at the lowest level considered safe according to the chosen level of protection. Hence, the third phase of the RA model is *exposure assessment*, where the legislator is preoccupied with controlling routes and levels of exposure to certain hazardous chemicals given that the hazardousness of chemicals is not subject to alteration whatsoever. Ultimately, the *risks* will be *characterised* in terms of nature, potency, and consequences of effects for humans and/or the environment.[64]

Risk management measures, ranging from authorisation and restriction of uses to a complete ban, can be promulgated – but only once the RA is concluded, the risks characterised, and the uncertainties appraised.

Second, as we shall see, policy assumptions and guesswork are not uncommon throughout what are considered to be purely scientific aspects of the risk appraisal process. Indeed, they take place in the preliminary stages of RA and, as a consequence, there seems to be no plausible reason that would prevent regulators for their part from engaging earlier on in the RA process.

If REACH truly is to operate on a precautionary basis in the pursuit of the high levels of human health and environmental protection aim, as its Article 1 states, then policy discourse and analytic considerations should be anticipated and accommodated during the scientific process of RA. Most importantly, the policy goals and considerations thus anticipated shall be of a different nature from the methods (mainly mathematical) already used by scientists to estimate safety standards. As the two reports from the European Environmental Agency (EEA) demonstrate, numerous examples of chemicals such as DDT, PBCs, Bisphenol A, etc. were tested and dealt with in terms of risk control under the existing test methods and scientific protocols. Yet, the consequences for human health and the environment deriving from their authorised uses under the existing laws have been catastrophic.[65] Nanoscale chemicals, as the second of these reports also indicates, seem to be following the same pattern in terms of late and non-tailored regulatory response. Even though the available information on nanotoxicity is studded by uncertainty, sufficient scientific data exist as to warrant action on the regulatory plan. Still, if any suggestion is to be provided on how to break the vicious circle of poor regulatory response to chemical risks,[66] it ought to be based on a proper understating of the regulatory regimes concerned with the control of chemicals risks.

The rest of this chapter is hence focused on elaborating on *how* and *why* regulators making use of RT to frame their health environmental protection measures often seem to grope around in the dark. Understating the role of uncertainty in RA is a mandatory starting point. Given that uncertainty affects the understating of chemicals' harm, it is important to underline once more that risk assessment, understood as the process that estimates the probability that certain harmful effects might occur following exposure to chemical hazards, can be *qualitative* or *quantitative* in nature.[67] The choice between the two methods depends on the availability and quality of data. The quantitative assessment is mainly based on mathematical calculations and inference models, whereas the qualitative one may involve the classification of data into weight-of-evidence categories[68] and include considerations such as the severity of the risk. More precisely, hazard identification, risk characterisation, and *uncertainty analysis* represent the domains within the RA process where *qualitative* methods can be applied.[69] With this in mind, the constitutive elements and paradigms of regulatory toxicology as used in RA are analysed in light of nanotechnology developments. Before that, a last crucial remark: although

Table 7.1 Comparison of human and environmental risk assessment

Human	Ecological
Protect one species – humans.	Protects multiple species, including plants, invertebrates and animals.
Well-established guidance and procedures.	Newer field where guidance and procedures are still evolving.
Criteria are meant to be protective of the individual, including sensitive subpopulations.	Criteria are meant to be protective of populations or habitats.
All adverse effects are considered.	Only growth, reproduction, and mortality endpoints are considered.
Carcinogenic effects are considered.	Cancer is not considered an adverse effect.

Source: see note 70.

the scientific paradigms governing the assessment of human health and environmental (ecological) risks are the same (i.e. hazard characterisation, exposure estimation, dose-response, and RC), significant differences exist in the way these paradigms are implemented. This is so not only because eco-systems are highly complex yet poorly understood, but also because the goals of the environmental risk assessment are different from the human health ones. Table 7.1 summarises the main differences in this regard.[70]

Note that to these inherent differences and difficulties in the RA process, an ulterior layer of complexity and uncertainty is to be added for the case of nanoscale chemicals' risks.

Identifying, assessing, and characterising hazards

Within the four-pronged model of RA that REACH currently employs, the identification of hazards is a mandatory starting point. In regulatory terms, this means that an effective and efficient RA will be possible only *if* and *to the extent to which* the inherent properties of a chemical will be identified by expert toxicologists. A precondition for hazard characterisation is the identifi-cation of the physical-chemical properties which determine the *toxicokinetics* and the *pharmacokinetics*. The former studies the rate at which a chemical enters the body and its fate once the chemical is inside the organism, whereas the latter studies how the exposed organism deals with the substance in ques-tion in terms of absorption, distribution, and excretion (ADME). In addition, toxicokinetics can be combined with *toxicodynamics* in what is called a toxicokinetic-toxicodynamic (TKTD) model, used normally for the quanti-fication of ecotoxicity[71] and the hazardousness of a chemical in terms of environmental impact. The toxicokinetics and the pharmacokinetics of a chemical are largely determined – within the current models of regulatory toxicology – by solubility, *molecular size*, dissociation behaviour, and vapour pressure.[72] It is not the intention of this chapter to elaborate on difficult scientific details. Nevertheless, a basic explanation of such concepts serves the purpose of understanding the science behind REACH. Moreover, the discussion on such parameters has been at the centre of the regulatory efforts on nanotechnology at the EU level and the scientific discourse in this regard.

The ECHA provides extensive guidance on information requirements in REACH, the gathering of such information, and their evaluation in the context of hazard assessment, in accordance with the tonnage-based system described in Chapter 3.[73] Pursuant to Article 10 of REACH, the minimum standard information to be included in the registration dossier includes:

- substance identity;
- physico-chemical properties;
- exposure/uses/occurrence and applications;
- mammalian toxicity;
- environmental toxicity;
- environmental fate, including chemical and biotic degradation;
- human data;
- data from *in vivo* or *in vitro* studies that have not been generated in accordance with the latest adopted/accepted version of the corresponding (validated) test method or to good laboratory practice (GLP) (or equivalent) standards;
- (Q)SAR model outputs;
- SAR model outputs, read-across, and category approaches.[74]

The generation of data on the physicochemical properties of substances is one crucial starting point in the RA process. The understanding of chemicals' mode of toxic action has a direct bearing on the understanding of the risks posed for health and the environment and for the control of such risks through effective regulatory measures. Therefore it is important that this 'information searching strategy is as wide as possible'.[75] This means that in-house company and trade association files containing data on chemical manufacturing and use should be supplemented by other sources of information such as databanks and databases of compiled data; (Q)SAR models; and even published literature including primary papers, books, and monographs.[76] As in the case of nanomaterials, the scarcity of data is particularly problematic. As stated in Chapter 4, the generation of characterisation data for nanoscale chemicals through the use of conventional *in vivo* and *in vitro* testing methods and even the Q(SARs) ones, is, at best, very limited. In such a situation, the use of alternative sources of information on physicochemical properties becomes essential. It can be argued that the alternative sources are the only available source of information for understanding the nature and the toxicity profiles of nanoscale chemicals. But notwithstanding the ever-increasing amount of literature on the subject, little to no regulatory action is taking place that could adjust the legal-technical provisions to the special nature of nano-chemicals. Furthermore, pursuant to the REACH system, registrants have a general duty to collect *all relevant and available information* on the intrinsic properties of a substance, to assist in identifying hazardous properties, and to make recommendations about risk management measures.[77] This is true regardless of whether or not testing for a given endpoint is required for the specific tonnage level.[78] These legal indications would suggest a duty for manufacturers of chemicals to collect data on possible toxicological profiles of nanoscale chemicals, regardless of the quantity produced. Whether such data need to be submitted, either as a specific dossier or as part of the registration dossier for the bulk chemicals, is rather uncertain as nothing in REACH indicates the obligation to treat nanoscale chemicals as *new* for regulatory purposes. Specific testing on physicochemical properties (e.g. boiling point, water solubility, flammability, etc.) and other human health (e.g. irritation and corrosion, acute toxicity, mutagenicity, carcinogenicity, etc.) and environmental endpoints (e.g. aquatic toxicity, degradation/biodegradation, terrestrial bioaccumulation, etc.) is required for registration purposes, according to volume bands. For each endpoint, the ECHA has drafted long and detailed Guidance Documents.[79]

In case the empirical information on the hazardousness of a chemical is inconclusive, the *Weight of Evidence approach (WoE)* can be used. The WoE represents a qualitative dimension of the hazard characterisation phase, defined as 'the process of considering the strengths and weaknesses of various pieces of information in reaching and supporting a conclusion concerning a property of the substance'.[80] The WoE outcome is a score number evaluating the reliability, relevance, and adequacy of data. Logically, the effectiveness of the WoE approach depends, among other things, on the quality of such data, the nature and severity of the effects, and the relevance of the information for the given regulatory endpoint. The *Klimisch* score is an endpoint-specific method used in the WoE to evaluate the *reliability* of data. It consists of a scoring system assigned to the available information from toxicological and ecotoxicological studies in the following way:

1 Reliable without restrictions
2 Reliable with restrictions
3 Not reliable
4 Not assignable[81]

In addition to reliability, the evaluation of *relevance* and *adequacy* of the scientific information should follow. If inconclusive information from each single individual source does not allow for an evaluation as to whether a substance has or does not have a particular dangerous property, there might still be sufficient WoE from several independent sources of information to allow for a decision on the same point. This is the case when newly developed test methods or equivalent testing methods recognised on the EU level, are unable to clarify if a chemical has or does not have a certain property and need therefore to be supplemented by expert judgment on the evaluation of the information at hand. In addition, the WoE might be a way to reduce testing on vertebrate animals in particular, contributing to the 3R aim (reduce, refine, replace) of REACH with regard to animal welfare.[82]

There is, however, a flip side to the WoE approach. Decisions based on this approach depend heavily on expert judgment and are, as a consequence, exposed to issues related to impartiality, transparency, and ethical considera-tion. This also means that there is no such thing as a precise RA and that 'sci-entists will *always* differ in the conclusions they draw from the same set of data, particularly if they contain some implicit value judgments'.[83] It is there-fore of primary importance that decision-makers understand that this process is laden with assumptions and values.[84] Hence, it emerges that contrary to the popularised image of the RA phase as an exquisitely scientific endeavour, extra-scientific considerations and other judgments significantly influence the way scientific information is assessed and relied upon, including in the very first steps of the risk appraisal process.

Hazard identification can be a clear example of a qualitative assessment which combines data on humans or laboratory animals, ancillary information (e.g. structure-activity and pharmacokinetics), and the final 'weighting' of such information by expert toxicologists, in order to describe 'the full range of available information and the implications of that information for human health [and the environment]'.[85]

Once the (eco)toxicological hazards of a chemical have been identified, the registrant is also required to determine the *dose descriptor* for each adverse effect to human health and the environment. The dose descriptor 'is the term used to identify the relationship between a specific effect of a substance and the dose at which it takes place'.[86] It is an important parameter since it is used to derive no-effect threshold levels for human health and the environment, in the subsequent phase of dose-response relationship.[87]

But are the methods thus far described applicable for the identification and characterisation of nano-related hazards?

Nano-specific guidance on substance identification

It has already been stressed elsewhere in this book that the special nature of substances in nanoscale is posing particular challenges for the use of the exist-ing methodologies to generate toxicity data for decision-making purposes. In this regard, several scientific opinions from the EU's most prominent scient-ific bodies such as the SCENIHR, the JRC, and the EFSA's panels, have conducted a considerable amount of work in trying to elucidate those aspects of nanosubstances that determine their toxicity profiles, so as to help the EU legislature to design a tailored regulatory response. As early as 2006, the SCENIHR was mandated by the Commission to assess the validity of the existing testing methodologies for nanoscale chemicals. Significant knowledge gaps were identified by the SCENIHR with regard to the appropriateness of the application of said testing to nano-scale chemicals. Concerning physico-chemical properties, the opinion concluded:

> It is unclear at the present time the extent to which the toxicokinetics, the environmental distribution and fate of nanoparticles can be predicted from knowledge of their physicochemical properties.[88]

The opinion suggests that other physicochemical properties owed to the nanoscale, such as information on the number of nanoparticles and/or their surface area able to affect nanoparticles' behaviour and fate in the human body and in environmental media. Therefore, when identifying hazards, nano-related parameters ought to be taken into account. The opinion stated:

> In order to understand and categorize the mechanisms for nanoparticle toxicity, information is needed on the response of living systems to the presence of nanoparticles *of varying size, shape, surface and bulk chemical composition*, as well as the temporal fate of the nanoparticles that are subject to translocation and degradation processes. The typical path within the organ and/or cell, which may be the result of either diffusion or active intracellular transportation, is also of relevance. Very little information on these aspects is presently available and this implies *that there is an urgent need for toxicokinetic data for nanoparticles*.[89]

In a later opinion, the SCENIHR reinforced the idea that there is a need to understand and assess the nano-specific physicochemical properties and once again drew attention to the fact that

> the size distribution of the substance to be evaluated may greatly influence the final outcome, in particular as *the toxic potency is most likely to be greater at the lower end of the size distribution spectrum*.[90]

While the debate on the best way of characterising nanoscale chemicals from a hazardousness standpoint based on their peculiar physicochemical properties is an ongoing one, the methodologies and the GDs in REACH and else-where continue to operate primarily on the basis of existing test methods and characterisation parameters.

However, due to the emerging shortcomings, the ECHA guidance on the compilation of safety data sheets (SDS)[91] in REACH indicates that when basic physical and chemical properties information is filled out with regard to the 'appearance' of the chemical at hand, the following should be observed:

> In describing 'granulometry' further available and appropriate information on properties referred to in *the OECD-WPMN of nanomaterials such as size and size distribution, shape, porosity, pour density, aggregation/agglomeration*

*state, morphology, surface area (m2/mass), surface charge/zeta potential and crys-
talline phase* should be taken into account. The available and appropriate
information on the *specific surface area refers to the specific surface area by
volume which is derived as a ratio of the surface area by mass* and the relative
density can be added here where considered to be relevant. In particular
this subsection may be used to indicate substances or mixtures that have
nanoforms put on the market. If the substance is supplied as nanomaterial, this *may* be indicated in this subsection. E.g. physical state: solid
(nanomaterial).[92]

The EU represents perhaps the only legal system to have adopted such
detailed specific GDs for nanomaterials on the generation of specific data
for human health and environmental endpoints testing. How effective such
documents are in practice, is another question entirely. For the physicochemical properties,[93] the nano-specific appendix to the *Guidance on
Information Requirements and Chemical Safety Assessment* highlights a number
of limitations and difficulties in interpreting uncertain data. Regarding the
physicochemical characterisation of nanosubstances and based on the conclusion of RIP-oN 2, a crucial indication is that nano-specific parameters
such as shape, surface area, and particle size distribution (either on its own
or as a specific part of the granulometry information required for bulk
chemicals) should be provided.[94] What emerges from the document is that
the use of non-testing methods (*in silico*) for specific endpoints, i.e. for the
assessment of hazard for humans is yet to be established for nanomaterials.
Consequently, the use of such methods must be scientifically justified and
applied on a case-by-case basis only, normally in a WoE context.[95] What is
more, *in vivo* tests for generating the same data on nanoscale chemicals
present also problematic points.[96]

How, then, are registrants supposed to fulfil basic registration requirements
in REACH in such complete ignorance and practical infeasibility?

Moreover, as explained in this chapter, ecotoxicology is the area most
shrouded in uncertainty and ignorance in the RA of chemicals. Assumptions
and extrapolations are the rule in this field, and almost nothing is known on
how chemicals impact ecosystems; consequently, it is impossible to provide a
tailored and effective regulatory response to the protection of the environment in a holistic way. Reference to some nano-specific tests elaborated by
the OECD is made in the ECHA's latest nano-specific Appendixes to the
GDs in question, although strong limitations are contextually recognised.

Thus, albeit plausible, such EU initiatives aimed at understanding the toxicity mechanism for nanoscale chemicals have not yet reached a consolidation
level that would allow them to generate concrete and reliable data to be used
in the RA process for nanomaterials.

Dose-response relationship: is a nano-dose bringing regulatory toxicology to its knees?

It is precisely the likelihood of harm following exposure to chemical hazards that determines the emergence of risk.[97] Risk thus is a probabilistic expression of hazard. Probabilistic because not only 'there is no such thing as precise risk assessment'[98] but also because even when RA is supported by fairly accurate data, the toxicity screening is performed for one substance at a time and therefore chemicals cocktail effects or even impact on ecosystems are neither understood, nor tested. As we shall see, a number of value judgments and safety factors are adopted in trying to establish the *safe dose*, which determines 'the strong probability that adverse effects will not result from the use of a substance under specific conditions, depending on *quantity* and manner of use'.[99] It is important to note here that probability may be expressed quantitatively or in relatively qualitative ways.[100] In this way, the dose-response relationship estimates the relationship between dose or level of exposure to a substance, and the incidence and severity of an effect.[101]

The main aspects that the dose-response relationship investigates are acute toxicity and chronic toxicity. *Acute toxicity* measures the lethal dose at which half of the animals to which such dose has been administered die (hence the abbreviation as LD_{50}). The way the lethal dose is determined is a progressive process: the laboratory animals are exposed to a range of doses, from a very low to a medium and to a very high one that the animals cannot survive after the first administration.[102] Different LD_{50} for different endpoints are then considered in accordance with the exposure pathways such as oral LD_{50}, dermal LD_{50}, etc.[103] In REACH, oral acute toxicity is required for chemicals produced in quantities over 1 t/y, and for quantities above 10 t/y at least one other route of acute toxicity must be tested.[104] Logically, the higher the LD_{50} the lower the presumed toxicity. Generally in toxicology, a maximum dose for this purpose is usually set at 2 g of chemical for 1 kg of body weight.[105]

Chronic toxicity concerns the testing of the effects caused by repeated daily exposure via various routes, during the entire lifespan of the tested animals or during significant portions of it. Commonly used chronic and subchronic toxicity animal tests include the '28-day sub-acute test, the 90-day subchronic test and the lifetime chronic test'.[106] REACH imposed a legal duty to perform at least a 28-day sub-acute test for chemicals produced above 10 t/y. By digging deeper in the science behind the law of REACH, there remain no doubts as to the fact that serious toxicity data requirements are stipulated only for chemicals produced in quantities above 10 t/y.

A range of doses, from low to medium and high are used for chronic and subchronic toxicity testing and the aim of the dose-range is that of being able to establish a *no-observable-(adverse)-effect level* (NO(A)EL) also known as no-effect level (NEL).[107]

The determination of NOAEL in terms of human health and environmental protection is crucial given that the NO(A)EL value is used as a *point of departure* (POD) in the process of establishing safety levels for the determination of acceptable risk. These are referred to as *dose descriptors*. Yet, NO(A)EL calculations are based on laboratory animal testing from which the data will then be extrapolated and assessed for human health and environmental effects. There will be thus a persisting inherent uncertainty due to the model itself, for instance, to inter- and intra-species differences. For these reasons, once a NO(A)EL is derived by way of testing, a safety factor ranging between 10 and 10,000 is applied in order to derive DNELs, i.e. the level of exposure to the substance above which humans should not be exposed.[108] The same process is performed for environmental risks in order to derive PNECs, i.e. 'the concentration of a substance in any environment below which adverse effects will most likely not occur during long term or short term exposure'.[109] Safety factors,[110] once called *uncertainty factors* (UFs)[111] are numbers reflecting the estimated degree of uncertainty in the process of extrapolating data from laboratory testing models for humans and the environment.[112] In other words, safety factors[113] are crucial and radically determinant in the shaping of environmental and human health protection policies. They seek to remedy the narrowness of the testing methods with regard to the heterogeneity of the population affected, the effects on ecosystems, and the limits related to the use of animals of different species for obtaining the data that feed the NO(A)EL estimations.

With regard to the concept of dose, an important distinction between *threshold* and *non-threshold* chemicals is introduced.

Threshold chemicals

In the case of *threshold chemicals*, the dose-response relationship is represented by a monotonic curve expressing the (linear) relationship between the levels of exposure and the potential harm. For human health estimations, acceptable daily intake (ADI)[114] or derived no-effect levels (DNELs) are established.[115] DNEL, which is 'the level of exposure to the substance above which humans should not be exposed', is used in REACH. Health risks are regarded as *adequately controlled* in REACH when the exposure levels are kept below the established DNELs.[116]

$$DNEL= NO(A)EL/safety\ factor$$

Notice that the DNELs are different for different health effects and tested endpoints. In addition, they are influenced by exposure patterns – exposed population, e.g. workers, children, etc.; duration of the exposure; and route of exposure[117] – and of course by the reliability of initial laboratory data on the dose of reference (NO(A)EL). However, the data sets REACH establishes are still tonnage-based and, as shown earlier in this chapter, they become significant only for chemicals produced in quantities above 10 t/y. A better quality and greater amount of toxicity data would enable a better way of calculating a reliable NO(A)EL with a subsequent reduced level of inherent model uncertainty. However, the intra- and inter-species uncertainties remain. In order to remedy such uncertainties, a safety factor of 10 is often applied for each extrapolation $(10 \times 10 = 100)$[118] in toxicology. The data regarding nanotoxicity are scarce both in terms of laboratory animal testing and, especially, human clinical studies. As Chapter 4 demonstrated, non-animal testing such as Q(SAR) consisting of mathematical and computer modelling is simply not available or is non-reliable for nanoscale chemicals. It is hence not clear how the NO(A)EL will be established for nanoscale chemicals, and what safety factors are to be applied to confused data in order to match at least the safety levels established for bulk form chemicals. The SCENIHR has warned that 'special protocols may be necessary to detect the NO[A]EL for nanoparticle specific effects'.[119] Of note is the fact that a DNEL should be reconsidered any time the availability of more robust toxicological information allows for it. What adds to the uncertainty and the assumption-driven process thus far described is the fact that it may well be possible to identify more than one dose descriptor ($LD_{50,}$ $LC_{50,}$[120] NO(A)EL) for a given endpoint because data from more than one study might be available to determine dose. Expert judgment must be employed here, as it is not possible to know beforehand which dose descriptor is the more appropriate one for the endpoint-specific DNEL.[121]

When it comes to the *environmental* risks, REACH (but also other chemical legislation worldwide) operates in a similar logic. Today the term *ecotoxicity* is used to describe the assessment of chemicals risks on the different species in the environment. It requires expertise in toxicology, chemistry, and ecology.[122] Despite humans being part of ecosystems and therefore part of this assessment, the proper evaluation of environmental toxicity and risks is quite different from that of human health effects. Under REACH, the risks are deemed to be adequately controlled if *exposure* (NB not the actual risk level) is kept below the established-as-safe predicted no-effect concentrations or PNECs. The ECHA clarifies that the PNEC

> is the concentration of a substance in any environment below which adverse effects will most likely not occur during long term or short term exposure. The PNEC needs to be determined for each environmental sphere (aquatic, terrestrial, atmospheric, sewage treatment, food chain).[123]

As we shall see, the ecotoxicity testing is even more complex and difficult to perform and, as a consequence, is shrouded in far greater uncertainty than the one concerning human health effects. One unsurmountable hurdle to precise and accurate data is the diversity of species populating ecosystems. There are between 10 and 100 million species on earth, and 1.5 million of those species have been taxonomically classified.[124] The minimum ecotoxicological risk assessment required in chemicals legislation is that on *fish*, *daphnids*, and *algae* which Traas and Van Leeuwen define as 'a gross simplification of an ecosystem'.[125] Other decisions on what to test and what not, contribute to the severity of the uncertainty that characterises RA of environmental impacts of chemicals. Extrapolation of data here is not only an intra-species one but also a species-ecosystem one. Safety factors are also applied in order to derive PNECs values. In practice

> the protection of species and ecosystem function is assumed by establishing either the most sensitive species of the relevant toxicity data and applying *safety factors, or a relevant statistic of the toxicity data set*, such as a certain cut-off percentage p when the toxicity data are described by a theoretical distribution function; known as species sensitivity distributions.[126]

Hence, the assumptions and guesswork take place much earlier in the assessment of environmental risks, even in just choosing what species to test and what type of sensitivity to take into account. Only after that are safety factors applied in order to derive the PNECs that regulatory schemes require. Hence, in REACH, PNECs for different environmental compartments are expressed in the following way:

PNECs = NO(A)EL/safety factors[127]

To put it succinctly, major uncertainty − if not nearly total ignorance − is dominant when it comes to the assessment of environmental risks deriving from chemical exposure.

Just like in the case of DNELs, when it is not possible to derive the PNECs, *qualitative* approaches can be used. However, the qualitative assessment of environmental hazards is a far more long and technical procedure to explain in a law book and thus we refer to the pertinent ECHA's GD.[128]

Non-threshold chemicals

Always within the dose-response relationship phase of the RA scheme currently used in decision-making procedures under modern chemical laws, such as REACH, another category of chemicals is considered separately. This concerns the *non-threshold chemicals* and their non-monotonic (e.g. U-shape) dose-response curve (as opposed to the monotonic one of threshold chemicals).

Perhaps the most known example of non-threshold chemicals is that of some categories of *carcinogens*. For *genotoxic carcinogens*, it is *not* possible to calculate a NO(A)EL, given that any dose will give rise to the genotoxic risk; however, the *potency* of such effects increases as the dose increases. It derives that any exposure is associated with a risk and that risk at a given exposure shall be estimated following a linear extrapolation from dose-response *in vivo* human or animal data.[129] Carcinogens' classification − which includes human carcinogens, animal carcinogens and non-classifiable carcinogens due to lack of data − doesn't take into account the potency or the mode of action, or at best uses them as supporting arguments.[130]

The discourse on this class of chemicals is an ongoing one and the situation is rather different for *non-genotoxic carcinogens*. Here a NO(A)EL is thought to be possible to determine,[131] provided that there is information on the mechanism that determines the mode of action.

Statistically speaking, for non-threshold chemicals, an effect is always expected to occur. Hence, a risk number of 10^{-6} – which is currently the accepted risk value for carcinogenic pollutants – represents the probability of occurrence of additional cancer cases. In other words, it determines the incremental cases to occur above the background cancer incidence in the population[132] (currently estimated to 1 in 2 over a lifetime). However, the number itself does not tell the whole story because a 10^{-6} is not the same in terms of cancer risk for the 'average exposed person' and the person 'constantly exposed' to the chemical by living in a highly contaminated area or through food. For this class of chemicals, the specificities and the elements that clarify the *qualitative* assessment of the risks are as important as the numbers in the case of quantitative assessments of dose-response PNEC and DNEL values for threshold chemicals.[133]

Generally, when it is not possible to derive DNEL(s) for an endpoint – normally, either because test data are absent or because testing is not technically possible due to the properties of a chemical – the dose-response relationship has to be established *qualitatively (or semi-quantitatively)*. As stated above, this might be the case for non-threshold substances or for threshold substances for which the available data do not allow scientists to reliably identify a threshold (e.g. sensitisation and irrigation).

In REACH the *qualitative assessment* consists in the assessment of the likelihood that effects are avoided when implementing exposure scenarios. In such a process, emphasis is placed on assessing the adequacy of control of exposure in the human population of interest by using other information than a DNEL to *qualitatively* describe the potency of the health effect.[134] This is all aimed at controlling risks through exposure control, given that a safe quantity of exposure is not possible to quantify. The qualitative evaluation of the potency of the effects is then used to develop Exposure Scenarios and risk management measures (RMMs) for controlling exposures and thereby risks.[135] There is a growing number of studies on the possible genotoxic effects induced in cells following exposure to nanoparticles. The SCENIHR has concluded:

> The genotoxic effects of conventional particles are driven by two mechanisms – direct genotoxicity and indirect (inflammation-mediated) genotoxicity. *Nanoparticles may act via either of these pathways since they cause inflammation and can also enter cells and cause oxidative stress.* There is some evidence that the small size allows nanoparticles to penetrate into subcellular compartments like the mitochondria and the nucleus. The presence of nanomaterials in mitochondria and the nucleus opens the possibility for *oxidative stress mediated genotoxicity, and direct interaction with DNA*, respectively. For some manufactured nanomaterials genotoxic

activity has been reported, mainly associated to ROS generation, while for others contradictory results were obtained.[136]

This suggests that nanoparticles act primarily through indirect genotoxic mechanisms, which means they are hardly susceptible to NO(A)EL calculations.[137] And in any event, the metrics to be used to assess the eventual *potency* would need to be different from the mass-related (mg and g) ones adopted by REACH.

On the environmental side, potential PBT and vPvB nano-chemicals pose similar challenges. Such properties are to be assessed during the preparation of CSA/CSR in REACH. Regarding the possibility for nanoscale chemicals to display PBT properties, the SCENIHR has concluded:

> It should be noted that there exists *not only the potential for persistence of the nanoparticles themselves in the environment, but also residual persistence of the substance after the degradation of the particle.* The methodology should take this into account. The *appropriate metrics* that best describe the dose response relationship should be also be used to describe PBT.[138]

> It should also be noted that when discussing *biopersistence* of nanoparticles, there exists not only the potential for persistence of the nanoparticles themselves, but also the residual persistence of the substance after the degradation of the particle.[139]

> If *no quantitative risk characterisation* can be pursued, *it is recommended that a qualitative risk characterisation be conducted.* This would involve PBT assessment, which, as described, cannot be fully followed at present.[140]

The conclusion seems to be that it is impossible to perform a PBT and vPvB assessment of nanoscale chemicals in REACH, *both in qualitative and quantitative terms.* The metrics currently used are one of the major hurdles in this regard. It remains unclear how the REACH requirements – especially those triggering authorisation and restriction duties for chemicals displaying PBT properties – are to be applied in order for environmental risks to be assessed and managed under the current regulation. A shift within the parameters and the judgments employed in RA seems to represent the only valid alternative. It is no surprise, therefore, that the short nano-specific GDs[141] the ECHA has elaborated on dose-response assessment,[142] for both human health and the environment, do not provide any reliable method for the derivation of DNELs/PNECs for this class of chemicals. The current uncertainties and methodological shortcomings would call for such a *prevalently qualitative* approach. And in any event, until the metrics for characterising dose are updated so as to reflect the nano mode of toxic action, the concept of dose will not be able to function correctly for nanosubstances in the process of RA.

Exposure assessment

The conventional paradigm of risk assessment so far analysed describes risk as a function of both hazard and exposure, with the consequence that if one variable is controlled (or absent), so is the risk posed by the chemical at hand.[143] Like many chemicals regulations worldwide,[144] REACH operates through a number of regulatory triggers. As broadly explained in the previous chapters, one such fundamental trigger is the quantity of production: REACH's basic requirements apply for chemicals produced or imported in quantities ≥ 1 t/y. Greater quantities of production/import trigger larger data requirements on toxicity both on human health and the environmental impacts. Ecotoxicity data submission becomes significant for quantities ≥ 10 t/y and significantly increases for quantities ≥ 100 and ≥ 1,000 t/y.

Authorisation and restriction rules apply regardless of the quantity of production, but as Chapters 5 and 6 showed, quantity-related criteria nevertheless influence the administrative and procedural rules of the sub-phases that lead to authorisation/restriction, burdening authorities with the task of, for instance, proving significant widespread uses of the chemical in question.

Pursuant to Article 14(1)(4) of REACH, a CSA shall be performed and a CSR completed for all substances subject to registration produced in quantities ≥ 10 t/y. Importantly, a CSA is also required for all substances subject to authorisation, regardless of the quantity of production. The CSA process consists of three major steps: hazard assessment, exposure assessment, and the subsequent and final RA step, that of risk characterisation.[145] In this process 'exposure assessment is the process of measuring or estimating the dose or concentration of the substance to which humans and the environment are or may be exposed, depending on the uses of the substance'.[146]

Therefore, defining the conditions under which the substance is manufactured and used becomes critical for the determination of the exposure levels. REACH refers to these defined conditions as exposure scenarios. For each exposure scenario, the exposure levels for humans and the environment need to be determined, covering all the identified uses and life stages of a substance.[147] However, the ECHA's guidance on this point specifies that only if the registrant concludes in the hazard assessment that the substance meets the classification criteria as dangerous according to Directive 67/548/EEC or the PBT or vPvB criteria, will an exposure assessment *be required* to define the levels of exposure.[148] Otherwise, the registrant duties under the CSA[149] will be limited to a CSR containing just the basic available data on the toxicological profiles of the chemical in question. This is of primary legal relevance: the inversion of the onus of proof that REACH is supposed to substantiate is threshold-dependent: it operates only for chemicals produced in quantities greater than 10 t/y. What is more, even for chemicals produced in such quantities, only if a first screening of hazardous properties leads the registrant to conclude on the dangerousness of the chemical or its PBT/vPvB properties or dangerousness in light of Directive 67/548/EEC criteria, will an exposure assessment be performed. For other chemicals produced in smaller quantities, no data on exposure (and consequently on risk characterisation) are required to be provided by the producer/importer.

Therefore, only when a substance produced in quantities greater than 10 t/y meets the criteria to be classified as dangerous in accordance with the Directive 67/548/EEC provisions or displays PBT/vPvB criteria, an exposure assessment is required, entailing the following steps:

- *Development* of *exposure scenarios.* This consists of a set of information describing the conditions of manufacture and use of a substance, for all its identified uses and all the lifecycle stages resulting from the identified uses. The description of such conditions shall include information on operational conditions, e.g. duration and frequency of use, amount of substance employed, concentration of substance in a product and process temperature; and RMMs, e.g. local ventilation, air filtering systems, waste water treatment, and personal protection equipment. On the basis of this information, initial exposure scenarios might be built, allowing for an initial characterisation of risks. If the initial risk characterisation demonstrates the risks to be under control, the initial exposure scenarios will become the final ones. If risks are not controlled, a refinement of the CSA shall take place. The *refinement of the CSA* consists of the following steps: *improve the hazard assessment* by obtaining more data; *improve the exposure assessment* by ensuring that the exposure estimation is realistic and reflects the conditions of use defined in the initial exposure scenario; *improve the conditions of manufacturing* or use, e.g. by introducing more stringent risk management measures.[150]
- *Exposure estimation* is performed for any exposure scenario under development until the final exposure scenario is defined. The ECHA notes that given that exposure data are often scarce and limited to the workplace, tiered exposure estimation models[151] are used instead of actual measurements of exposure.

It results from the considerations on exposure that its estimation is often based on predictions and use of models that might be susceptible to under- or over-estimation. Moreover, when models are used, the initial data used to start the model going, ought to be fairly accurate and sufficient in order to allow for an as-accurate-as-possible estimation of exposure levels. Given the scarcity of data on nano-chemicals and the lack of a legal requirement to register them in REACH, this point of the RA process appears to be particularly problematic.[152] More so if it is considered that exposure scenarios are a primary tool for risk communication along the supply chain. If such scenarios cannot be built or are unrealistic, then the safety information flow along the supply chain will be seriously undermined, with potential negative consequences for the control of health and environmental risks.

As C.J. Van Leeuwen notes, 'exposure assessment is an uncertain part of risk assessment' principally for two reasons: because of the lack of information during the industrial release of the chemicals (*point-source-pollution*) and the effective presence of such chemicals in consumer products and the emissions thereof (*diffuse sources of pollution*).[153] The Commission services estimated in 2012 the quantity of nanomaterials on the market on a global level of 11.5 million tonnes, with a market value of roughly €20 billion.[154] According to the same document, carbon black accounted for around 85 per cent of total nanomaterials on the market and synthetic amorphous silica accounted for another 12 per cent.[155] According to another document from the SCENIHR, these two nanomaterials have been chemically synthesised using bottom-up methods for more than 60 years.[156] Therefore, the question arises: are such chemicals really that new? If they have been produced for more than half a century, data on their production, use, and distribution in terms not only of product application but also of geographic distribution of such products should be abundant.

A 2014 opinion from SCENIHR provides a better picture on the volumes of production and type of chemicals in nanoscale manufactured and marked today:

> The market is dominated by two very widespread commodity materials, i.e. *carbon black* (9.6 million t), and *synthetic amorphous silica* (1.5 million t). Other nanomaterials with significant amounts on the market include aluminium oxide (200 000 t), barium titanate (15 000 t), *titanium dioxide* (10 000 t), cerium oxide (10 000 t), and *zinc oxide* (8 000 t). Carbon nanotubes and carbon nanofibres are currently marketed at annual quantities of several hundreds of tonnes (other estimates go up to a few thousands of tonnes). *Nanosilver* is estimated to be marketed in annual quantities of around 20 tonnes. In addition, there is a wide variety of nanomaterials which are either still at the research and development stage, or which are marketed only in small quantities, mostly for technical and biomedical applications.[157]

All such nanomaterials have already drawn regulatory attention on the EU level. Carbon nanotubes were denied exemption from registration and evaluation in REACH pursuant to Annex IV, where substances for which sufficient information is known are considered to cause minimum risk because their intrinsic properties are listed. This is due to the asbestos-like behaviour of carbon materials in nanoscale.[158] The *titanium dioxide*[159] and *synthetic amorphous silica*[160] cases saw the ECHA's request of information on the nanoform rejected, after the BoA annulled such decisions, following an appeal initiated by major producers of such chemicals. As to *nano silver*, the long debate on if and how to regulate it – principally in light of the environmental toxicity concerns the substance poses – little of substance is taking place on the EU level (see Chapter 6). What emerges clearly from the SCENIHR estimations is the fact that certain nano-chemicals have a long and well-established history of production and use. Interestingly, these data are the result of voluntary disclosure as a result of the collaboration with industry as to date – with the exclusion of EU regulations regarding food additives, FCMs, cosmetics, and biocides – there are no legal obligations that impose a duty to test and assess the nanoscale of a given chemical.

Concluding on exposure assessment, it is relevant to point out here that one of the main limitations to the assessment of exposure is the impossibility of calculating a single predicted environmental concentration (PEC). Whereas for health risk assessment, different routes of exposure are usually taken into account in order to establish a comprehensive exposure expressed in maximum daily intake, for ecotoxicity, this is not possible. Therefore, different PECs might be calculated for individual environmental compartments such as water, air, and soil; a general PEC is currently not possible to calculate.[161]

Risk characterisation

The next and final stage of RA in REACH explains what use the legislators make of the dose descriptors and the DNELs/PNECs values this way derived, in order to establish if risks for humans and the environment are adequately controlled or if they are deemed to be unacceptable and hence in need of regulatory measures in the form of authorisation or restriction. During risk characterisation, all the data this far generated are interpreted and evaluated in order to estimate the incidence and severity of the adverse effects likely to occur to humans and/or environmental media due to actual or predicted exposure to a certain chemical.[162] It is also at this point of the RA that assumptions, uncertainties, and inaccuracies of data generated are weighted carefully by using expert judgment.

In one of the WHO's most authoritative formulations, risk characterisation is defined as

> the *qualitative and, wherever possible, quantitative determination of the probability* of occurrence of adverse effects of the agent under defined exposure conditions.[163]

In chemical laws today, risk characterisation can be *quantitative, qualitative*, or *semi-quantitative* in nature. Before analysing the first two of these categories as used in REACH, it is important to stress here that the qualitative element ought to be always included in the RC. This is so because even in the case where numeric values can be obtained (e.g. RC risk quotients), qualitative information on methodology, working assumptions, and alternative interpretation, should always be presented to risk managers.[164] In other words, including the qualitative evaluations of the numeric values established through testing methods and computer modelling, helps to contextualise and understand the relative reliability of such data. As we shall see, REACH endorses instead a *mainly quantitative* approach to risk characterisation as a general rule, while allowing also for semi-quantitative and qualitative RC in special cases. Just like for exposure assessment and in accordance with Article 14(5) of REACH, the obligation to carry out an RC is triggered only if the previous steps of the CSA[165] demonstrated that the substance meets the criteria for classification as dangerous in accordance with Directive 67/548/EEC or has PBT/vPvB properties.

Quantitative RC in REACH

REACH stipulates that risks are considered to be *adequately controlled* when

a   the exposure levels estimated … do not exceed the appropriate DNEL or the PNEC, *and*,
b   the likelihood and severity of an event occurring due to the physicochemical properties of the substance … is negligible.[166]

Cleary, departing from the WHO/IPCS indications, REACH endorses as a general rule a *quantitative* (called also deterministic) approach to RA, which seeks to estimate the likelihood of adverse effects occurring in humans or in the environment due to exposure (actual or predicted) to a given chemical.[167] Following such an approach, RA should yield quantifiable levels of risk – known also as risk characterisation ratios (RCRs) – by comparing exposure levels (NO(A)EL or PEC) to *no effect levels* (DNELs and PNECs) for all endpoints and all stages in the life-cycle of a chemical, for humans and for the environment respectively.[168] Put differently, the risks in REACH are regarded as adequately controlled when the RCRs for human health and the environment are below one.[169]

Specifically, the *environmental* risk characterisation ratios are yielded by the PEC/PNEC fraction for each environmental compartment. If such ratio is greater than one,[170] then the risks are considered *not* adequately controlled and RMMs must be adopted or further testing performed.[171] In addition, the higher the PEC/PNEC ratio, the higher the risks for the ecosystem and the higher the need to consider precautionary measures. As the ECHA guidance explains, the calculation of PEC is shrouded in structural uncertainty connected to the environment that is being taken into account (local, regional), sources of pollution/release, etc. Similarly, the way the PNEC is derived is also a product of predictions, assumptions, and conjectures. The result will be that in any case, uncertainty and ignorance will be part of the model and, as a result, the ratio of PEC/PNEC will always carry such uncertainty. Indeed, one of the leading experts in regulatory toxicology, Prof. Van Leeuwen, when speaking about uncertainty in environmental RA, states:

> Inadequacies of models include a fundamental lack of knowledge concerning underlying mechanisms, failure to consider multiple stresses, responses of all species, extrapolation beyond the range of observations, and instability of parameter estimates. In fact two related types of

uncertainties can be distinguished: quantifiable uncertainties (the 'known unknowns') and undefined uncertainties that cannot be described or quantified (the 'unknown unknowns'). The *PEC/PNEC approach is an example of such 'unknown unknowns'*.[172]

Is the author suggesting that in terms of environmental toxicity the science behind the law is dominated by ignorance? If so, what is the purpose of regulatory actions which are completely dependent on ... ignorance? How is REACH supposed to provide reliable data that legitimate actions in terms of risk regulation? Although the discussion on uncertainty is much more complex and requires an elaborated analysis which looks at uncertainty through various lenses – historical, sociological, epistemological, philosophical, and especially statistical – it appears that the existence of a deep fallacy in ecotoxicity testing is not fully understood by the public by at large or even by regulators perhaps.

Uncertainties surrounding PNECs derivation are even more accentuated than those of the DNELs. The main difficulties are related to the need to extrapolate from laboratory test results to the level of a complex ecosystem. It can be argued that for environmental RCR the qualitative approach should always accompany any attempt to quantitatively characterise risks, given the intense use of guesstimations and value judgments in the process.

Qualitative RC in REACH

Importantly, REACH contemplates also a *qualitative* RC option which comes into play when a deterministic/quantitative approach is either not possible because of the lack of data, or because the substance in question exhibits modes of toxic action which are not well understood or do not respond to the 'dose-makes-the-poison' golden rule of regulatory toxicology. As a consequence, for such chemicals it is often not possible to derive DNEL or PNEC values of a given endpoint.[173] For human health risks, REACH sets forth three examples when RCR ratio is not possible:

1   A substance exerts its effects by a threshold mode of action, but the available data still don't allow for a reliable identification of the threshold, like for the endpoints of sensitisation and irritation.
2   A substance exerts its effects by a non-threshold mode of action. Here the default assumption is that risk will manifest even at very low doses and hence a safe threshold cannot be established, like CMR substances.
3   Test data for one or more endpoints are simply absent.[174]

Therefore, quantifying risks of such substances is not possible and a qualitative approach is used instead. CMR substances are classical examples of chemicals which trigger a purely *qualitative* approach to risk characterisation. In relation to such chemicals, the ECHA specifies:

In a *strictly qualitative* approach (for e.g., genotoxic substances (i.e. non–threshold mutagens) without information on in vivo carcinogenicity) *estimation of specific levels of risk for a given exposure pattern is not possible and emphasis is placed on assessing the adequacy of control of exposure in the human population of interest* (e.g. workers, consumers, or humans exposed indirectly via the environment). The *qualitative risk characterisation approach* operates with more *qualitative measures for the potency of the substance used for developing exposure scenarios with appropriate risk management measures (RMMs)* and operational conditions (OCs). It is based on the principle that the more severe the nature of the hazard, the stricter the RMMs/OCs needed. This approach, in particular for high hazard substances is to some extent similar to the *ALARA-principle (as-low-as-reasonably-achievable)* originally used in the area of radiation protection.[175]

Nanoscale chemicals seem to reflect all three points above for which qualitative RA is warranted, given the scarcity and paucity of data on their human health impact is almost total according to EFSA's and SCENIHR's opinions. It is therefore unfortunate that the amendment proposed by the EU Parliament did not find the necessary support to be incorporated in REACH, so that nanoscale chemicals could be listed, alongside CMR, PBT/vPvB, and EDCs, as substances subject to authorisation (see Chapter 2). Bringing nanoscale chemicals under the authorisation rules would have also signified that a qualitative risk assessment would have been required by REACH for this class of chemicals.

Be this as it may, this chapter argues that a *qualitative* risk characterisation ought to be followed in the case of nano-chemicals. The ECHA explains:

> The process steps for a qualitative assessment are very similar to those of a quantitative assessment. The main differences are that the *hazard assessment conclusions are based on hazard qualitative description and potency considerations rather than DNELs (there is no 'threshold' level)*, and the *risk characterisation is developed by justification rather than calculation of a risk characterisation ratio.*[176]

The description of the qualitative RC, which mirrors the analytic–deliberative approach endorsed by the 1996 NRC Report, appears to be a more suitable alternative for dealing with highly uncertain substances like the nanoscale ones.

Similar considerations can be made for *qualitative environmental risk characterisation*. In their specific guidance, the ECHA clarifies that the document in question

> is mainly a guidance on how to quantitatively assess the effects of a substance on the environment by determining the concentration of the substance below which adverse effects in the environmental sphere of concern are not expected to occur. This concentration is known as

Predicted No-Effect Concentrations (PNECs). *If it is not possible to derive the PNEC then this shall be clearly stated and fully justified such as for the air compartment where only a qualitative assessment is normally possible.*[177]

It is not the aim of this chapter to go into very technical details of complicated formulas. However, it is relevant to state once more that the whole process of environmental risk characterisation is shrouded by deep uncertainties, even for the conventional chemicals. The application of assessment factors that range from 10 to 10,000 are common procedures in this phase. Yet, for chemicals like those displaying PBT/vPvB properties, a PEC or PNEC cannot be derived, and a qualitative risk characterisation becomes imperative. If it is not possible to determine PNEC and DNEL a qualitative characterisation of the effects expected to be caused by the chemical should be performed as part of the CSR.[178] As the ECHA puts it:

> The objective of the qualitative [environmental] risk characterisation will be to assess the level of control over the risks generated by the substance. Operational conditions and risk management measures will be directed to *minimise emissions and exposure to the environment.*[179]

Generally speaking, overall justification for using a qualitative approach for characterising risk rests on the assumption that numerical estimates are only as good as the set of data they are based on, or as Van Leeuwen effectively puts it: 'garbage in, garbage out'.[180] As shown, the risk for such a scenario in the case of nanotoxicity data is high. The switch to a qualitative approach would be advisable for nano-chemicals as doing so would allow for a discursive-based analysis. This would arguably lead to a clearer acknowledgement of the limits of science and the use of contextual value judgments, cultural preferences, and precaution assumptions, already in the framing of the risk issues the RA is set to investigate. Instead of deriving numeric values on the toxicity profiles of a chemical, the qualitative characterisation of risk asks the following questions:

- How extensive is the database supporting the risk assessment?
- Does it include human epidemiological data as well as experimental data?
- Does the laboratory data base include test data on more than one species?
- If multiple species are tested, do they all respond similarly to the test substance?
- Are extrapolations being made from more or less sensitive varieties, species, and endpoints?
- What are the data gaps, the missing pieces of the puzzle?
- What are the scientific uncertainties?
- What science policy decisions are made to address these uncertainties?
- What working assumptions underlie the risk assessment?
- What is the overall confidence level in the risk assessment?

All of these qualitative considerations are essential to deciding what reliance to place on a number and to determining potential risk.[181] The answer to a great part of these questions for nanoscale chemicals would clearly result in the awareness that very little is known on the nature, the potency, and the effects of their toxic mode of action. The following section illustrates why.

Risk assessment for nanoscale chemicals: what is currently possible?

In a recent study, the Danish EPA tried to calculate the PEC and PNEC values for some nanomaterials thought to be of particular environmental concern, including nano silver. Due to the scarcity of data, the PEC/PNEC findings were limited to the freshwater compartment.[182] The Report attributes the 'serious limitation for the precision of the modelling of the environmental concentrations and in most cases conservative (worst-case) estimates' to the difficulty to obtain data on the quantity of nanomaterials produced and released in Denmark.[183]

As an EU member, Denmark has fully implemented the REACH framework and has been in the forefront for stricter chemicals risk management therein.[184] However, when it comes to chemicals in nanoscale, Denmark seems to struggle with the gathering of data essential to national studies on environmental impacts of such chemicals. It can be speculated, then, that the REACH machinery is not helping in generating data on this class of chemicals.

In the case at hand, the Report concluded that for some of the studied nano-chemicals a PEC/PNEC was not possible to establish for soil, air, and other environmental compartments such as marine environment. The obtained values hence concerned exclusively the freshwater environmental media. The Report holds:

> The current regulatory paradigm is that in principle the existing risk assessment methodologies are applicable to ENM [engineered nanomaterial]. This means that, *at present, no nano-specific arguments are included in the estimation methods for PNEC estimation, i.e. that it is possible to extrapolate from effect concentrations obtained in the laboratory to concentrations protective for the environment by dividing with an assessment factor. It is, however important to note that the validity of the fundamental assumption, i.e. that PNECs for ENMs can be estimated as though they were dissolved chemicals, has not been evaluated.* Given the range of nano-specific concerns discussed by Lützhøft et al. (2015) *it is at present not possible to claim that the use of the current approaches ensure that organisms will be protected at concentrations below the derived PNEC.* In other words, specific circumstances related to ENMs, which differ from conventional chemicals, could likely affect the validity of the approach for deriving PNEC in an unpredictable manner (Baun et al., 2009).[185]

In other words, the PNEC values were calculated on mass-based exposure considerations and, as such, did not take into account nano-specific properties. Yet again, the underlying fallacy of the REACH system is stressed here: the assumption (derived by the regulatory toxicology underpinning the REACH provisions) that dose, expressed in function of mass, is the pivotal feature of toxicity and that the dose-toxicity correlation is a linear one.

More in detail the Report states:

> *Regarding the estimation of PNEC values for nanomaterials the major gap is the lack of underlying proper data suited for risk assessment.* There is a general lack of reliable data, in the sense that despite a wide range of tests have been performed according to accepted international guidelines (or modification thereof), they *cannot be fully trusted to yield accurate and conservative estimates of the toxicity of an ENM.* This is by far due to varying exposure conditions during the ecotoxicological testing, which is a violation of the underlying assumption of constant exposure concentration, leading to constant organism concentrations and further to constant target location/ organ concentrations.

> Another factor, common for most of the ENMs, which influenced the adequacy of the studies already performed for regulatory risk assessment, was the general *lack of material characterisation, especially measurements of the dose metric during and at the end of the test, but in fact also for basic data on inherent properties, e.g. for material identification and characterisation.*

> *Finally, it should be emphasized that the PNEC estimations given throughout this report are based on the assumptions that 1) the current test methods are applicable to nanomaterials, and 2) that the current extrapolation methodologies are valid for nanomaterials. Both of these assumptions are questionable* (for a further discussion of this see Lützhøft et al., 2015). When ENMs are tested in standard ecotoxicity tests the validity criteria of monotonous concentration-response curves and stable exposure conditions are challenged due to the behaviour of ENMs in testing media and in different test concentrations. The links between transformed states of the ENMs (e.g. dissolved or agglomerate forms) and biological effects are at present unknown. However, it is known that transformation during testing influence the test results. For PNEC estimation by application of an AF this constitutes a major problem for the validity of the extrapolation from standardized tests, since environmental effects may occur at lower concentrations than those used in the standardized tests. Thus, it is questionable whether the PNEC established by application of an AF will indeed be protective for organisms in the environment.[186]

In a previous report recalled also by the Danish EPA Report in question, Lützhøft et al. had warned:

The values Environmental effects of engineered nanomaterials reported here should therefore be taken as indicative for the order of magnitude for the PNEC given the current regulatory recommendations for PNEC estimation and not be used as the definitive protective concentration for the environment.[187]

Notwithstanding the difficulties in testing nanosubstances, this report suggested that some nanoscale materials such as silver and titanium dioxide present concerning ecotoxicity profiles.[188] Such indications ought to have been taken into account for the regulatory process of such materials under REACH.[189] What clearly emerges here, though, is the urgent and fundamental need to generate data circa the environmental fate of nano-chemicals. In the case of nano-chemicals it is unclear how reliable data are to be produced, if the currently employed models for generating them are ignorance-prone ones. Specifically for nanomaterials, the SCENIHR, already in 2007 stated:

> Risk characterisation methodology recommended in the Technical Guidance Documents can be followed for nanoparticles, *if and only if PECs and PNECs can be calculated with confidence*. These are *not generally available at present, negating the possibility of a full quantitative risk characterisation as presently required and defined in the Technical Guidance Document*.[190]

The RIP-oN 3 conclusion best explicates why it is unlikely that the current toxicology machinery would apply to nano-testing, stating:

- It is in principle possible to determine PNEC using the *present methodology*. However, *by doing so the particle behaviour of nanoparticles is neglected and it is inherently assumed that nanoparticles behave like dissolved (organic) chemicals*.
- The assessment factors were originally intended not only to cover the uncertainty related to the amount of available data, but also factors like inter- and intraspecies differences and extrapolations from laboratory to field. The value of the assessment factors are based on regulatory practice and empirical knowledge on ecotoxicological effects of chemicals. Since there is no history for evaluation of nanomaterials, *it is at present not possible to claim that the use of the presently available assessment factors will ensure that species will be protected at concentrations below PNEC*.
- The extent that these factors influence the ecotoxicological impact of nanomaterials is unknown. Currently, *even the scientific evidence for these factors is contradictory and varies from nanoparticle to nanoparticle* (Baun et al., 2009). *This impedes the reliability and interpretation of the available ecotoxicity data the direct use of the reported LC50, EC50 and NOEC for PNEC assessment*.[191]

RIP-oN 3 basically claims that the metrics that are used in traditional toxicology are unlikely to work for nanomaterials due to the fact that the toxic behaviour of the latter class of chemicals depends upon other criteria than mass alone.

The Report continues:

> It is important to note that there are *other parameters which can act as modifiers of the toxicity*, including particle size, size distribution, density, surface modification, aggregation/agglomeration state and shape, *but these parameters would not generally be considered as scalable quantities and do not appear to conform to the current use of the term 'metric' under REACH, and were therefore not considered further in relation to the metric issue.*[192]

The Report hence 'blames' the REACH text for its lack of any sort of reference to metrics and parameters which, according to expert scientists, would better serve the scope of analysing the toxicological profiles of nanoscale chemicals. The question of the right metrics to be adopted when testing nano-chemicals can be considered as the Achilles' heel of the regulatory issues on risks to humans and the environment posed by nanotoxicity. Similar considerations to those on PNECs were made by RIP-oN 3 with regard to the calculation of the DNELs for nanoscale chemicals under the current GDs. Of particular emphasis is the fact that the amendments to the REACH Annexes, coming into force in 2020, do not foresee any change to the metrics currently used and endorsed by the text of REACH, including the minimum threshold of 1 t/y that will continue to apply also for nanomaterials or the use of mass-based unities to determine toxicity in the process of risk assessment.

Here it can be concluded that the *quantitative* risk assessment model operating in REACH through the determination of acceptable PNECs and DNELs levels, which, in turn, represent the very essence of the *adequately controlled* risks concept and the safety consideration, is not possible for nanoscale chemicals. A qualitative assessment should be always necessary.

As it was shown so far, uncertainty is everywhere in risk assessment. It is endemic, it is natural, and to some extent unavoidable. However, it is important for decision-makers to understand the nature, the degree, and the consequences of such uncertainty in terms of safety implications. Modern laws like REACH therefore provide for the account of uncertainties. The following will investigate how effectively the models for uncertainty analysis are accounting for informing better decision-making, especially concerning nanoscale chemicals.

The uncertainty analysis in chemicals law: historical background and main features

Given that in recent times uncertainty documentation has become an important part of risk assessment, uncertainty analysis has become a mandatory feature of chemical safety dossiers in the EU and beyond.[193]

Uncertainty can be broadly defined as the assessor's lack of knowledge[194] and is owed both to the parameters assessed in a given system of analysis and to the models used in such analysis. Hence, what is referred to as *total uncertainty*[195] is the sum of *variability* and *uncertainty stricto sensu*. As noted above, the uncertainty analysis has been regarded as another part of the RA process where the qualitative approach to risk is not only possible but necessary in order to enable effective decision-making. Uncertainty analysis (UA) complements the RC step of the RA by ideally including a full discussion of uncertainties associated with the estimates of risk.[196] Another important role of a UA is that of 'revealing whether the point estimate used to summarize the uncertain risk is "conservative", and if so, to what extent'.[197]

The root of the tradition to account for uncertainty in RA can be traced back to Chapter 19 of the UNCED *Agenda 21*, which called for an environmentally sound management of toxic chemicals. A 'significant strengthening of both national and international efforts' was indicated as a major goal in this regard.[198] The Strategic Approach to International Chemicals Management (SAICM) global policy framework was adopted during the 2002 World Summit on Sustainable Development and in 2006, and the harmonisation and sound-management goal was reaffirmed. Hence, in order to foster a harmonised approach to the assessment of risks deriving from exposure to chemicals, the WHO launched the International Programme on Chemical Safety (IPCS). The IPCS offers guidance on a number of chemicals RA aspects[199] including the specific *Guidance Document on Uncertainty and Data Quality in RA*.[200] The first part of said Guidance deals with uncertainty analysis in exposure assessment.[201] It suggests a tiered approach to such analysis by using both qualitative and quantitative (hence both deterministic and probabilistic) methods, stipulating ten guiding principles to be followed in such analysis.[202] Although the document is not legally binding in nature, it has constituted a reference point for risk assessors and regulators worldwide.

For example, the ECHA has drafted, as part of *Guidance on Information Requirements and Chemical Safety Assessment*, Chapter R.19 which deals specifically with the UA.[203] The need to perform a UA and include it in the RA process is owed to the awareness on the inherent and inevitable uncertainties existing in the way RA is conceptualised. Therefore, uncertainty is owed both to risk models in use and the quality of data serving as inputs into the formulas therein.[204]

Currently, there are two ways of dealing with uncertainty, depending on whether the risk models embed a deterministic approach or rather a probabilistic one to risk assessment. Also, it must be recalled that both the deterministic and the probabilistic models can be used to elucidate the uncertainties embedded in the formulas though which quantitative RA operates. REACH employs both modes for UA purposes and the following offers an overview on what that means, also with regard to nanomaterials.

Uncertainty analysis in REACH

So far this chapter has shown that the translation of the legal language of REACH in scientific terms reveals a broad, intertwined, and uncertainty-shrouded array of toxicological considerations. This kind of epistemic uncertainty undoubtedly affects the way decisions on the management of such uncertain risks are made.[205] What the analysis so far conducted highlighted though, is that far from being a domain of purely scientific rigour, free from subjectivity, the RA phase – which is where science is put at the service of law, at least in providing the elementary and presumably solid knowledge framework which the law, in a second moment, is called to flesh out in accordance with the societal and democratic processes – is a natural harbour of uncertainty. Such uncertainty is to some degree unavoidable because of the epistemological limits of science.[206] Also, in areas such as that of regulatory toxicology, additional uncertainty is created by the models used in experiments and the multiple variables and methodologies therein. Scientists, and in this case, toxicologists dealing with risks posed by complex chemicals, normally incorporate uncertainty in their experimental data. One way of doing that, is the use of safety factors (SFs). Yet, exposure uncertainties are not tackled by SFs.[207] It is hence relevant here to introduce a more detailed understanding of the way uncertainty is dealt with under the REACH rule of law.

If a dose-response relationship can be established during exposure assessment, then risks can be *quantified* (PEC/PNEC or NO(A)EL/DNEL ratios). The role of exposure assessment is to provide information about the *distribution* of expected magnitude of exposure, its source and routes, and the individuals of a population that are exposed.[208] However, the likelihood or frequency of exposure is a difficult concept to explain objectively, although an attempt is made to quantify it using empirical statistics.[209] This leads to the need to understand the fine distinction between *uncertainty* and *variability* in the data generation process, since its consequences on the regulatory plan are all but negligible, especially precaution-wise speaking.

Uncertainty is defined as 'imperfect knowledge concerning the present or future state of an organism, system, or (sub)population under consideration'.[210] Uncertainty evaluation should account for qualitative, quantitative, descriptive, and prognostic aspects of knowledge limits in assessing and measuring exposure.[211] *Variability* refers instead to the heterogeneity of the studied parameters such as 'the natural variations in the environment, exposure paths, and susceptibility of subpopulations'.[212] It cannot be controlled neither by the exposure assessor or the decision-makers;[213] thus it affects the accuracy of a statement [about risk].[214] It derives that *variability* cannot be eliminated and thus prompts the regulatory toxicologist to adjust her protective measures when a certain level of safety is to be attained or maintained,[215] due for instance, to regulatory requirements. As Sir David Cox, one of the most prominent living statisticians, puts it:

Variability is a phenomenon in the physical world to be measured, analysed and where appropriate explained. By contrast, uncertainty is an aspect of knowledge.[216]

Therefore, it is crucial to keep in mind that the uncertainty which needs to be analysed as part of the RA process is a combination of variability (called also 'aleatory uncertainty') and of 'epistemic/fundamental' uncertainty.[217] The analysis of such uncertainty is of primary relevance not only in terms of risk assessment but in the realm of risk communication too. UA outcomes can greatly determine not only the overall reliability of the results yielded by the RA but also the way such results shall be dealt with in the presence of residual uncertainty – uncertainty that was not possible to eliminate statistically. As previously explained in this chapter, decision on chemicals regulation are essentially decisions on controlling exposure, given that the hazardousness of a chemical cannot be altered whatsoever.[218] It becomes hence imperative for regulators to properly understand the *uncertainty* (and *variability*) analysis in order to be able to evaluate what kind of risk is incumbent and how best to respond to it.

The pre-REACH system made use of a largely deterministic approach to RA and uncertainties were not explicitly quantified.[219] In such a model, uncertainties were arbitrarily considered in assessment factors or worst-case assumptions and were only applied in exposure, effects, and risk characterisation as a (pre)cautionary measure.[220] An example is the assignment of safety factors to derive the PNECs. Such factors would be reflected in the PEC/PNEC ratio representing the RCR quotient. The outcome of such a ratio will be a simple 'yes/no' answer to the question of whether the risks are deemed to be adequately controlled. However, the degree of conservatism is in this case unknown.[221]

REACH builds on this approach by adding at the same time probabilistic elements to the analysis of uncertainty. The ECHA suggests a stepwise approach to uncertainty analysis in REACH, which starts with a 'basic qualitative' approach and continues, if appropriate, with a more complex deterministic and probabilistic analysis.[222] Because REACH delegates a good part of the RA to industry, it is particularly necessary to have a proper and transparent treatment of uncertainty in the appraisal of chemicals risk.[223] The *tiered approach* suggested for uncertainty analysis in REACH takes as a starting point the acknowledgement that uncertainties in hazard/exposure assessment and risk characterisation can be divided into three main categories:

1 Scenario uncertainties

Uncertainty of this type is linked to the inaccuracy of specific scenarios according to the identified uses of a substance, including descriptive errors (e.g. wrong or incomplete information) or errors of assessment (e.g. choice of the wrong model).

2 *Model uncertainty*

Mathematical and other models are used in RA. Since laboratory models represent a simplification of reality, they inevitably conceal some degree of uncertainty owed, among other things, to the extrapolation and use of the model outside the domain for which it was developed.

3 *Parameter uncertainty*

Parameter uncertainty concerns the uncertainty linked to the specification of numerical values – measurement errors; sample uncertainty; selection of data, i.e. choice of dose descriptor; extrapolation of alternative data, e.g. (Q)SAR, *in vitro* testing, and read-across methods. This kind of uncertainty is common if data are lacking or are insufficient.[224]

The ECHA stipulates that UA is recommended when the RCR is close to the regulatory trigger value (above or below an RCR of *one*). In this case the need to perform a UA might derive either by the factual use of non-standard methods for characterising risk, or simply because the registrant wants to perform a UA to improve the RC. Hence, in case of an RCR close to or above one, and/or use of non-standard no-guideline methods to assess risk, the registrant might choose to explain in the CSR what uncertainty was encountered and explain it in qualitative terms.

Given that serious uncertainties are involved in each stage of the RA of nanomaterials, a UA would be advisable for 'testing' every RCR that might have been derived for nanoscale chemicals.[225] Moreover, in the case of nanoscale chemicals, all three types of uncertainties will accompany the assessment of risks under the existing REACH test methods and the ECHA's pertinent GDs. The peculiar and poorly understood (eco)toxicological profiles of such chemicals do indeed exacerbate all three types of uncertainty, inherent to the assessment in chemical risk in general. The mode of delivery of nano-chemicals in the test systems needs to be supplemented/modified/replaced to ensure that they reflect the relevant exposure scenarios.[226] In addition, perhaps the most acknowledged problematic parameter in nanotoxicity, i.e. the characterisation of dose, adds to scenario uncertainties. For nanoscale chemicals, parameter uncertainty is nearly absolute, thus making the use of alternative methods such as (Q)SAR and read-across nearly pointless for the mitigation of uncertainties. Finally, all these types of uncertainties are nested into a broader framework of uncertainty: that of models used in RA. Those models are considered to be inappropriate for tackling and assessing nano risks and in need of modification in accordance with the new developments of nano-science.[227]

Hence a number of pertinent questions, naturally emerging at this point, would be the following: is the uncertainty analysis in its current articulation in REACH able to remedy the endemic and total uncertainty characterising every single step of RA for nano-chemicals? Isn't there rather a risk that the general uncertainty deriving from the insistence to apply existing methods/ models also for this class of chemicals (regardless of their strong limitations and very disputable feasibility) will only be ignored and obscured by the propagation of the idea that the current uncertainty analysis in REACH can apply also for nanoscale chemicals? Further, wouldn't this at the end create a vicious circle of uncertainty and ignorance that decision-makers would find difficult to break through precautionary acting?

Lastly, transparency on the RA process is also essential for civil society and the communities that might be affected by uncertain risks. The right to know suggests that the concerned individuals should be able to enjoy access to transparent and complete information on the state of knowledge, including the assumptions and the quality of data used in a decision to manage risk in a certain way rather than in another. It can be speculated that if it was clearly communicated to the consumer that the nano-enriched products they use in everyday life are tested – if at all – through methods not designed for that class of chemicals, with the consequence of exposing them and the environment that surrounds them to unknown and potentially catastrophic risks, perhaps the attitude towards such products would be different.

This book seeks to contribute to the elucidation of this aspect in the hope that consumer awareness will provide the propellant force for the adoption of truly precautionary measures on nanoscale chemicals.

An example of alternative models for dealing with widespread uncertainty for nanosubstances

Rarely has the precautionary principle been invoked so early in the R&D process and from such a variegated group of stakeholders, as has been in the case of nanotechnology and the products of its applications. As the American Industrial Hygiene Association (AIHA) has recently suggested:

> Both the nanomaterial hazard and risk of exposure (as well as the level of *uncertainty* about each) should be considered when selecting controls. When uncertainty about hazard and/or exposure risk exists, a *precautionary approach* is recommended.[228]

As stated early in this chapter, the hazardousness of a chemical cannot be controlled or managed as such. Therefore, the only option left in the case of particularly hazardous chemicals is that of controlling exposure. The AIHA report in question offers a hierarchy of control exposure for nanomaterials. At the top of this hierarchy there is the option of eliminating or reducing hazard/exposure. What is relevant for the approach to RA suggested in this chapter is the fact that AIHA suggests: 'For *best results*, consider *exposure prevention* and *control measures early in the planning of experiments, development of products, and design of manufacturing processes*, so that appropriate controls can be planned and selected.'[229] In order to obtain optimal protection, the report is suggesting not only measures to control and prevent exposure but, most notably, that such prevention and control be *anticipated* as early as in the experiment planning phase. Clearly, a genuinely precautionary approach here involves action as early as the embryonic phases of the RA.

A report from the Institut de recherche Robert-Sauvé en santé et en sécurité du travail (IRSST), a leading occupational health and safety research centre in Canada, explains why the PP is a desirable strategy in reducing workplace exposure:

> There is still no consensus, however, on a measurement method for characterizing occupational exposure to nanomaterials, making *quantitative risk assessment difficult if not impossible* in many situations. As a result, a *precautionary approach* is recommended to minimize worker exposure.[230]

> Though general trends are emerging suggesting a variety of toxic effects, it is clear that toxicity is product-specific. Given the resulting uncertainty, and the *virtual impossibility of obtaining all the information necessary for adequate assessment of a product's toxicity, a precautionary approach based on strict preventive measures to achieve minimum exposure remains the best method of protecting workers* and preventing the development of occupational disease.[231]

The report offers a useful scheme on how the approach for toxicity assessment could incorporate precaution.

It is clear from this scheme that precautionary action in the RA phase is strictly connected to the level of uncertainty and, logically, to the knowledge gap that gave way to such uncertainty in the first place. In this logic, a quantitative RA – which is the principal method used in REACH except for particular cases, e.g. for SVHCs – is feasible only when sufficient knowledge allows for risk to be fully assessed and quantified. As knowledge levels decrease, uncertainty becomes more pronounced and traditional RA methods ought to be supplemented with alternative testing, e.g. (Q)SARs. Up to this point, determination of safety standards is supposed to be still possible (i.e. determination of safe doses and adequately controlled risks). However, as toxicity data availability and quality decrease further, the RA methods change from quantitative to qualitative. Qualitative methods that REACH foresees, for instance in the case of chemicals having PBT or vPvB properties, are more aimed at reducing or preventing exposure, as the determination of safe exposure is not possible because of the impossibility to quantify risk.

Given the great uncertainty characterising nanomaterials, the IRSST report, in line with other authoritative opinions in merit, suggests that 'control banding' is the approach most commonly recommended for assessing

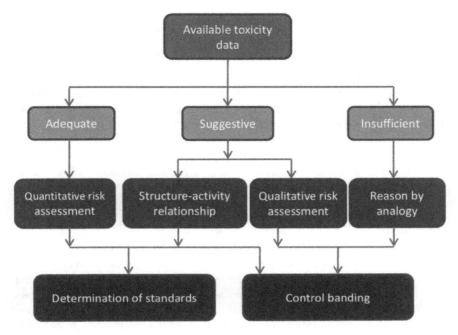

Figure 7.1 Proposed approach for toxicity assessment.[232]

Source: This figure was published in Ostiguy, C., Debia, M., Roberge, B., and Dufresne, A. (2015). Best practices guidance for nanomaterial risk management in the workplace (Report n°R-899). Montréal, QC: IRSST.

nanomaterial-related risks.[233] This method basically suggests a flexible and progressive approach to risk control, where the starting point for highly uncertain risks is that of qualitative assessment, applied for each component of RA.[234] Necessarily, value-based and discursive methods ought to be used in this case in order for precaution to be implemented. Once this has led to better knowledge on the risks associated with nanomaterials, a transition towards semi-qualitative and finally quantitative methods can take place.

An important conclusion can be drawn here: for an effective and genuinely precautionary regulatory process, the inversion of the onus of proof shall take place very early in the process of data generation. For highly uncertain risk and ignorance to some extent, the only feasible way to operationalise such an inversion is through making the producers of nano-chemicals responsible for actually generating data on toxicity.

And as shown in this chapter, the only way to reasonably operate such an inversion, is to abandon the artificial and misleading idea that traditional/ quantitative RA methods can be employed in the case of nano-chemicals or other classes of chemicals, such as EDCs, whose risks cannot be appraised and quantified because of the current loopholes and inadequacies of both science and law.

REACH scientific essentials in need for review

The many difficulties that can be encountered in the RA and RM of complex chemicals, are effectively summarised in the following passage which is important to cite here in its entirety, given also that it is authored by one leading expert in the area of toxicology:

> In the regulatory process, risk assessment will never provide 'the correct answer' and risk management will never provide 'absolute' solutions. To assume otherwise would be to accept that there will be no further changes in the knowledge, views, values, rights and duties accepted by society and its individual members over time.
>
> The multiple uncertainties in risk assessment mean that it is possible for its conclusions to be attacked from both sides. Arguments over whether or not assumptions in risk assessments are scientifically valid often amounts to debate about whether it is better to err on the side of 'false positives' (if there is an error, it is more likely to be a false indication of *danger) or 'false negatives' (if there is an error, it is more likely to be a false indication of safety). Those who might be harmed by the substance being assessed will generally favour false positives; those who would gain from the substance will generally favour false negatives. Different groups often interpret the results from the same study in different ways.*
>
> Risk assessment can be most useful when those who rely on it to inform the risk management process understand the context, its nature and its limitations, and use it accordingly. This means that *decision-makers must at least understand that the process is assumption and value laden*; that they are aware what assumptions were used in the assessment in question, and what values they reflect. They must also be aware that the *risk estimate is expressed as a range, with a given certainty that the true average lies within that range*; that variability is expressed to the degree that it is known; and that uncertainties can be reduced but often at high cost.
>
> Managing risks implies management of the simplicity-complexity dilemma. Risk managers must take all these factors into account when making a decision, along with political and economic factors which are not related to the risk assessment. *Wisdom and knowledge are a prerequisite for informed decision-making*. Risk management of chemicals is an international challenge. Frameworks differ in scope and depth and continue to undergo dramatic changes. *New challenges will continue to arrive.*[235]

Based on these observations, it is possible to envisage a few preliminary suggestions on how to address the main shortcomings of some of the most crucial techno-scientific foundations of REACH, in order to improve their application to nanoscale chemicals.

Testing methods and the science of the law

As shown in this chapter, REACH takes a predominantly quantitative approach to RA, with a rather marginal role assigned to the qualitative method. In a paper on the impact of the treatment of epistemic uncertainty in environmental fate models and the consequences of this treatment for regulatory strategies, the authors concluded that 'non-probabilistic treatment of uncertainty resulted in more conservative (read safe) chemical regulation'.[236] As Vose points out, 'the biggest uncertainty in a risk analysis is whether we started off analysing the right thing and in the right way'.[237] Concerning nano-chemicals in REACH, the starting off of the risk analysis begins with considering and treating nano-chemicals in the same way as the traditional bulk chemicals. Nothing in REACH requires nanosubstances to be considered *new* under the law and science framework that REACH puts in place; this does not seem to be the right way to start. Hence, the risk appraisal is done namely by entrusting the existing toxicity testing methodologies with the task of addressing risks which, by design, they are unable to address. The slowness of the EU regulator to thoroughly review and amend some core legal and technical concepts in REACH is hence seriously undermining any potential of the legislation to ensure high levels of human health and environmental protection for highly concerning chemicals such as nanoscale and endocrine disrupting ones. A silver lining might be offered by the newly adopted nano-amendments to the REACH Annexes and the hope that the specific nano-requirements thereof will initiate a process of data generation specific to the nanoform. Nevertheless, such improvement might still be too little (the legal text of REACH will keep being nano-silent as no reform is undertaken in that regard), too late (the nano-amendments will come into force in 2020, well after the final registration 2018 deadline and it will in any case take time before the data generation process based on such new requirements takes hold within REACH).

Further, in terms of testing strategies REACH is less revolutionary than it looks. It is true that with the adoption of the regulation, data requirements for the *existing* substances introduced in 1981, will certainly increase compared to the previous situation where virtually no data existed. However, for new chemicals, the data set required by REACH is even lower and less rigorous than that of the pre-REACH law on the new substance, defined as those produced after 1981![238] Suffice it to mention here that for chemicals produced in lower quantities, 1–10 t/y, the data required by REACH will not even be sufficient for the initial characterisation of inherent properties,[239] which as we saw, constitute the indispensable and necessary starting point in any RA process. What REACH brought along was a shifting from the (mainly) hazard-based model of chemicals risk control to the (mainly) risk-based model in place today. However, the levels of protection of the environment and human health are weakened precisely by this new feature. Risk-based models assume that risk of chemicals can be understood, measured, and controlled (mainly by controlling exposure).[240] Only if this foundational assumption is accepted as true, can the REACH burdening of industry with risk assessment tasks and data generation duty of unprecedented extent for EU chemicals (but perhaps global) be seen as revolutionary. If, on the contrary – and as in the case of nanoscale chemicals and EDCs that depart from the idea that risk can be controlled by controlling the dose of exposure – this assumption cannot be expected as true, the model adopted by REACH appears less revolutionary.

In addition, the burden shift on industry is an alleviated one compared to the one borne by authorities in the pre-REACH era, where the task to assess and test chemicals risks was triggered at a 10 kg threshold, with further in-depth testing following for greater volumes of production.[241] In practical terms, the current threshold for the assessment of chemicals is that of 10 t/y where the duty to provide a CSR is triggered. Consequently, the threshold has been increased by a factor of 100, allowing industry to get away with virtually no substantial testing data for quantities below 10 t/y. It is uncertain how many of the 100,000 chemicals registered as existing by 1981 are still produced and placed on the EU market. Some estimations calculate that among 30,000 and 70,000 chemicals are still in production and that 20,000 of them are marketed in quantities between 1 and 10 t/y[242] – thus escaping the proper REACH regime in terms of testing and data generation. Hence, the bone thrown to advocates of stricter regulation of chemicals was that of imposing a CSR requirement (and the relative data generation and testing obligations) that would apply only to 10,000 out of 30,000 chemicals.

It has thus been already noted that 'the objectives of REACH cannot be achieved under the current risk assessment approach'.[243] The pitfalls of the REACH system for chemicals produced under a certain threshold (10 t/y) are thus coupled with a more general problem in the way risk assessment is con-ceptualised as compared to the previous chemicals laws, that is:

> Whereas the former legislation on new and existing substances required a comprehensive risk assessment and a risk characterisation (RC) for all rel-evant toxicological effects, REACH requires a RC for the leading health effect (i.e., the toxicological effect that results in the most critical DNEL) for a given exposure pattern (duration, frequency, route and exposed human population) associated with an exposure scenario (ES). It is to be noted that one exposure pattern can fit to more than one ES.[244]

The case of nano-chemicals is bringing precisely these systemic fallacies into the spotlight. For nanoscale chemicals simply cannot be made to fit into a system that suffers an alarming range of lacunas and oversights, owed not only to the epistemic limits of knowledge, which are common for newly developed chemicals, but, and perhaps more so, to the legal approach in tackling such limitations and knowledge gaps. Nano-related risks are asking the legislator to face up to the fact that thick uncertainty and ignorance permeates (especially, but not exclusively) ecotoxicological testing. Such limitations are nothing new. They have always been there and are to be attributed in part to the nature of the scientific understanding of chemicals harm, which more often than not, lags behind the R&D and commercialisation of such chemicals.

However, while the generation of more knowledge (e.g. with the entry into force of the nano-amendments to the REACH Annexes) and the adoption of new methodologies might contribute to the understanding of the nano toxic modes of action, this is no guarantee that all uncertainties will be removed. Therefore, legal principles that allow decision-making before complete scientific proof is obtained, represent the only way to prevent harm from occurring or at least for minimising harm. The PP but also the substitution principle, both enshrined in EU environmental law, are examples in this regard. Still, part of the limitations and the consequent inaccuracies in environmental and human health data generation, are owed to obsolete test methods and to certain fossilised concepts that rule regulatory toxicology, such as that of the existence of a safe dose expressed in function of mass. Both sources of limitations seem to demand one action on the regulatory plan: anticipation of precautionary thinking and acting already in the risk assessment phase. The kind of knowledge-limitation encountered in the process – risk, uncertainty, ignorance, and ambiguity – shall determine the potency of precautionary acting, the point in time in the regulatory process, and the measures, including necessary banning, to be adopted in this regard.

Issues of definition and dose-related considerations

One way to take precautionary action could be to reconsider the accuracy and adequacy of the definition of what is to be considered a nanosubstance. Some suggestions can be found in the EFSA and the SCENIHR opinions in this regard, where an upper limit of 500 nm is recommended, derogating to the 1–100 nm size range adopted by the Commission Communication on the definition of the term nanomaterial. Other precautionary considerations can be found in the Communication itself, which states that in case of nano-chemicals known to be of a hazardous nature – like multiple forms of carbon nanotubes (CNTs) – the size limit set between 1 and 100 can be derogated. Yet, the Communication is not binding in nature and the definition of nanomaterial endorsed in the document can become of legal relevance only by being incorporated in other specific legislation. This has already happened in the biocides, the pesticides, the cosmetics, and the novel foods regulations area. Nevertheless, doubts on the legitimacy of similar transpositions still remain.

The case of EDCs offers relevant insights in this regard. The delay of the Commission in adopting a definition for EDCs under the biocide regulation was sanctioned by the General Court for breaching Article 265 of the TFEU. The case was brought in front of the Court by Sweden which sought and obtained a declaration from the Court on the fact that the Commission has unlawfully refrained from laying down rules for the definition of EDCs.[245] The court held that

> *the Commission cannot rely on the fact that the scientific criteria which it had proposed were the subject of criticism,* in summer 2013, *on the ground that they had no basis in science and that their implementation would affect the internal market.* The existence of that criticism is irrelevant to the fact that the Commission had an obligation to act before 13 December 2013 by adopting the delegated acts referred to in the regulation.

> The regulation reflects the balance desired by the legislature between an improvement in the functioning of the internal market by the harmonisation of the rules concerning the placing on the market and use of biocidal products, on the one hand, and the preservation of a high level of protection of human and animal health and the environment, on the other. In the exercise of the powers delegated to it by the legislature, the Commission cannot call that balance into question. In those circumstances, the fact that the regulation also seeks to improve the functioning of the internal market cannot, on any bases, alone, call into question the clear, precise and unconditional obligation on the Commission to adopt the delegated acts, nor allow the Commission to abstain from their adoption.[246]

What can be deducted from the words used by the Court is the fact that by failing to implement the scientific criteria functional to the adoption of a definition on what constitutes an EDC, the Commission is impairing the balance the biocide regulation seeks to strike between the functioning of the internal market and that of high levels of human and environmental health protection. The reluctance of the Commission to act upon definition issues – as demonstrated by the utterly delayed update to the 2011 Recommendation on the definition of the term 'nanomaterial' – appears to hinder the attainment of the high levels of protection aim, as testing and assessment of the environmental and human health impacts of such chemicals is not possible without a definition, whereas the commercialisation and use of consumer goods can take place (as is currently the case) even in the absence of a definition and specific regulation.

Although definitional issues are of crucial relevance, they are only one hallmark in the chain of technical and legal concepts that upholds the human and environmental protection aim of REACH. It is true that REACH has operated a general overhaul of the legal text of chemicals law on the EU level, bringing along at least some consistency and uniformity of rules both for data generation and risk management measures. However, the regulation brings only minor and superficial updates to test methods, with the consequence that risk assessment under REACH today follows the same paradigm as 30 years ago.[247] Hence, the acclaimed REACH revolution might not be a revolution from within but rather just a renovation to the legal facade instead. In addition, a new definition of what is to be considered a nano-chemical (or an EDC), without a contextual modification of the testing methodologies used for assessing the new hazards posed by such chemicals, would result in an empty provision;[248] defining nanomaterials on the basis of their specific properties, i.e. surface area and number size distribution, while leaving untouched the concept of nano-dose in toxicology, would be a hoax because to admit that the toxicological profiles of a chemical are owed to other parameters than mass and still employ mass in dose-response relationship testing, makes no sense in terms of human health and environmental protection. Therefore, besides an appropriate definition, the concept of dose needs to be revised, and with it the dose-response relationship curves. The ECHA's position in this regard is that for what it concerns exposure assessment, the available and currently used models, 'are not always *tuned* to and *calibrated* for' nano-chemicals exposure situations.[249] Such instability is attributed primarily to the fact that they operate through parameters that are not yet validated for nanomaterials, therefore the actual model estimates 'are inaccurate'.[250] Vague suggestions are given on how to perform field measurements for generating data to be used in risk characterisation.[251]

Hence, neither the revision of the scientific principles nor the legal provisions alone are likely to improve the regulatory status of nano-chemicals in REACH. A contextual evolution of both these aspects of REACH, to take place through a constant dialogue between toxicology findings and legal norms design, is necessary if modern chemicals risks are to be tackled and curtailed in the pursuit of the high levels of protection aim.

Adaptive risk regulations?

In the absence of predictive environmental exposure models that generate quantitative results, the ECHA suggests the use of alternative evaluation frameworks and *adaptive risk management*.[252] The International Risk Governance Council held an international conference on *Planning Adaptive Risk Regulations* at the University College London, in January 2016. The main objective of the conference was to bring together representatives of different interests in the field of nanotechnology, in order to encourage discussion and creative thinking on how regulation can accommodate rapid technological development. Flexibility in regulation design was identified as a desirable means for guaranteeing legal coverage for new and emerging risks without hindering innovation.[253] However, flexibility alone would create uncertainty for industry and investors alike, therefore, the participants of the conference held that such a feature has to be embedded in the law and 'must also be planned'.[254] It was unclear what such flexibility would imply for the legal plan. It appeared more as a call for further relaxation of the few existing legal requirements in order to 'skip' ignorance and uncertainty rather than handle them. As one of the speakers, Dame Anne Glover, former Chief Scientific Adviser to the EU Commission, noted:

> To support business investment in new technology, regulation needs to be clearly defined but often the evidence underpinning the policy is not certain and may be continually evolving, especially in areas of new technology. The challenge is to develop an *evidence-based* process where uncertainty can be included in policy formation in a way that does not reduce the confidence of business who may wish to invest in novel technology.[255]

Dame Glover strategically uses the term 'evidence-based' instead of 'proof-based'. One reading of such use can be that regulations should be *informed by* and *based on* scientific evidence. Given that sound science and absolute certainty are not possible, the use of science in regulation should not be abused either by delaying risk regulation or by inflating it when unnecessary. If properly applied, the legal principle of precaution can be successfully employed to avoid this double abuse of science, and guide decision-making in face of uncertainty.

Summing up

This chapter dealt in detail with the science of REACH. The REACH framework operates a redistribution of the onus of proof and the burden of generating the data needed to control and manage chemicals risk for human health and the environment. However, as this chapter tried to demonstrate, this redistribution is a significant one only when compared to the previous situation where 99 per cent of chemicals in circulation had virtually no data on their toxicity. It has been argued that the situation was created by the hazard-based criteria used by regulatory standards chemicals law *and* the disproportionate burden placed on the regulator as a consequence. Therefore, REACH operates *mainly* on risk-based criteria, albeit in a better distributed onus of proof, where industry is also required to be at the forefront of the data generation process. However, what REACH failed to do was reconsider its own upholding of scientific foundations. As with most of the modern laws ruling over complex matters, REACH is necessarily nested in a set of scientific principles and methods that supposedly ensure that the legal decisions are underpinned by rational scientific considerations. Consequently, the legal text of REACH is an articulation in policy terms of the findings of regulatory toxicology informing chemicals policies. What nanotechnology and EDCs are putting under the spotlight is the fact that it is the precisely the underlying science that is primarily responsible for the inadequacy of the legal response to environmental challenges posed by these new and complex chemicals.

Even more concerning in light of the early understandings on the toxicity mode of nano-chemicals, is that for chemicals under 1 t/y not even registration or notification is now required. It is relevant to mention here that REACH still foresees the hazard-based criteria for the Authorisation and the Restriction phase. However, as Chapters 5–6 showed, this is serving the aim of high levels of environmental and human health protection only partially: in the case of Authorisation, the hazard-based criteria play an important role, although exposure criteria tied to volumes of use and production are still crucial, burdening this way the authorities with the task of generating data. As far as Restriction is concerned then, its procedures are directly inherited from the pre-REACH system where it is for regulatory bodies to demonstrate unacceptable risks in case a restriction is to be issued. REACH as a whole hence endorses a wig-wag version of precaution: Registration and Authorisation are imprinted by a stronger precautionary spirit, whereas Evaluation and Restriction are basically inherited from the pre-REACH system. However, even in the precautionary driven phases, the concept of mass-based dose and the correlated thresholds for triggering a given set of legal requirements, strongly undermine the materialising of a genuinely precautionary ruling.

Against this backdrop, an ideal scenario would be the following: the onus of proof ought to rest with the risk producers (i.e. industry) while the approach to the regulation of such risk ought to be prevalently *hazard-based* – at least for highly complex and uncertain chemicals like the ones in nanoscale. The audacity (and thus, controversy) of this ideal scenario is that it advances the idea that even a potential moratorium/ban should be among the possible regulatory options for nanotechnology and the products of its applications.

Notes

1 Elizabeth Fisher, 'Risk and Environmental Law: A Beginner's Guide' in Benjamin J. Richardson and Stephan Wood (eds), *Environmental Law for Sustainability: A Reader* (Hart Publishing 2006) 97, 97, emphasis added.
2 Council Regulation (EC) 440/2008 laying down test methods pursuant to Regulation (EC) No. 1907/2006 of the European Parliament and of the Council on the Registration, Evaluation, Authorisation and Restriction of Chemicals (REACH) [2008] OJ L142/1.
3 This definition is by H. Paul A. Illing and Timothy C. Marrs, 'Regulatory Toxicology' in Bryan Ballantyne, Timothy C. Marrs, and Tore Syversen (eds) *General and Applied Toxicology: Vol. 6* (3rd edn, Wiley 2009) 2527.
4 Franz-Xaver Reichl and Michael Schwenk (eds), *Regulatory Toxicology* (Springer 2014) 1.
5 REACH establishes that risks are considered to be adequately controlled when in accordance with section 6.4 of Annex I. Scott clarifies that:

Annex 6.4 states that a risk will be considered to be adequately controlled if the exposure levels do not exceed the appropriate DNEL or PNEC, and if the likelihood and severity of an event occurring due to the physicochemical properties of the substance is negligible.

See J. Scott, 'REACH and the Evolution of EU Administrative Law', Comparative Administrative Law conference 7–9 May, Yale Law School, 12. Available at www.law.yale.edu/academics/papers.htm accessed 27.06.2016, footnote 57.

6 A different approach is taken for certain classes of chemicals, such as non-threshold ones, as will be shown further in this chapter.
7 Helmut Greim, 'Aims and Mission of Regulatory Toxicology' in Franz-Xaver Reichl and Michael Schwenk (eds) *Regulatory Toxicology* (Springer 2014) 3, 12.
8 P.J. Bert Hakkinen, Asish Mohapatra, and Steven G.G. Gilbert (eds), *Information Resources in Toxicology* (4th edn, Academic Press 2009) 1343.
9 Greim (n 7) 4.
10 NRC, *Risk Assessment in the Federal Government: Managing the Process* (National Academies Press 1983).
11 Ibid. 7, emphasis added.
12 Ibid. 148, emphasis added.
13 Ibid. 148, emphasis added.
14 Ibid. 3.
15 Ibid. 18.
16 Ibid. 3.
17 NRC 1983 (n 10) 4.
18 Wrongly so because it is stated elsewhere in the document that: 'Risk assessment is an analytic process that is firmly based on scientific considerations, *but it also requires judgments to be made when the available information is incomplete.* These judgments inevitably draw on both scientific and policy considerations.' NRC 1983 (n 10) 48, emphasis added.
19 NRC, *Understanding Risk: Informing Decisions in a Democratic Society* (National Academy Press 1996).
20 The Royal Society, *Risk: Analysis, Perception and Management – Report of a Royal Society Study Group* (Royal Society, London 1992).
21 NRC 1996 (n 19) ix.
22 Perhaps it is of relevance here to mention the fact that this second report was commissioned to the Committee on Risk Characterization, Commission on Behavioral and Social Sciences and Education, whereas the Red Book from 1983 was prepared by the Committee on the Institutional Means for Assessment of Risks to Public Health, Commission on Life Sciences.
23 NRC 1996 (n 19) 25.
24 Ibid. 186.
25 Ibid. 14. Note that, still, judgments beyond science are not excluded *in toto*. It is hence difficult to sustain that the science/democracy dichotomy advocated in such report is hermetic and with no room for manoeuvre. It is certainly a rigid one, and yet not totally impermeable to the infiltration of policy judgments.
26 Ibid. 20.
27 Elizabeth Fisher, *Risk Regulation and Administrative Constitutionalism* (Hart Publishing 2007) 13.
28 Klinke and Renn propose also an analytic–deliberative approach to risk regulation; see in general Andreas Klinke and Ortwin Renn, 'Precautionary Principle and Discursive Strategies: Classifying and Managing Risks' (2001) 4:2 Journal of Risk Research 159.
29 Ortwin Renn, Andrew Stirling, and Ulrich Müller-Herold, 'The Precautionary Principle: A New Paradigm for Risk Management and Participation' (2004) 3 Working Papers IDDRI 1, 19.

30 Franz-Xaver Reichl and Michael Schwenk (eds), *Regulatory Toxicology* (Springer 2014) 1.
31 Ibid. 1.
32 For a short account on this, see W. Lenz, 'A Short History of Thalidomide Embryopathy' (1988) 38 Teratology 203.
33 Horst Spielmann, 'International Regulation of Toxicological Test Systems' in Franz-Xaver Reichl and Michael Schwenk (eds), *Regulatory Toxicology* (Springer 2014), 182.
34 Except for Brazil, China, and India. Ibid. 181.
35 Ibid. 182.
36 REACH foresees that ecotoxicological and toxicological tests shall be carried out in accordance with the provisions laid down in Council Directive 2004/10/EC on the harmonisation of laws, regulations and administrative provisions relating to the application of the principles of good laboratory practice and the verification of their applications for tests on chemical substances [2004] OJ L50/44 (GLP directive) or other accepted international standards. See REACH recital (37) and Article (13).
37 Spielmann (n 33) 182.
38 What exactly constitutes soft law, is widely debated among legal scholars. However, the definition assigned to the term here is the broad one encompassing both non-binding norms with legal relevance and binding norms with a soft dimension. See in this regard: Fabien Terpan, 'Soft Law in the European Union: The Changing Nature of EU Law' (2015) 21 European Law Journal 68, 71.
39 Pierre-Marie Dupuy, 'Soft Law and the International Law of the Environment' (1990) 12 Mich. J. Int'l L. 420, 424.
40 Spielmann (n 33) 183.
41 'OECD and EU Test Guidelines' (*ECHA*) http://echa.europa.eu/support/oecd-eu-test-guidelines accessed 20.02.2019.
42 The notice has the following formulation:

> This document contains guidance on REACH explaining the REACH obligations and how to fulfil them. However, users are reminded that the text of the REACH Regulation is the only authentic legal reference and that the information in this document does not constitute legal advice. The European Chemicals Agency does not accept any liability with regard to the contents of this document.

43 Article 263(1) TFEU foresees that: 'It shall also review the legality of acts of bodies, offices or agencies of the Union intended to produce legal effects vis-à-vis third parties.'
44 Joanne Scott, 'In Legal Limbo: Post-Legislative Guidance as a Challenge for European Administrative Law' (2011) 48 Common Market Law Review 329, 331.
45 Steven Vaughan, *EU Chemicals Regulation: New Governance, Hybridity and REACH* (Elgar 2015) 93.
46 Ibid. 96.
47 Available at http://echa.europa.eu/web/guest/guidance-documents/guidance-on-information-requirements-and-chemical-safety-assessment accessed 19.02.2019.
48 See: Case A-008–2015 *Evonik v ECHA* [2015]; Case A-009–2015 *Iqesil SA v ECHA* [2015]; Case A-010–2015 *Rhodia v ECHA* [2015]; Case A-011–2015 *J.M. Huber v ECHA* [2015].
49 ECHA 'Guidance for Identification and Naming of Substances under REACH and CLP' (ECHA-16-B-37.1-EN May 2017) 36.
50 'REACH Guidance for Nanomaterials Published' (*ECHA/NA/17/12*) https://echa.europa.eu/-/reach-guidance-for-nanomaterials-published accessed 20.02.2019.

51 See: ECHA, 'Appendix 4: Recommendations for Nanomaterials Applicable to the Guidance on Registration' (Draft, January 2017).

52 Ibid. 8.

53 Commission, 'General Report on the Operation of REACH and Review of Certain Elements Conclusions and Actions' (Staff Working Document) 8 SWD (2018) 58 final Part 1/7, 41.

54 Ibid. 114.

55 Council Regulation (EC) 440/2008.

56 An 'endpoint' is defined as an effect observed in a toxicity study. These particular effects are selected because they are biologically significant and indicate a health and/or environmental concern. Theresa L. Pedersen, 'Dose-Response Assessment' (*ExtoxNet*, September 1997) http://extoxnet.orst.edu/faqs/risk/dose.htm accessed 19.02.2019.

57 See: Commission Regulation (EU) No. 260/2014 of 24 January 2014 amending, for the purpose of its adaptation to technical progress, Regulation (EC) No. 440/2008 laying down test methods pursuant to Regulation (EC) No. 1907/2006 of the European Parliament and of the Council on the Registration, Evaluation, Authorisation and Restriction of Chemicals (REACH)[2014] OJ L81/1.

58 'OECD Chemical Studies Show Way Forward for Nanomaterial Safety' (*OECD*) www.oecd.org/chemicalsafety/news-nanomaterial-safety.htm accessed 19.02.2019, emphasis added.

59 Ibid.

60 'Testing Programme of Manufactured Nanomaterials – Dossiers and Endpoints' (*OECD*) www.oecd.org/chemicalsafety/nanosafety/dossiers-and-endpoints-testing-programme-manufactured-nanomaterials.htm accessed 19.02.2019.

61 For nano silver see OECD, 'Series on the Safety of Manufactured Nanomaterials No. 53. Dossier on Silver Nanoparticles' (ENV/JM/MONO(2015)16/PART4, 14 December 2015). 8; For SWCNTs see OECD, 'Series on the Safety of Manufactured Nanomaterials No. 70 Dossier on Single-walled Carbon Nanotubes (SWCNTs) (ENV/JM/MONO(2016)22, 7 July 2016) 8.

62 See: '11,500-page OECD Dossiers on 11 Nanomaterials are of "Little to No Value" in Assessing Risks' (*CIEL*, 2017) www.ciel.org/news/11500-page-oecd-dossiers-11-nanomaterials-little-no-value-assessing-risks/ accessed 20.02.2019.

63 Walter Aulmann and Nathan Pechacek, 'Reach (and CLP): Its Role in Regulatory Toxicology' in Franz-Xaver Reichl and Michael Schwenk (eds), *Regulatory Toxicology* (Springer 2014) 785.

64 See Nertila Kuraj, 'Complexities and Conflict in Controlling Dangerous Chemicals: The Case of Regulating Endocrine Disruptors in EU Law', in Eléonore Maitre-Ekern, Carl Dalhammar, and Hans Christian Bugge (eds), *Preventing Environmental Damage from Products: An Analysis of the Policy and Regulatory Framework in Europe* (CPU 2018) 285–286.

65 EEA, 'Late Lessons from Early Warnings: The Precautionary Principle 1896–2000' (Environmental issue report No. 22 2001) and EEA, 'Late Lessons from Early Warnings: Science, Precaution, Innovation' (No. 1/2013).

66 Stephen Breyer, *Breaking the Vicious Circle: Toward Effective Risk Regulation* (Harvard University Press 1993).

67 NRC, *Science and Judgment in Risk Assessment* (National Academies Press 1994) 26.

68 Ibid. 311.

69 Ibid. 26–27.

70 Leah D. Stuchal and Stephen M. Roberts, 'Risk Assessment of Chemicals' in Bryan Ballantyne, Timothy C. Marrs, and Tore Syversen (eds) *General and Applied Toxicology: Vol. 6* (3rd edn, Wiley 2009) 2674.

71 'Mechanistic Effect Models for Ecotoxicology' (*Ecotoxmodels*) www.ecotoxmodels. org/toxicokinetic-toxicodynamic-models/ accessed 19.02.2019.

72 Hans-Uwe Wolf and Michael Schwenk, 'Importance of Physical-Chemical Properties for Toxicological Risk Assessment' in Franz-Xaver Reichl and Michael Schwenk (eds) *Regulatory Toxicology* (Springer 2014) 521.

73 See ECHA, 'Guidance on Information Requirements and Chemical Safety Assessment Part B: Hazard Assessment' (ECHA-11-G-16-EN, December 2011).

74 ECHA, 'Guidance on Information Requirements and Chemical Safety Assessment Chapter R.3: Information Gathering' (ECHA-2011-G-12-EN, December 2011)1–2.

75 Ibid. 2.

76 Ibid.

77 REACH, Article 12(1), recital 17.

78 REACH, Annex VI, Step 1 – Gather and Share Existing Information.

79 Available at: https://echa.europa.eu/guidance-documents/guidance-on-information-requirements-and-chemical-safety-assessment accessed 01.03.2019.

80 ECHA, 'Practical Guide 2: How to Report Weight of Evidence' (ECHA-10-B-05-EN, 24 March 2010) 2.

81 ECHA-11-G-16-EN (n 73) 7.

82 REACH, Annex XI, section 1.2.

83 C.J. Van Leeuwen, 'General Introduction' in C.J. van Leeuwen and T.G. Vermeire (eds), *Risk Assessment of Chemicals: An Introduction* (Springer 2007) 5.

84 Ibid. 29.

85 NRC 1994 (n 67) 363.

86 ECHA, 'Guidance in a Nutshell Chemical Safety Assessment' (ECHA-09-B-15-EN, 30 September 2009) 10. Note that this document has been rendered obsolete. Nonetheless, this book finds the conceptual references in the old document still useful for illustrating the general variables involved in RA. See: https://echa.europa.eu/documents/10162/13655/pg_sme_managers_reach_coordinators_en.pdf/1253d9f9-d1f04ca8-9e7a-c81e337e3a7d accessed 23.01.2019.

87 Ibid., ECHA-09-B-15-EN.

88 SCENIHR, 'Modified Opinion (After Public Consultation) on the Appropriateness of Existing Methodologies to Assess the Potential Risks Associated with Engineered and Adventitious Products of Nanotechnologies' (10 March 2006), 51.

89 Ibid. 21, emphasis added.

90 SCENIHR, 'Opinion on the Appropriateness of the Risk Assessment Methodology in Accordance with the Technical Guidance Documents for New and Existing Substances for Assessing the Risk of Nanomaterials' (21–22 June 2007) 35.

91 Safety data sheets are an information tool foreseen by REACH in case certain hazardous information needs to be passed down the supply chain. See: https://echa.europa.eu/safety-data-sheets accessed 01.03.2019.

92 ECHA, 'Guidance on the Compilation of Safety Data Sheets' (ECHA-15-G-07.1-EN, November 2015) 77, emphasis added.

93 ECHA, 'Guidance on Information Requirements and Chemical Safety Assessment, Appendix R7–1 Recommendations for Nanomaterials Applicable to Chapter R7a – Endpoint Specific Guidance' (ECHA-17-G-16-EN, May 2017).

94 Ibid. 14.

95 ECHA-17-G-16-EN (n 93) 55.

96 Ibid. 54.

97 Van Leeuwen 2007 (n 83) 3.

98 Ibid. 5.

99 Ibid. 2, emphasis added.

100 NRC 1996 (n 19).

101 Van Leeuwen 2007 (n 83) 4.

102 Joseph Plamondon, *Underlying Foundation of Science Used in the Regulation of Industrial Chemicals* (Smithers Rapra 2009) 7.
103 Ibid.
104 T.G. Vermeire et al., 'Toxicity Testing for Human Health Risk Assessment' in C.J. van Leeuwen and T.G. Vermeire (eds) *Risk Assessment of Chemicals: An introduction* (Springer 2007), 240.
105 Plamondon (n 102) 7.
106 Vermeire et al. 2007 (n 104) 244.
107 Sven Ove Hansson, *Setting the Limit: Occupational Health Standards and the Limits of Science* (Oxford University Press 1998) 10.
108 ECHA-09-B-15-EN (n 86) 11.
109 Ibid. 12.
110 ECHA used the term 'assessment factor'.
111 Illing and Marrs (n 3) 2533.
112 Van Leeuwen 2007 (n 83) 5.
113 Safety factors are defined as: 'Numerical adjustment used to extrapolate from experimentally determined (dose–response) relationships to estimate the agent exposure below which an adverse effect is not likely to occur.' See WHO/IPCS, 'Risk Assessment Terminology' (2004) 10.
114 'Estimated maximum amount of an agent, expressed on a body mass basis, to which individuals in a (sub)population may be exposed daily over their lifetimes without appreciable health risk.' WHO/IPCS, 'Risk Assessment Terminology' (2004) 10.
115 ECHA-09-B-15-EN (n 86) 11–12.
116 Aulmann and Pechacek (n 63) 792.
117 ECHA-09-B-15-EN (n 86) 12.
118 Greim (n 7) 10. The 100-fold expressed NOAEL is also called margin of exposure (MOE) or margin of safety (MOS).
119 SCENIHR 2007 (n 90) 31.
120 Lethal Concentration (LC) refers to the concentration of a chemical in environmental compartments, e.g. air and water. It is in other words the equivalent of the LD values for environmental toxicity testing. Therefore, the concentrations of the chemical in air/water that kills 50 per cent of the test animals during the observation period is the LC_{50} value.
121 ECHA-11-G-16-EN (n 73) 32.
122 T.P. Traas and C.J. Van Leeuwen, 'Ecotoxicological Effects' in C.J. van Leeuwen and T.G. Vermeire (eds), *Risk Assessment of Chemicals* (2nd edn, Springer 2007) 281.
123 ECHA-09-B-15-EN (n 86) 12.
124 Traas and Van Leeuwen 2007 (n 122) 282.
125 Ibid. 282.
126 Ibid. 283, emphasis added.
127 Note that the NO(A)EL here refers to environmental exposure. The NEL can also be used in formula instead of the NO(A)EL.
128 Available at: https://echa.europa.eu/guidance-documents/guidance-on-information-requirements-and-chemical-safety-assessment accessed 02.03.2019.
129 Greim (n 7) 10.
130 Ibid. 14.
131 Although see Ellen Silbergeld, 'The Uses and Abuses of Scientific Uncertainty in Risk Assessment' (1986) 2 Natural Resources & Environment 17.
132 Dorothy E. Patton, 'The ABCs of Risk Assessment: Some Basic Principles Can Help People Understand Why Controversies Occur' (1993) 1 EPA Journal 10, available at: http://people.bethel.edu/~kisrob/hon301k/readings/risk/RiskEPA/riskepa1.html accessed 20.02.2019.

133 Ibid.
134 ECHA-11-G-16-EN (n 73) 30.
135 Ibid.
136 SCENIHR, 'Risk Assessment of Products of Nanotechnologies' (19 January 2009) 9.
137 Greim (n 7) 12.
138 SCENIHR 2007 (n 90) 50, emphasis added.
139 Ibid. 50, emphasis added.
140 Ibid., emphasis added.
141 See ECHA, 'Guidance on Information Requirements and Chemical Safety Assessment Appendix R8–15 Recommendations for Nanomaterials Applicable to Chapter R.8 Characterisation of Dose [Concentration] – Response for Human Health' (ECHA-12-G-09-EN, May 2012) 12; 'Guidance on Information Requirements and Chemical Safety Assessment Appendix R10–2 Recommendations for Nanomaterials Applicable to Chapter R.10 Characterisation of Dose [Concentration] – Response for Environment' (ECHA-12-G-10-EN, May 2012) 6.
142 For the bulk chemicals see ECHA, 'Guidance on Information Requirements and Chemical Safety Assessment Chapter R.8: Characterisation of Dose [Concentration]-Response for Human Health' (ECHA-2010-G-19-EN, November 2012) 195; 'Guidance on Information Requirements and Chemical Safety Assessment Chapter R.10: Characterisation of Dose [Concentration]-Response for Environment' (May 2008) 65.
143 Qasim Chaudhry, Hans Bouwmeester, and Rolf F. Hertel, 'The Current Risk Assessment Paradigm in Relation to the Regulation of Nanotechnologies' in Graeme A. Hodge, Diana M. Bowman, and Andrew D. Maynard (eds), *International Handbook on Regulating Nanotechnologies* (Edward Elgar 2012) 126.
144 Exception being made for New Zealand where the obligation to assess risks is quantity-independent and thus triggered by the sole act of production/import of the chemical. See S. Rocks et al., 'Comparison of Risk Assessment Approaches for Manufactured Nanomaterials' (Defra project, CB403 Final report, 2008) 4.
145 ECHA-09-B-15-EN (n 86) 5.
146 Ibid. 5.
147 Ibid.
148 Ibid. 13.
149 It must be recalled here that for substances produced in quantities above 10 t/y, as part of the registration dossier, a CSR must be prepared, containing, among other data, a preliminary CSA.
150 ECHA-09-B-15-EN (n 86) 14.
151 The used models are ECETOC TRA10 model for workers and consumer exposure estimation, available at www.ecetoc-tra.org accessed 22.10.2016 and EUSES model11 for environmental exposure estimation, available at www.ecb.jrc.it/euses accessed 22.10.2016; ECHA-09-B-15-EN (n 86) 17.
152 ECHA-09-B-15-EN (n 86) 15.
153 Van Leeuwen 2007 (n 83) 4.
154 Commission, 'Second Regulatory Review on Nanomaterials' (Communication) COM (2012) 572 final 3.
155 Ibid. 3, footnote 8.
156 SCENIHR, 'Scientific Basis for the Definition of the Term "nanomaterial"' (6 July 2010) 23.
157 SCENIHR, 'Opinion on Nanosilver: Safety, Health and Environmental Effects and Role in Antimicrobial Resistance' (10–11 June 2014) 20, emphasis added.
158 'Carbon Nanotubes That Look Like Asbestos, Behave Like Asbestos' (*PEN*, 19 May 2008) www.nanotechproject.org/news/archive/mwcnt/ accessed 21.02.2019.

159 Case A-011–2014 *Tioxide Europe and Others v ECHA* [2014].
160 Case A-015–2015 *Evonik and Others v ECHA* [2015] and Case A-014–2015 *Grace GmbH & Co. KG v ECHA* [2015].
161 Van Leeuwen 2007 (n 83) 4.
162 Ibid. 5.
163 WHO/IPCS, 'Guidance Document on Characterizing and Communicating Uncertainty in Exposure Assessment' (2008) 1, emphasis added.
164 NRC 1994 (n 67) 365.
165 Which, according to Article 14(3) of REACH, consist of: '(a) human health hazard assessment; (b) physicochemical hazard assessment; (c) environmental hazard assessment; (d) persistent, bioaccumulative and toxic (PBT) and very persistent and very bioaccumulative (vPvB) assessment'.
166 REACH, Annex I, Section 6, para 6.4.
167 C.J. Van Leeuwen, B.G. Hansen, and J.H.M. De Bruijn, 'The Management of Industrial Chemicals in the EU' in C.J. van Leeuwen and T.G. Vermeire (eds), *Risk Assessment of Chemicals: An Introduction* (Springer 2007) 536.
168 Ibid. 536.
169 See ECHA, 'Guidance on Information Requirements and Chemical Safety Assessment Part A: Introduction to the Guidance Document Reference' (ECHA-2011-G-15-EN, December 2011) 2.
170 Van Leeuwen, Hansen, and De Bruijn 2007 (n 167) 536.
171 See in general the explanation provided in ECHA, 'Principles for Environmental Risk Assessment of the Sediment Compartment: Proceedings of the Topical Scientific Workshop' (ECHA-14-R-13-EN, May 2014) 10.
172 Van Leeuwen 2007 (n 83) 22, emphasis added.
173 ECHA-2010-G-19-EN 2012 (n 142) 3.
174 Ibid.
175 Ibid. 4–5, emphasis added.
176 ECHA, 'Practical Guide 15: How to Undertake a Qualitative Human Health Assessment and Document it in a Chemical Safety Report' (ECHA-12-B-49-EN, November 2012) 2, emphasis added.
177 ECHA, 'Guidance on Information Requirements and Chemical Safety Assessment Chapter R.10: Characterisation of Dose [Concentration]-Response for Environment' (2008) 7, emphasis added.
178 REACH, Annex I, section 6.5, 260.
179 ECHA-09-B-15-EN (n 86) 18.
180 Van Leeuwen 2007 (n 83) 20.
181 Van Leeuwen 2007 (n 83) 20.
182 Jesper Kjølholt et al., *Environmental Assessment of Nanomaterial Use in Denmark* (The Danish Environmental Protection Agency 2015) 9.
183 Ibid.
184 For instance, the Danish EPA has been working closely with the ECHA in order to prepare the necessary dossier required by REACH's Annex XV for the restriction of hazardous chemicals. The efforts are aimed at restricting four phthalates DIBP, DBP, BBP, and DEHP in articles, because the risks posed by such chemicals to human and environmental health cannot be adequately controlled. Such a dossier was to be submitted by 8th January 2016. Denmark initially came up with the idea of restricting such chemicals nationally but the Commission reacted through a communication from 2014, stating that restriction is harmonised on the EU level by REACH and thereby Member States cannot derogate with stricter national measure. See 'Echa and Denmark to Prepare Phthalates Restriction' (*CW*, 11 March 2015) https://chemicalwatch.com/23104/echa-and-denmark-to-prepare-phthalates-restriction accessed 03.03.2019.
185 Kjølholt et al. (n 182) 80, emphasis added.

186 Ibid., emphasis added.
187 Hans-Christian Holten Lützhøf et al., *Environmental Effects of Engineered Nanomaterials, Estimations of Predicted No-Effect Concentrations (PNECs), Environmental Project No. 1787* (The Danish Environmental Protection Agency 2015) 45.
188 Kjølholt et al. (n 182) 74.
189 See Chapters 4–6 on the status of nano silver and nano TiO_2 within the process of substance evaluation and the struggle to get past the simple CoRAP listing.
190 SCENIHR 2007 (n 90) 9/52/60, emphasis added.
191 R.A. Aitken et al., 'Specific Advice on Exposure Assessment and Hazard/Risk Characterisation for Nanomaterials under REACH (RIP-oN 3) – Final Project Report' (JRC, RNC/RIP-oN3/FPR/1/FINAL 2011) 91–92.
192 Ibid. vii.
193 Michael Schumann, Ozkaynak Haluk, and Alexandre Zenié, 'Uncertainty Analysis in Exposure Assessment: Relevance for Regulatory Toxicology' in Franz-Xaver Reichl and Michael Schwenk (eds), *Regulatory Toxicology* (Springer 2014) 379.
194 David Vose, *Risk Analysis: A Quantitative Guide* (3rd edn, Wiley 2008) 49.
195 Ibid. 49; the term 'uncertainty' used in this section refers to the *total uncertainty* expressing both variability and uncertainty in chemicals RA.
196 NRC 1994 (n 67) 27.
197 NRC 1994 (n 67)167.
198 Agenda 21: Programme of Action for Sustainable Development, 1992–06–14, UN GAOR, 46th Sess., Agenda Item 21, UN Doc A/Conf.151/26 (1992), Chapter 19, para 19.3.
199 'Harmonization Project Publications' (*WHO*) www.who.int/ipcs/publications/methods/harmonization/en/ accessed 22.02.2019.
200 WHO/IPCS, 'Uncertainty and Data Quality in Exposure Assessment, Harmonization Project Document No 6' (2008).
201 WHO/IPCS, 'Guidance Document on Characterizing and Communicating Uncertainty in Exposure Assessment' (2008).
202 Ibid. xii–xiii.
203 ECHA, 'Guidance on Information Requirements and Chemical Safety Assessment Chapter R.19: Uncertainty Analysis' (ECHA-12-G-25-EN, November 2012).
204 Stuchal and Roberts (n 70) 2670.
205 See in general Muhammad S. Iqbal and Ullrika Sahlin, 'Treatment of Epistemic Uncertainty in Environmental Fate Models – Consequences on Chemical Safety Regulatory Strategies' (2012), emphasis added, available at http://lnu.diva-portal.org/smash/get/diva2:556538/FULLTEXT01.pdf accessed 21.02.2019.
206 See in general Amanda Guillan, 'Epistemological Limits to Scientific Prediction: The Problem of Uncertainty' (2014) 4 OJPP 510.
207 ECHA-11-G-16-EN (n 73) 31. Here the term *assessment factors (AF)* is used instead.
208 Schümann, Haluk, and Zenié (n 193) 378.
209 Rolf Hertel, Michael Schwenk, and H. Paul A. Illing, 'Current Role of the Risk Concept in Regulatory Toxicology', in Franz-Xaver Reichl and Michael Schwenk (eds), *Regulatory Toxicology* (Springer Berlin Heidelberg 2014) 497.
210 WHO/IPCS, 'Risk Assessment Terminology' (2004) 15.
211 Schümann, Haluk, and Zenié (n 193) 378.
212 Ibid. 378.
213 Ibid.
214 Hertel, Schwenk, and Illing 2014 (n 209) 497.
215 Ibid. 497.
216 In Vose (n 194) 47.

217 Ibid. 48.
218 Schümann, Haluk, and Zenié 2014 (n 193) 379.
219 F.A.M. Verdonck, P.A. Van Sprang, and P.A. Vanrolleghem, 'Uncertainty and Precaution in European Environmental Risk Assessment of Chemicals' (2005) 52 (6) IWA 227, 229.
220 Ibid. 229.
221 Ibid. 230.
222 The ECHA explains the actions to be followed in each step of the tiered approach this way:

> *Level 1 – Qualitative assessment* Level 1 treats all uncertainties qualitatively. For qualitative analysis, it is proposed to list the different sources of uncertainty and or variability. These sources can be classified in order to identify the main uncertainties and ways to refine the CSA. Uncertainties assessed at Level 1 may be communicated by listing or tabulating them, together with an indication of their direction and magnitude. … In addition, it will generally be desirable to give a more detailed discussion in the text of the more important uncertainties, and of their combined effect on the assessment outcome. … *Level 2 – Deterministic assessment* Uncertainties assessed at Level 2 (deterministic) generate alternative point estimates, by making a series of reasonable worst-case assumptions for the determination of the exposure and by the use of varying factors for the determination of the hazard. Reasonable worst case assumptions can be incorporated in different ways, e.g. built into the exposure model, based on expert judgment ('I have never observed a factor X lower than Y') or on a quantitative measure (e.g. 95th percentile estimates for use as input data for modelling of environmental exposure). Deterministic approaches can be thought of as a simplified sensitivity analysis. … *Level 3 – Probabilistic assessment* Uncertainties assessed at level 3 (probabilistic) include a probabilistic assessment of those uncertainties which appear critical to the outcome of the chemical safety assessment. Probabilistic approaches enable variation and uncertainty in effects and/or exposure and the resulting risk to be quantified, mainly by using probability distributions instead of fixed values in risk assessment. The results of a probabilistic risk assessment (PRA) are also shown as distributions. This allows the assessor to see the most likely impact (expressed as the RCR), but also within which ranges. This could potentially provide a better basis for making decisions about further iterations of the CSA. In addition, output from a probabilistic assessment will often include a sensitivity analysis, identifying major contributors to variability and uncertainty in the estimated exposure. Note however that Assessment Factors will be derived and fixed according to the TGD.
>
> ECHA-12-G-25-EN (n 203) 15

223 Verdonck, Van Sprang, and Vanrolleghem (n 219) 233.
224 ECHA-12-G-25-EN 2012 (n 203) 8–9.
225 Ibid. 12.
226 SCENIHR, 'Opinion on the Appropriateness of Existing Methodologies to Assess the Potential Risks Associated with Engineered and Adventitious Products of Nanotechnologies' (SCENIHR/002/05 2005) 60.
227 See among others SCENIHR 2009 (n 136).
228 AIHA, 'Personal Protective Equipment for Engineered Nanoparticles' (24 October 2015) 2, emphasis added, available at www.aiha.org/government-affairs/Documents/Personal%20Protective%20Equipment%20for%20Engineered%20Nanoparticles_Final.pdf accessed 20.02.2019.
229 Ibid. 2.

230 Claude Ostiguy et al., 'Best Practices Guidance for Nanomaterial Risk Management in the Workplace' (2nd edn, Report R-899, 2015) 27, emphasis added.
231 Ibid.13, emphasis added.
232 Ibid. 27.
233 Ibid.
234 Specifically:

> In control banding, hazards are identified and allocated to bands (hazard bands) based on current knowledge of the nanomaterials involved and conservative assumptions about missing information. These hazard bands are combined with estimations of occupational exposure potential (exposure bands) to infer a risk level. For each risk level, there is a corresponding appropriate minimum control technology. The application of this approach requires expertise in chemical risk assessment and management …
>
> Ostiguy et al. (n 230) 28

235 Van Leeuwen 2007 (n 83) 28–29.
236 Iqbal and Sahlin (n 205), emphasis added.
237 Vose (n 194) 35.
238 Magnus Breitholtz et al., 'Improving the Value of Standard Toxicity Test Data in REACH' in Johan Eriksson, Michael Gilek, and Christina Rudén (eds) *Regulating Chemical Risks: European and Global Challenges* (Springer 2010) 886.
239 Christina Rudén and Sven Ove Hansson, 'Registration, Evaluation, and Authorization of Chemicals (REACH) Is but the First Step – How Far Will It Take Us? Six Further Steps to Improve the European Chemicals Legislation' (2010) 118 Environ Health Perspect. 6, 9.
240 See in general Kuraj (n 64).
241 Commission, 'Strategy for a Future Chemicals Policy' (White Paper) COM (2001) 88 final 6.
242 G. Lind, 'The Only Planet Guide to the Secrets of Chemicals Policy in the EU: REACH – What Happened and Why?' (Inger Schörling 2004)16; COM (2001) 88 final, 15.
243 G. Schaafsma et al., 'REACH, Non-testing Approaches and the Urgent Need for a Change in Mind Set' (2009) 53 Regulatory Toxicology and Pharmacology 70, 70.
244 ECHA-2010-G-19-EN 2012 (n 142) 2.
245 General Court of the European Union, Press Release No. 145/15 'Judgement in Case T-521/14 Sweden v Commission' (16 December 2015) 1, emphasis added.
246 Ibid. 1–2, emphasis added.
247 Breitholtz et al. (n 238) 85.
248 See Kuraj (n 64).
249 ECHA, 'Human Health and Environmental Exposure Assessment and Risk Characterisation of Nanomaterials: Best Practice for REACH Registrants' (Third GAARN meeting Helsinki ECHA-14-R-10-EN, 30 September 2013) 7.
250 Ibid. 7.
251 Ibid.
252 Ibid.
253 IRGC, 'Planning Adaptive Risk Regulation' (conference proceedings materials 2016).
254 Ibid.
255 Ibid. 9.

8 Concluding remarks and the way forward

Recap of the main arguments

The aim of this concluding chapter is to sum up the major findings of the research analysis developed in the attempt to answer the core question(s) that constitute the object of this study. Given that such analysis spanned different disciplines, in line with the interdisciplinary methodology this book employs, the main findings are chapter-specific. Therefore, the intent of the present chapter is to bring together the different layers of understanding generated in each realm of the analysis in order to deliver a comprehensive outlook on the investigated problems and, to the extent possible, indicate further lines of inquiry.

The main question this book aimed at answering was: *Does REACH, as it currently stands, appropriately and exhaustively cover nanoscale substances so that high levels of human health and environmental protection are ensured also for this class of chemicals?*

In answering this question, the book looked at the way a complex and modern legal endeavour like REACH articulates and addresses the concept of chemical risks and, particularly, its built-in element of uncertainty. While it provided a detailed analysis of REACH provisions in general, the focus was on how such provisions apply to nanoscale substances.

By setting the backdrop against which the analysis of this study is developed, the *first chapter* demonstrated why nano-chemicals are unlike anything else. It illustrated how those very features that make nanosubstances so attractive for their uses in different consumers' products are the features responsible for a number of health and environmental risks, including the potential destruction of the biosphere and the collapse of human civilisation beyond a point of non-return.[1] The trust placed on the revolutionary nature of nanoscale chemicals is so great that they are considered to be a *key enabling technology* (KET), able to further the advancement of solutions to some of the most pressing global problems, ranging from effective medical treatments and clean-up of contaminated sites, to employment, technological progress, and increase of the general well-being. By confronting the potential risks with the acclaimed benefits, Chapter 1 tried to contextualise the discussion revolving around nanosubstances' risk, stressing the fact that any regulatory initiative, including REACH, should not disregard the dual nature of nano-applications and nano-chemicals as one example of it.

Chapter 2 elaborated on the history of the adoption of the REACH Regulation, showing how uncertainty and ignorance about chemicals harm was what spurred the REACH reform in the first place. The toxic ignorance created by a fragmented and inconsistent set of requirements in the pre-REACH period, created a situation where there existed no data on the toxicity of 99 per cent of some 100,000 chemicals produced and used in the EU. The main problem with the pre-REACH directives, as Chapter 2 showed, was that they stipulated a set of differentiated provisions on toxicity testing and a data generation depending on whether chemicals were produced before or after 1981. The arbitrary criterion of the date of production resulted in the grandfathering of the majority of chemicals, regardless of their risks. This resulted in the lack of any incentive for producers to search for and replace dangerous chemicals with safer alternatives. The consequences in terms of health and environmental effects of this unfortunate regulatory and policy choice have been deleterious. Governmental and NGO reports, on both sides of the Atlantic, have pointed out an increase in the number of health-related issues such as allergies and sensitisation, linked to exposure to complex man-made chemicals. A number of alarming environmental problems, ranging from the poisoning of vital resources to the loss of biodiversity and disruption of biological processes, were also pointed out in such reports. Hence, REACH had the unprecedented task of remedying the toxic ignorance by eliminating the burden of the past (i.e. the grandfathering system) and grappling with the consequent burden of the present, in which the authorities had to demonstrate a risk before regulatory measures could be adopted.

However, in trying to solve such burdens, the EU legislature did not take into account the regulatory needs of the rapidly emerging field of nanotechnology. Despite numerous calls from both the scientific and academic world, the amendments suggested by the EU Parliament, requiring an explicit inclusion of nanosubstance as SVHCs under the most precautionary-driven phase of REACH, that of Authorisation, did not make it beyond the first draft of REACH. As a result, the current nano-silent text of REACH gave way to what this book calls 'the burden of the very small', i.e. the extremely difficult task of regulating nano-risks under laws that are not designed with the nano-related specificities in mind. As can be clearly understood by the parallel development of the law and science on nanotechnology during the REACH negotiation process (see the Appendix to this book), the failure to bring nano-chemicals under the Authorisation grid represents one of the most egregious missed opportunities in REACH. This is confirmed by the fact that once REACH came into force in its current nano-silent version, it took the EU legislature more than one decade to pass a few nano-specific amendments to some of the REACH Annexes. The missed momentum on nanotechnology has consequences beyond the EU area since, as shown in Chapter 2,

REACH is affirming itself as a global standard-setter, able to export its model of regulation to third countries, like Turkey, and eventually, to such countries' commercial partners. While these countries are likely to benefit from the improvement of chemical risks understanding and control that a framework like REACH enables, they will also most likely 'inherit' the suboptimal regulation of nanoscale chemicals that comes from including nano-provisions only in the Annexes but not in the legal text of REACH.

The failure to include nano-chemicals in REACH in general and under its Authorisation phase in particular, led to the current situation of legal uncertainty – if not complete legal void – on the status of nanosubstances in REACH. The difficulties of capturing nanoscale chemicals under the regulatory grid of a nano-silent and technologically neutral statute like REACH, were elucidated by the detailed analysis of the Regulation, developed in *Chapters 3–6*. The analysis of the four phases of REACH, which can be considered as quasi-autonomous yet organically connected regulatory programmes, yielded a number of shortcomings and bottlenecks, which were not necessarily exclusive to nano-chemicals regulatory issues. The main finding was that the shift from hazard-based to risk-based criteria in the regulatory model of REACH creates an illusory idea of the reversion of the burden of proof on industry. In the pre-REACH system, hazard, rather than risk, triggered regulatory action, although the burden of providing data on toxicity in order to justify a ban or a restriction on the use of a given substance was entirely on the regulating authority. REACH advances the idea that it is for the industry to demonstrate safety ('No data, no market') in order to gain access to the EU market. However, contrary to the previous system where regulatory action was triggered at 10 kg/y of production, in REACH, substantive data requirements are triggered only at 10 t/y. As a consequence, a great number of substances produced in lower quantities will escape the REACH requirements, thus creating a situation similar to that of the previous system where certain chemicals were commercialised without data on their toxicity. The assumption informing such regulatory choice is the idea that the greater the quantity of production, the greater the exposure of humans and the environment and the greater the risks to be regulated. However, as the case of EDCs and nanoscale chemicals demonstrates, lower quantitates do not necessarily equate with lower or negligible risks. In addition, the overly bureaucratic and cumbersome procedures of each of the four phases of REACH, most notably the one of Authorisation, make the adoption of effective and prompt risk measures difficult in practice. In general, Chapters 3–6 found that the tiered system through which REACH operates, based on the idea that the dose makes the poison, is highly problematic. Like the cases of nanoscale chemicals and EDCs demonstrate, the toxic mode of action of complex modern chemicals is *not* related to the concept of a quantity-expressed dose. Therefore, grandfathering low volumes of production of such chemicals from the REACH obligations is worrisome from a health and environmental protection standpoint.

This was also the argument of *Chapter 7*, which demonstrated why grand-fathering chemicals produced in low volumes such as EDCs and nanosubstances is worrisome also from a *scientific* point of view. This chapter was premised on the idea that any analysis on the success or failures of toxic regulations in addressing and curtailing health and environmental risks posed by chemical substances, depended to a great extent on the underlying scientific foundations that informed such regulations. Therefore, in Chapter 7, the legal provisions of REACH were viewed through regulatory toxicology lenses. One of this book's arguments is that the mastering of the law alone is unlikely to provide any guidance for navigating and understating REACH's complexity and its implications in terms of human health and environmental protection. This is the reason why delving into the science of toxicology that informs the REACH provisions was seen as a necessary and important step of this book. Therefore, in order to answer the main research question on the effectiveness of REACH for tackling and curtailing nano-risks, the regulatory toxicology paradigms upon which the REACH norms rest, have been assessed. In this way, the model of risk assessment that underpins and informs the risk management choices in REACH, was deconstructed. This part of the book sought to make explicit the science-policy choices that REACH amply employs. Importantly, Chapter 7 showed what the concept of 'adequately controlled risk', which is REACH's benchmark of safety, actually means in the realm of toxicology. Far from being a purely scientific and a value-free endeavour, toxicology just like any other 'exact' or 'natural' science is a value-laden, highly subjective and, to some extent, a socially constructed activity. The use of safety factors, probabilistic models, and sometimes sheer 'guesstimations' are, as shown, common practice in the assessment of chemicals' toxicity. The analysis on the methods and protocols used in toxicology demonstrated that it would be virtually impossible to provide scientific data to risk managers if the endemic uncertainty and the knowledge gaps were not bridged through extra-scientific considerations. But while the use of these science-policy elements is not a problem per se, the concealing of their use is. Keeping the risk managers outside the risk assessment process and failing to explain in clear and direct terms what a given RC ratio or safety factor means within the scientific theory or model used to assess risks, can convey a false sense of safety on the regulatory plan. In other words, deferring the task of providing clear-cut regulatory answers to science, without having a grasp on the epistemological limits of science as a discipline, is highly dangerous, especially if consolidated by means of legal instruments that are supposed to reduce and control potentially catastrophic risks. Chapter 7 found that the problems with the lack of transparency and participation (of both risk managers and the general public) in the science-policy choices used in risk assessment, are a common feature of chemical regimes. What nanosubstances (and EDCs before them) are causing is precisely this: a raised awareness on the existence of extra-scientific considerations that can strongly condition the outcome of a certain regulatory process. In such situations of uncertainty about the nature and magnitude of (nano-)risks there exists a principle of law that can be applied without waiting for a causal link between the hazardous chemical/technology (nanotechnology/nanosubstances) and the prospected risks to be firmly established by science: the precautionary principle.

This book only briefly elaborated on the place of precaution as a central principle of EU environmental law, instead deferring the main discussion on the nature and reach of precaution in such realms to a vast and ever-growing scholarship. The book did, however, advance the suggestion that for modern and complex chemicals, precaution, usually seen as a risk management tool, ought to be anticipated in the risk assessment phase. Chapter 7 showed how this is not only possible, but desirable. Further, it showed how the need for a transparent, inclusive, and democratic decision-making process is even more acute in the case of nanotechnology, where risks are not only poorly understood and almost impossible to assess, but also of a potentially infinite magnitude. Additionally, risk managers should have a proper understanding of the risk assessment data they use as a basis for their precautionary measures. To this end, risk assessors should also be required to disclose the underlying assumptions made when generating data for risk-regulation purposes. In other words, the conjectures, default assumptions, and probabilistic models should be made explicit in an open and constant dialogue with risk managers.

Only if risk managers have a proper understating of the way science operates will the element of precaution in the sense of anxiety, worry, and concern for human and environmental health be triggered. This in turn might lead to solicitude, devotion, and attentiveness with regard to the issue warranting regulatory action. In other words, this would be a way of taking *Care* in precaution. Thus, the daunting task of regulating nanosubstances in REACH and beyond lies precisely in the fact that the unprecedented risks posed by such chemicals make it virtually impossible for risk managers to overlook the scientific foundations of the law and their implications for decision-making. Importantly, nanosubstances challenge the golden rule of regulatory toxicology: 'the dose makes the poison'. Overall, nanosubstances simply escape the paradigmatic rules and concepts through which toxicology currently operates. By advancing the idea that there are chemicals for which no safe dose of exposure exists, nanosubstances and EDCs suggest that in order to protect human life and ecosystems from deleterious and perhaps irreversible risks, a phasing out and/or a total ban in production and use might be the only acceptable regulatory option.

In other words, nanosubstances' status in REACH brings under the spotlight the numerous inherent flaws of regulatory toxicology, which are arguably to blame for many environmental and health problems faced today. However, unlike for conventional chemicals, uncertainties concerning nanotoxicity cannot be covered or remedied by the use of safety factors or probability calculations, because even the basic data on nanotoxicity are missing. Hence the case of nano-chemicals risk denounces a structural problem of REACH: while the Regulation renovated the legal facade of chemicals legislation, a contextual overhaul of the upholding scientific platform of REACH, i.e. regulatory toxi-cology, did not take place with the review of the legal norms.

Current state of the art: the insufficiency of the sole Annex modification and the need for a thorough legislative overhaul

As noted earlier in this book, it took the Commission 11 years[2] to draft and approve changes to the REACH Annexes. The delay caused indignation and even outrage among the ECHA, and several MSs and NGOs, which deplored the Commission's 'maladministration of governance'.[3] In fact, the amend-ment of the REACH Annexes, aimed at ensuring 'further clarity on how nanomaterials are addressed and safety demonstrated in registration dossiers',[4] ought to have been presented, by way of a draft implementing act, by December 2013. Why such delay then? It must be recalled that the Commis-sion had launched a comprehensive REACH Implementation Project on Nanomaterials (RIP-oN) as early as 2009. Three Reports were produced as a result. The RIP-oN 2[5] & RIP-oN 3[6] concerning *Information Requirements* and *Chemical Safety Assessment*, respectively, led to the adoption of nano-specific Appendixes to the pertinent ECHA's GDs analysed in this book. The RIP-oN 1 concerned the Achilles' heel of the regulatory process on nanoma-terials both in REACH and beyond, i.e. substance identification.[7] To that end, the object of RIP-oN 1 was thus 'to evaluate the applicability of existing guidance and, if needed, to develop specific advice on how to establish the substance identity of nanomaterials'.[8] The failure to adopt this report came as a consequence of a strong disagreement between the involved stakeholders about the criteria to be used for the identification of nanomaterials pursuant Article 3(1) and Annex VI Section 2 of the REACH. Consequently, the per-tinent GD in question, although updated in 2017, still offers no guidance on the identification of nanosubstances.[9]

Furthermore, that the delay in amending the REACH Annexes, was owed in good part to the decision from the Commission to perform an Impact Assessment (IA) despite the fact that the REACH directive does not stipulate any requirement to perform an IA in order for the Commission to adopt new amendments. The IA is a form of in-house information gathering, which allows for the generation of evidentiary support to be used in decision-making. Hence, IA is, whenever it is conducted, a preliminary step aimed at informing and aiding decision-making but never substituting it.[10] A decision of the CJEU on EDCs seems to validate the thesis that the IA should be clearly required by the provisions of the regulation which is going to be modified by Commission intervention (and this was not the case for REACH). What is more, according to this ruling, even if an IA is clearly mandated by the legislative act, the Commission cannot derogate the deadline set for the adoption of (the delegated) acts it is assigned to adopt in accord-ance with the delegating regulation.[11] Notwithstanding such judgment, the

Commission went its own way and only in February 2016, published an Inception Impact Assessment on 'Possible amendments of Annexes to REACH for registration of nanomaterials'.[12] A public consultation followed and finally the amendments were approved in late 2018 and are to come into force in 2020. However, this book's conclusion is that such amendments – commendable as they are in the situation of total uncertainty created by the lack of any reference to nanotechnology in the current text of the Regulation – are insufficient to ensure that nanoscale chemicals are *appropriately and exhaustively* regulated in REACH. The arguments in support of this claim are as follows:

1   The amendments to the Annexes were adopted before the Commission could agree on an update to the 2011 Recommendation on the definition of the term 'nanomaterial'. Hence, the changes to the Annexes incorporate the 'old' definition of 2011 and this will remain the case even after an updated definition is formally adopted, most likely in 2019.

2   Such 'decoupling' of legislative reviewing processes (that of REACH's Annexes on the one hand, and that of the 2011 Recommendation on the other) risks creating further uncertainty on the regulatory plan, despite some experts claiming that the changes to the definition are unlikely to create significant problems for the fulfilment of the duties imposed on nano-producers by the new REACH Annexes.[13] While this remains to be seen, another shortcoming of this digressive timeline lies in the fact that neither the Annexes' modifications nor the updated definition were adopted in time for the last registration deadline of May 2018. This means that *phase-in* substances in nanoscale meeting the criteria for being registered under this last tier are extremely unlikely to have been registered as such, as there was virtually no specific obligation for registrants to do so.

3   Further, the changes to the Annexes with regard to the characterisation of nanosubstances, despite being clearly premised on the 2011 Recommendation with regard to the definition of the term 'nanomaterial', in fact make use of the term 'nanoform', which is not the same as 'nanomaterial'. As a result, uncertainties persist within the approved amendments concerning, for example, whether different nanoforms of the same substance will need to be characterised on a strictly case-by-case basis (e.g. nano silver of 20 nm and nano silver of 30 nm of dimensions). This might result in further uncertainties, including the use of certain alternative testing such as (Q)SARs and grouping and read-across.

4   The ECHA GDs containing nano-specific Appendixes, are non-binding in nature. Therefore, the powers of the ECHA to request additional information specific to the nano-form must come from the legal text of REACH in order to be legitimate and enforceable. The annulments of the ECHA decisions requesting additional information on the nanoform within the current nano-silent text of REACH and Annexes, have clearly

established this. The BoA ruled out the possibility of the ECHA requesting what REACH does not mandate the Agency to request. Moreover, the BoA ruled that the ECHA cannot use terms that are nowhere defined ('nanosubstance' is not defined in REACH yet, and is not defined in the ECHA GDs either), as this would create legal uncertainty for registrants. Lastly and most importantly, the BoA annulment of the SAS decision indicated that the mere fact of a substance being in nanoform is not equivalent to it being of concern. The outcome of such decisions leaves little room for doubt that the language of the legal text of REACH is binding and cannot be expanded or interpreted in a totally discretionary way by the ECHA. Also, the BoA made it perfectly clear that concerns about risks related to the nanoform are not formally delineated as such under the REACH framework, placing thus the burden of proof on the authorities seeking to curtail such risk.

5   In light of the above, residual perplexities are likely to remain as to whether once the approved amendments come in to force in 2020, the ECHA will be able to request any information it deems necessary on the nanoform and the related risk profiles. This is so because Article 3 of REACH, where the definition of substance is contained, as well as the other Articles, will remain nano-silent. An intervention in the binding legal text of the Regulation would have provided greater legal certainty as to the legal duties to test and assess nanosubstances separately from their bulk counterparts and, eventually, from different nanoforms as well.

6   Perhaps the greatest drawback of this decade-long amendment process is the specification in all the new amendments to the REACH Annexes of their applicability to the 'nanoforms covered by registration'. This means that the minimum threshold of 1 t/y will remain unchanged even after 2020, with the consequence of a conspicuous quantity of nanomaterials produced in lower volumes, still slipping through the new and tighter regulatory grids of the nano-specific Annexes. If it is considered that nanosubstances' toxicity is not a direct function of quantity (of exposure) expressed as a function of mass, this regulatory choice is clearly worrisome; it breaks with the ambition of REACH to ensure a high level of human and environmental protection.

7   As a consequence of the above, the only regulatory option for tackling and curtailing the risk of nanosubstances produced in quantities lower than 1 t/y is that of Authorisation. However, as shown, internal sub-phases of Authorisation link back to some consideration on volumes of production and risk criteria, something which makes the employment of this procedure particularly burdensome for the ECHA and the MSs to apply to nanomaterials. In other words, even with the changes to the REACH Annexes, the current situation and the related difficulties will continue to persist for low-volume nanosubstances that are not covered by registration.

8   Finally, it must be recalled that test methods able to assess the specific risk of nanomaterials are still generally lacking. Progress on this front is slow

and costs are considerable. Therefore, even with the new nano-specific duties clearly stated in the amended REACH Annexes, it remains obscure how the law is to remedy the uncertainty currently prevailing in the scientific domain, i.e. that of nanotoxicity. As explained, the progress of law and science taking place on parallel tracks and with different speeds, still constitutes one crucial hindrance to the tortuous process of bringing nano-risks under the REACH system. There is hence a need for the disciplines to communicate and coordinate their efforts in attaining tailored and cutting-edge regulatory options for risks of potentially infinite impact such as those posed by nanotechnology and the products of its application.

When the above points are considered, the modifications to the Annexes appear less revolutionary and future-proof, and instead have a high risk of becoming obsolete in a very short time.[14] An intervention on the legal text of REACH and the nano-specific reformation of its main Articles such as those on substance definition, minimum thresholds, and substances of equivalent concern, remains the only alternative for affording proper regulatory coverage to nanoscale chemicals under the massive structure of REACH.

It is the final argument of this book that in order for REACH to live up to the Commission's claim that it sets the best possible framework for the risk management of nanomaterials, a proper and comprehensive overhaul and review of its key legal concepts is needed. In other words, the 're-opening of the can of worms',[15] as some have labelled the process of renegotiation of the REACH framework for the inclusion of nano-specific norms in the legal text of the Regulation, is necessary.

Further reflections and one suggestion

As has been demonstrated, REACH is called to regulate a Janus-faced technology, and to do so by striking the right balance between the acclaimed wonderful benefits and uncertain unprecedented risks that nanotechnology brings. Whether nanotechnology is some sort of panacea for all the troubles that afflict modern life or, rather, a Pandora's Box containing all the evils of the world, remains to be seen.

Yet, the case of asbestos' tragic history of regulation demonstrates that the alluring promises that new materials and technologies hold, can easily obfuscate the need for a sober and holistic evaluation of the new risks involved. The tendency to magnify future and imagined benefits, while underestimating or even ignoring concrete risks, has been plaguing chemicals risk regulation since the eve of the Second Industrial Revolution. As mentioned, two reports from the European Environmental Agency, the 2000 *Late lessons from early warnings: the precautionary principle 1896–2000* and the 2012 *Late lessons from early warnings: science, precaution, innovation*, demonstrate such a tendency. Said reports are a collection of cases where law clearly failed to understand and address risks early enough and with enough normative and scientific care as to keep harms within acceptable levels for human health and the environment. The common denominator in all the EEA cases is the misinterpretation and misuse of the precautionary principle. The history of the poor regulation of dangerous chemicals – such as DDTs, benzene, lead in petrol, vinyl chloride, asbestos 17α-ethinyloestradiol – can be seen as examples where the essence of precaution has been betrayed. In its core meaning, the principle of precaution requires proactive measures aimed at avoiding unacceptable risks, even when scientific uncertainty does not allow for a clear evaluation of the magnitude of such risk, or for the establishment of the causal relationship between the hazard and the risk in question.

Therefore, this book concludes that the failure to act in a precautionary manner falls short of the moral responsibility to *Care*, which according to Hyginus and Goethe is the very essence of the human being and of the web of life supporting and nurturing its time on the planet. *Care*, this final chapter argues, is not some romantic concept to be found in fables. Rather, it is a quintessential element of precaution as the root of the German *Vorsorgeprinzip*, namely *Sorge*, clearly indicates. As such, *Care* can be conceptualised as the moral responsibility of regulators to adopt precautionary measures so as to avoid irreversible risks. In other words, precautionary decision-making that is based on *Care* can be used as an effective legislative tool to control, prevent, and, when necessary, ultimately halt the production, use, and environmental dispersion of hazardous chemicals. However, such version of precaution is still not substantiated on the EU level for cases of nanoscale chemicals.

What is more concerning, unlike in the GMO case, where the public opinion played an important role in the normative choices for controlling health and environmental risks, in the case of nanotechnology, little or no information at all is available to the average consumer on what exactly is at stake. For instance, there is no information on the fact that one possible consequence of the Faustian bargain in obtaining the great power of nanotechnology might be the destruction of the biosphere.[16] So while the dreamed-for benefits are highly acclaimed and stated in various scientific and policy documents, silence envelops the main risks we might run, including that of erasing human civilisation.

Hence it is hard not to see a parallel between the great promises of nanotechnology and the dizzying numbers on its market turnovers – including prospected benefits in terms of employment, environmental remedies, and healthcare solutions – and Faust's contemplation of the grandness and benevolence of his work:

> Such teeming would I see upon this land.
> On acres free among free people stand.
> I might entreat the fleeting moment
> Oh tarry, yet, thou art so fair![17]

However, here Faust is blind because he has scorned Sorge (*Care*) and refused to recognise her power; his vision is thus oblivious to the reality that the canal whose deepening he thinks he is directing is actually his own grave dug by Lemures.

In light of such consideration, this book sees the story of previous regulatory failures in controlling deleterious risks of chemicals together with the partial reform of the REACH Annexes only, as a refusal of the law to acknowledge *Care* as an inseparable element of life. The Faustian narrative demonstrates that the striving for certain goals (i.e. economic development and technological revolutions), while 'shutting out a sometimes worrisome and painful concern for people and institutions, results in terrible external and internal harm'.[18] Given that some kind of caring is manifested in everything humans do,[19] the observation on the lack of an element of care in the legislative models, which purport to offer a plausible response to environmental risks posed by dangerous chemicals, is worrisome. The question that *Sorge* (*Care*) poses to Faust, 'Hast du die Sorge niegekannt?' (Have you ever known Care?), if posed with regard to legal instruments dealing with chemicals risk, is likely to receive, just like in the case of Faust, a negative answer. However, *Care* has two primordial meanings, which are interrelated and to some extent inseparable: on the one hand, it means anxiety, worry, and concern, and on the other, solicitude, devotion, and attentiveness, with connotations of responsibility, trusteeship, and protection.[20] The precautionary principle, as a philosophical principle of care even before a principle of environmental law, carries both the elements of 'worrying about' and 'solicitude' and 'devotion' about the future. Nonetheless, the way the principle is employed today falls short of these rich semantic attributes and their potential expressions in the legal realm.

Therefore, the answer to the main research question can be but a negative one. The current REACH framework does *not* effectively and exhaustively address the risks posed by the chemicals in nanoscale. The analysis developed over the preceding chapters tried to thoroughly substantialise such conclusion. Based on the recap of this book's argument in the previous section, it is not difficult to view each of the identified legislative and conceptual flaws of REACH in this regard as a lack of care.

Transparency and participation, this book holds, are essential to the creation of that worrisome concern about the future, which is one of the essential elements of precaution understood as *Care*. It is thus important in the case of nanotechnology to trigger the element of worry and anxiety about the future in order to spur precautionary action. By trying to shed some light on the many flaws of the science used as a legitimate basis for decisions (not) taken on nano-chemicals, this book sought to trigger that important element of concern that can spur adequate changes in REACH and beyond. Ultimately, this book contends that precaution understood as *Care* can give rise to a new approach to the regulation of risks that can harm humans and the environment in an unprecedented and irreversible way. This suggestion is elaborated in the following and last section.

Precaution as Statesman's Care under the imperative of responsibility

It is the final argument of this book that, when placed at the centre of the precautionary decision-making process concerning nano-risks, the element of *Care* can lead to the adoption of what Hans Jonas called 'the imperative of responsibility'.[21]

Jonas suggested that in situations of persistent uncertainty concerning catastrophic risk, an imaginative 'heuristics of fear' (e.g. the destruction of the biosphere) replacing the projections of hope (e.g. revolution in medicine, chemistry, and general well-being by use of nanotechnology) must tell us what is at stake and what to beware. For Jonas, it is precisely the magnitude of such stakes, coupled with the insufficiency of our predictive knowledge, that should lead 'to the pragmatic rule to give the prophecy of doom priority over the prophecy of bliss'.[22] He offers a new imperative that should illuminate regulators' actions when faced with highly uncertain and potentially catastrophic risks, the *imperative of responsibility*, which he formulates as follows:

> 'Act so that the effects of your action are compatible with the permanence of genuine human life'; or expressed negatively: 'Act so that the effects of your action are not destructive of the future possibility of such life'; or simply 'Do not compromise the conditions for an indefinite continuation of humanity on earth'; or, again, turned positive: 'In your present choices include the future wholeness of Man among the objects of our will.'[23]

Jonas suggests that when regulators are faced with enduring uncertainty on technologies that might have irreversible consequences, *caution* 'is the better part of bravery and surely a command of responsibility'. In such a situation, the recourse to caution includes the options of renouncing risky technology. Nanotechnology has been considered as capable of causing the collapse of global systems.[24] The scenario of collapse has been described as a condition 'where civilisation collapses to a state of great suffering and does not recover, or a situation where all human life ends'.[25] Similar risks have been envisaged for the environment, i.e. an 'ecological collapse on ecosystems where an ecosystem suffers a drastic, possibly permanent, reduction in carrying capacity for all organisms'.[26] While the debate on nano-related risks is an ongoing one, the risks so far envisaged seem to correspond to situations that would fall under the imperative of the responsibility domain.

Therefore, restrictive measures, ranging from moratoriums and/or bans either on nanotechnology or specific products of its applications, should at least be up for discussion among the different precautionary measures available to legislators to control nano-risks.

Nothing seems to prevent the suggestion that the pursuit of such a critical technology must be renounced, as Jonas argues, not only because the promise of a wonderful life[27] nanotechnology brings 'if ever attained, it could not last, but more so because already the road in that direction leads to disaster'.[28]

Notes

1 See on this D. Pamlin, S. Armstrong, and S. Baum (eds), *12 Risks That Threaten Human Civilisation: The Case for a New Risk Category* (Global Challenges Foundation 2015).
2 See 'REACH Annex Nano Revision "Not Future Proof"' (*CW*, 7 November 2017) https://chemicalwatch.com/60918/reach-annex-nano-revision-not-future-proof accessed 22.02.2019.
3 Ibid.
4 Commission, 'General Report on REACH Accordance with Article 117(4) of REACH and Article 46(2) of CLP, and a Review of Certain Elements of REACH in Line with Articles 75(2), 138(2), 138(3) and 138(6) of REACH' COM (2013) 49 final, 12–13.
5 S.M. Hankin et al., 'Specific Advice on Fulfilling Information Requirements for Nanomaterials under REACH (RIP-oN 2) – Final Project Report' (JRC, RNC/RIP-oN2/FPR/1/FINAL 2011).
6 R.A. Aitken et al., 'Specific Advice on Exposure Assessment and Hazard/Risk Characterisation for Nanomaterials under REACH (RIP-oN 3) – Final Project Report' (JRC, RNC/RIP-oN3/FPR/1/FINAL 2011).
7 JRC, 'REACH Implementation Project Substance Identification of Nanomaterials (RIP-oN 1) – Advisory Report' (AA N°070307/2009/D1/534733 2011).
8 Ibid. 8.
9 ECHA 'Guidance for Identification and Naming of Substances under REACH and CLP' (ECHA-16-B-37.1-EN May 2017), 36.
10 'Guidelines on IA' (*Commission*) http://ec.europa.eu/smart-regulation/guidelines/ug_chap3_en.htm accessed 21.02.2019.
11 Judgment in Case T-521/14 *Sweden v Commission* [2015] ECLI:EU:T:2015:976.
12 Commission, DG ENV, 'Possible Amendments of Annexes to REACH for Registration of Nanomaterials' (Inception Impact Assessment), AP 2014/ENV+/013 2016, 3.
13 See 'Small Things Are Finally in REACH' (*CW*) https://chemicalwatch.com/67610/small-things-are-finally-in-reach accessed 06.12.2018.
14 On such concerns see: 'REACH Annex Nano Revision "Not Future Proof"' (n 2).
15 'REACH Review: Re-opening a Can of Worms?' (*EurActiv*, 12 March 2012) www.euractiv.com/section/science-policymaking/video/reach-review-re-opening-a-can-of-worms/ accessed 22.02.2019.
16 Bill Joy, 'Why the Future Doesn't Need Us' (*Wired*) 4 January 2000 www.wired.com/2000/04/joy-2/ accessed 13.5.2019.
17 This is the translated version used in Bruce Rich, *Mortgaging the Earth* (Beacon Press 1994) 104.
18 Warren T. Reich, 'History of Care' (*Georgetown University*) http://care.georgetown.edu/Classic%20Article.html accessed 22.02.2019.
19 Ellis Dye, 'Sorge in Heidegger and in Goethe's Faust' (2009) 16 Goethe Yearbook 207, 215.
20 Rich (n 17) 318.
21 Hans Jonas, *The Imperative of Responsibility: In Search of an Ethics for the Technological Age* (University of Chicago Press 1984).
22 Ibid. x.
23 Ibid. 11.

24 See Pamlin, Armstrong, and Baum (n 1).
25 Ibid.
26 Ibid.
27 Or even immortality, as some claim, if its use as an enabling technology for the development of synthetic biology is considered. See in general: Henk van den Belt, 'Playing God in Frankenstein's Footsteps: Synthetic Biology and the Meaning of Life' (2009) 3 Nanoethics 257.
28 Jonas (n 21) 191.

Appendix

Nanotechnology considerations during REACH's legislative process of adoption

Relevant European documents regarding nanotechnology	REACH negotiation progress	Nano-specific/relevant amendments in REACH
December 2002 FP6 includes nanotechnologies and nanosciences among top priorities areas of R&D for the period (2002–2006)	**February 2001** The White Paper on a new strategy for a future EU chemical policy is published	The WP contains no reference to nanotechnology. Minimum threshold to trigger registration: 1 t/producer/importer/year
June 2003 UK Royal Commission calls for the implementation of a new chemical law based on the precautionary and the substitution principles. The RC disagrees with the White Paper decision to increase the tonnage requirement for registration under REACH from 10 kg to 1 t/y, calling it an 'unjustified' choice.	**October 2003** The REACH legislative proposal is adopted (COM(2003) 644 final)	Nanosubstances are absent from the proposed legislative text. The tonnage threshold of 1 tonne per manufacture per year is reaffirmed as the minimum amount to trigger the application of the new chemical law.
November 2003 The Commission adopts *A European Initiative for Growth* indicating nanotechnologies, specifically nanoelectronics, as one of the most prominent and crucial areas of research and funding, expected to boost EU economy and growth in the near future.	**December 2003** The REACH proposal is being debated in Council (2003/0256(COD))	No discussion on nano-related norms is taking place.

Relevant European documents regarding nanotechnology	*REACH negotiation progress*	*Nano-specific/relevant amendments in REACH*
March 2004 DG SANCO of the Commission holds a workshop on RA issues related to nanoparticles. The exposure of consumers to nanoparticles through product use is officially recognised. The forthcoming REACH is indicated as a legislative tool already in need of revision. The 1 t/y criterion for registration is deemed inappropriate in addressing nano-chemicals. **July 2004** The Royal Society and Royal Academy of Engineering publishes *Nanoscience and Nanotechnologies: Opportunities and Uncertainties*, one of the earliest and most comprehensive scientific studies of merit. The Report states that nanoparticles' toxicity is determined by different factors compared to the bulk materials. Size, greater surface area, and reactivity enable a deeper penetration of cellular and sub-cellular levels and should be taken into account when evaluating exposure. Size alone is not sufficient.	**September 2004** Committee referral is announced in Parliament, first reading/single reading phase (2003/0256(COD)). **December 2004** The REACH proposal text is undergoing its next Council debate stage 2003/0256(COD).	Nanotechnology is not contemplated. The 1 t/y minimum threshold for registration is maintained and, in addition, a proposal to ease the requirements on the information to be supplied for substances produced in quantities 1–10 t/y is proposed. The Council calls for a general need to pursue a high level of human and environmental protection while ensuring the competiveness of the EU enterprises, especially the SMEs. Though the Council stresses the need to prioritise the registration of substances of very high concern from a very early stage, no mention is made of nanotechnology and nanosubstances.
June 2005 The Commission adopts 'Action Plan for Europe 2005–2009' (COM(2005) 243) on nanotechnology. Relevant legislation shall be amended to accommodate nanotechnology, with particular attention to regulatory triggers such as thresholds. Toxicity, exposure, risk assessment, and labelling thresholds are some of the indicated potential targets. REACH is deemed potentially capable of dealing with nanoparticles produced 'in very high volumes'.	**November 2005** The Parliament should adopt its position on the first reading of the REACH draft.	The 1 t/y minimum threshold is maintained. An explicit mention of substances in nanoform is still lacking in the text of the draft. The draft is silent on nanotechnology.

Relevant European documents regarding nanotechnology	*REACH negotiation progress*	*Nano-specific/relevant amendments in REACH*
September 2005 First Scientific Opinion from SCENIHR is published. REACH's criteria and triggers are deemed inappropriate for dealing with nanosubstances. The need to review REACH emerges clearly.	**November 2005** The Parliament adopts its first reading draft. The text is debated in the Council, which will adopt its position in June 2006.	The draft in question is silent on nanotechnologies and is built on the general definition of 'chemical substance'. The minimum threshold criterion of 1 t/y is maintained as the principal trigger for registration.
March 2006 SCENIHR publishes a modified Opinion (after public consultation) on the appropriateness of existing methodologies to assess the potential risks associated with engineered and adventitious products of nanotechnologies. The need to carefully consider the differences between nano and conventional bulk chemicals is stressed.	**October 2006** Committee recommendation tabled for plenary, second reading (ordinary legislative procedure). Draft of the Parliament on a legislative resolution based on the Council position. FINAL A6–0352/2006	For the first time a reference to nanotechnology is included in the proposed amendments, justifying it on the basis of the SCENIHR Opinion of March 2006. Amendments (24), (79), (87), (161), and (165) modify the legislative draft so as to explicitly include the reference to nanosubstances, specific tonnage considerations, and general subjection to the Authorisation phase and the prioritisation process therein.
During **2006** SCNEIHR was presumably working on the Opinion requested by the Commission on 'The appropriateness of the risk assessment methodology in accordance with the Technical Guidance Documents for new and existing substances for assessing the risks of nanomaterials'. The Opinion was going to be published in June 2007.	**December 2006** The final act is signed and published in the Official Journal. The Regulation will come into force in June 2007.	Any reference to nanotechnology and nanosubstances was withdrawn already from the resolution adopted by the Parliament in its second reading stage P6_TC2-COD(2003)0256. The final legal rule of REACH is silent on nanotechnologies and is built on the general definition of 'chemical substance'. The minimum threshold criterion of 1 t/y is maintained as the principal trigger for Registration.

Index

Page numbers in **bold** denote tables, those in *italics* denote figures.

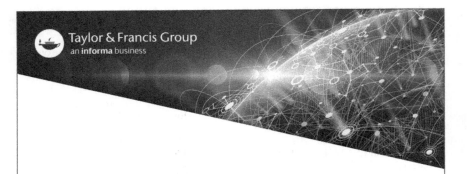